Discrete Methods in Epidemiology

DIMACS

Series in Discrete Mathematics
and Theoretical Computer Science

Volume 70

Discrete Methods in Epidemiology

James Abello
Graham Cormode
Editors

Center for Discrete Mathematics
and Theoretical Computer Science
A consortium of Rutgers University, Princeton University,
AT&T Labs–Research, Bell Labs (Lucent Technologies),
NEC Laboratories America, and Telcordia Technologies
(with partners at Avaya Labs, HP Labs, IBM Research,
Microsoft Research, and Stevens Institute of Technology)

American Mathematical Society

This DIMACS volume presents the proceedings from the DIMACS workshop on Data Mining and Epidemiology held at the DIMACS Center, Rutgers University, March 18–19, 2004.

2000 *Mathematics Subject Classification.* Primary 92D30; Secondary 68R01.

Library of Congress Cataloging-in-Publication Data

Discrete methods in epidemiology : DIMACS Workshop, Data Mining and Epidemiology, March 18–19, 2004, DIMACS Center, Rutgers University/James Abello, Graham Cormode, editors.

p. cm. — (DIMACS series in discrete mathematics and theoretical computer science; 70)

"Volume grew out of the activities of the DIMACS Working Group on Data Mining and Epidemiology"—Acknowledgement p.

Includes bibliographical references and index.

ISBN 0-8218-3754-0 (alk. paper)

1. Epidemiology—Congresses. 2. Epidemiology—Mathematics—Congresses. 3. Computer science–Congresses. I. Abello, James M. II. Cormode, Graham, 1977- III. DIMACS Workshop, Data Mining and Epidemiology (2004 : Rutgers University) IV. DIMACS Working Group on Data Mining and Epidemiology (2004 : Rutgers University) V. Series.

RA651.D57 2006
614.4—dc22 2005057092

AMS softcover ISBN 978-0-8218-4379-6

♾ The paper used in this book is acid-free and falls within the guidelines
established to ensure permanence and durability.
Visit the AMS home page at `http://www.ams.org/`

10 9 8 7 6 5 4 3 2 1 12 11 10 09 08 07

Contents

Foreword

The DIMACS working group on Data Mining and Epidemiology held a meeting on March 18-19, 2004 at Rutgers University. We would like to express our appreciation to James Abello, Graham Cormode, Kenton Morgan and David Ozonoff for their efforts to organize and plan this successful conference.

The meeting was part of the 2002-2007 Special Focus on Computational and Mathematical Epidemiology, and was organized by one of a number of special focus research groups called "working groups" as part of the special focus. We extend our thanks to Martin Farach-Colton, Sunetra Gupta, Donald Hoover, David Krakauer, Simon Levin, Marc Lipsitch, David Madigan, Megan Murray, S. Muthukrishnan, David Ozonoff, Fred Roberts, Burton Singer and Daniel Wartenberg for their work as special focus organizers.

The meeting brought together researchers who approach the study of epidemiology from a variety of disciplines, some applied and some theoretical. These included computer scientists, mathematicians, statisticians, and biologists together with both descriptive and analytical epidemiologists. The goal of the meeting as well as of this volume is the exploration of cross-disciplinary approaches to the study of epidemiology.

DIMACS gratefully acknowledges the generous support that makes these programs possible. Special thanks go to the National Science Foundation, New Jersey Commission on Science and Technology, Office of Naval Research, Alfred P. Sloan Foundation, Burroughs-Wellcome Fund, and to DIMACS partners at Rutgers, Princeton, AT&T Labs - Research, Bell Labs, NEC Laboratories America, and Telcordia Technologies, and affiliate partners Avaya Labs, HP Labs, IBM Research, Microsoft Research, and Stevens Institute of Technology.

Fred S. Roberts
DIMACS Director

Robert Tarjan
Co-Director for Princeton

Preface

Faced with the question of the intended audience for a collection such as the one assembled here, we have been asking ourselves the following questions:

(a) What is epidemiology? Who is an epidemiologist?

(b) What are the flavors of epidemiology?

(c) What are the types of questions epidemiologists work on?

Dave Ozonoff provided to us the following quote by Rothman that sheds some light on possible answers to the questions posed above:

> "Unfortunately, there seem to be more definitions of epidemiology than there are epidemiologists. Some have defined it in terms of its methods. While the methods of epidemiology may be distinctive, it is more typical to define a branch of science in terms of its subject matter rather than its tools... If the subject of epidemiologic inquiry is taken to be the occurrence of disease and other health outcomes, it is reasonable to infer that the ultimate goal of most epidemiologic research is the elaboration of causes that can explain patterns of disease occurrence."

In general terms, epidemiology deals with populations rather than individuals. One of its goals is to study the frequency of occurrences of health related events. It has a major but not exclusive concern with causes and determinants of disease patterns in populations. The premise is that a systematic investigation of different populations can identify causal and preventive factors. Epidemiology is an observational rather than an experimental science. Sample questions take the form of:

- Does population exposure to x increase the risk of a disease w?
- Are dietary supplements $\{x, y, z\}$ beneficial in lowering the risk of malady w?
- Do behavioral interventions reduce risk behaviors?

We have observed that occurrence measures, causal inference and study designs play prominent roles in the daily endeavors of a typical epidemiologist. Descriptive and analytical epidemiology are two overlapping flavors of this discipline.

Descriptive epidemiology attempts to describe patterns of disease according to spatial and temporal information about the members of a population. These patterns are described by tabulations or summaries of surveys and polls or by parametric or non-parametric population models. Models are in general global descriptions of the major part of a data set. Patterns on the other hand are local features of the data that can be described by association rules, modes or gaps in density functions, outliers, inflection points in regressions, symptom clusters, geographic hot spots, etc. Some epidemiologists appear more interested in local patterns rather than in global structure. This raises questions of how "realistic" certain patterns are.

Analytical Epidemiology attempts to explain and predict the state of a population's health. A typical goal is to summarize the relationship between exposure and disease incidence by comparing two measures of disease frequency. These comparisons may be affected by chance, bias and by the presence or absence of an effect. This explains naturally why statistical methods play a major role in Epidemiology since bias is a central preoccupation of its practitioners. Bias means a systematic error that results in an incorrect or invalid estimate of the measure of association. This can create or mask associations. Selection and information bias are two of the main bias types. In particular, selection shall be independent of exposure if the purpose of the study is to explain the relationship between exposure and disease occurrence. In summary, one of the central themes in analytical epidemiology is to understand the roles of bias, chance and real effect in the understanding of populations health.

To evaluate the role of chance, statistical hypothesis testing and estimation appear to be the tools of choice. On the other hand, generative models offer a way to describe infectious disease dynamics. Since disease patterns are of primary interest, data mining algorithms and detection of rules for pattern formation have a lot to offer. Classification and taxonomies are useful tools to develop predictive models. In general we believe that some questions addressed by epidemiologists benefit from viewing them in a mathematical and algorithmic context. This volume is a first attempt to bridge the gap between the two communities. Its main emphasis is on discrete methods that have successfully addressed some epidemiological question. We begin by providing introductory chapters, on some of the key methods from discrete data mining by a selection of researchers in this area; and on descriptive epidemiology by D. Schneider. These collect, in a digested form, what we believe are among the most potentially useful concepts in data mining and epidemiology.

Next there are two chapters reporting work in epidemiology that suggest a discrete, analytical approach: Shannon on challenges in molecular data analysis, and Hirschman and Damianos on a system for monitoring news wires for indications of disease outbreaks. The remainder of the volume draws out further some of the key areas in the intersection between epidemiology and discrete methods. The technique of formal concept analysis, and the amazing depth of mathematical structure that arises from it is explored in chapters by Ozonoff, Pogel and Hannan, and Abello and Pogel. The dynamics of disease transmission can be modeled in a variety of ways, but often involves setting up systems of differential equations to model the ebb and flow of infection, as demonstrated by Desai, Boily, Mâsse and Anderson, and Vázquez, in the context of quite different problems. Eubank, Kumar, Marathe, Srinivasan and Wang study massive interaction graphs and give results by a combination of combinatorial methods and simulation; Abello and Capalbo focus on properties of graphs generated by an appropriate random model; while Hartke takes a combinatorial model of disease spread on tree graphs. Finally, we see two applications of Support Vector Machines to epidemiological data sets, from Li, Muchnik and Schneider (using breast cancer data from the SEER database) and from Fradkin, Muchnik, Hermans and Morgan (using data on disease in chickens). Some other potential areas of interest that we have not touched in this collection relate to patient confidentiality, coding and cryptography and multiscale inference.

We hope the volume helps to foster cooperation between epidemiologists, computer scientists and mathematicians. We believe this will help elucidate the main algorithmic and mathematical issues. In a relatively brief period of time we noticed a variety of interconnections between the disciplines, far richer than we ever dreamed of. We trust that the papers included here are a good indicator of the possibilities that discrete mathematical thinking can offer to a variety of epidemiological questions.

James Abello
Graham Cormode
Piscataway, NJ, 2005

Acknowledgments

This volume grew out of the activities of the DIMACS Working Group on Data Mining and Epidemiology. This working group is part of the Special Focus on Computer Science and Epidemiology funded by NSF EIA Grant 02-05116. The themes of the working group and associated events can be accessed by visiting `http://dimacs.rutgers.edu/Workshops/WGDataMining/` and `http://dimacs.rutgers.edu/SpecialYears/2002_Epid/episeminars.html`.

The papers appearing in this volume are chiefly the results of interactions promoted by the working group. The editors want to express their appreciation to the DIMACS staff for their assistance with the logistics of organizing meetings of the Working Group, the DIMACS directorate for the funding, the members of the DIMACS Computational Methods Group for their insightful talks, Dave Ozonoff and Dona Schneider for sharing their epidemiological expertise, F. Roberts, T. Imielinski, Apostolos Gerasoulis, S. Muthukrishnan, and S. Sudarsky for their continued support.

All the speakers at meetings of the working group, contributing authors, the many anonymous referees of chapters, and working group participants deserve special credit for helping in one way or another make this volume possible.

J. Abello, DIMACS and Ask.com
G. Cormode, DIMACS and Bell Labs — Lucent Technologies

DIMACS Series in Discrete Mathematics
and Theoretical Computer Science
Volume **70**, 2006

Selected Data Mining Concepts

James Abello, Graham Cormode, Dmitriy Fradkin, David Madigan,
Ofer Melnik, and Ilya Muchnik

ABSTRACT. In this multi-authored chapter, we introduce six key techniques from data mining that have been succesfully applied to epidemiological data analysis.

- *Cluster Analysis* is an unsupervised learning technique that takes large collections of data points and attempts to identify *clusters* of similar points. More formally, it tries to create clusters to optimize various mathematical properties, such as minimizing the maximum spread of each cluster, or minimizing the sum of the spreads. A variety of algorithms have been proposed to create clusters from a data set, including k-means, hierarchical clustering, and expectation maximization.
- *Association Rules* have become one of the central tools in transactional data mining. They can also be applied as a way of looking for correlations and associations within epidemiological data.
- *Support Vector Machines* are a popular *classification method* which produce linear classifiers in the form of cutting hyperplanes, which divide the space into positive and negative examples. Through the so-called "kernel-trick" it can also produce non-linear rules by projecting the data into a different space.
- *Statistical Techniques* are a bedrock of epidemiological study, through sampling, hypothesis testing, experiment design, and inference techniques. An important suite of methods draw on Bayesian inference, giving more interpretable confidence bounds and simpler model fitting.
- *Boosting* is a very influential technique for "boosting" the quality of classifier-based methods by varying the emphasis put on examples to focus the classification method on the "harder examples". The output of a number of rules is then combined by taking a weighted majority vote. The method has been extended to a wide variety of settings, and applied to a large number of different scenarios.
- *External Memory Algorithms* are needed when the volume of data being processed exceeds the internal (fast) memory of the machine, and means that some data must reside on external (slow) memory, ie disks. Such methods give deep insights into the structure and properties of the underlying algorithms.

2000 *Mathematics Subject Classification.* Primary 62-07 Statistics — Data analysis; Secondary 68W01 Algorithms – General.

The first two authors thank Fred Roberts for his continued support. We also thank the National Science Foundation and DIMACS for making this collaboration possible.

Dr. Muchnik's work was supported through NSF grant CCR 0325398.

A. Cluster Analysis

Graham Cormode

1. Introduction

The notion of 'clusters' is a very natural one, and occurs frequently in discussions of epidemiology. We hear about 'cancer clusters', areas where the number of reported cancer cases within an area or group of people exceeds the expected amount. Such clusters lead to investigation of possible carcinogens or explanation for greater susceptibility amongst certain groups.

When thinking about clusters, people most often think of geographical clusters—the image of "pins in a map" is a resonant one. In fact, this approach has its roots in the very foundation of epidemiology. The famed work of John Snow in 1854 was to plot cases of cholera on a map of London, and to observe that these were centered around certain water pumps. Thus the result of this early instance of clustering was to produce a hypothesis on the source of the cholera cases, which was subsequently verified. The evolution of this early success in visualizing data has been the development of sophisticated GIS systems, which can rapidly plot a variety of data on top of maps in many ways.

However, not all data is geographic in nature. Patient admission records contain large numbers of variables of different types: geographic (home address, work address); time (date of birth, duration of symptoms); categorical (existing medications, socio-economic indicators); textual (physician's notes); and numeric (patient readings, such as heart rate, blood pressure etc.). We would also like to cluster such data in order to find patterns of similarity that can lead to new hypotheses. It is no longer possible to plot such high dimensional and heterogeneous data on a chart and visually pick out clusters. Instead, we turn to data mining approaches to take the data and find the clusters therein.

We will focus on the data mining methods used to produce these clusters, but there are many other aspects of the problem surrounding this that we only touch on.

- **Data Collection.** Data Collection is a major hurdle for any data mining task. Designing experiments and enrolling volunteers to get a significant study group can be a major commitment. Sometimes data mining is characterized as "data dredging": taking existing data sets collected for some other purpose and 'dredging' them for new information. Even this approach is fraught: since the data was not collected with the current goal in mind, there may be relevant attributes missing. Important information about the collection method may have been lost. It may be necessary to fuse together multiple data sets, and done without sufficient care this can lead to erroneous conclusions. Lastly, there are myriad issues of privacy and consent: subjects may have agreed to their data being used in one study, but do not want it to be used for innumerable others. Issues of individual privacy also mean that some attribute values (home address, date of birth) may be omitted, randomly perturbed by a small amount, or otherwise changed. Data users need to be aware of all these effects before drawing conclusions from the data.

- **Data Cleaning.** No data set is perfect. At the very least, one can expect missing values for some attributes, some errors in transcription or data input, and duplicate entries. Dealing with these issues is a topic of major study in itself [**1**]. Sometimes, a received data set has already been 'cleaned'. Perhaps 'scrubbed' is a better term: missing values are sometimes filled in with average values, or values copied from similar looking records. Values outside "sanity bounds" (ages greater than 120, pulse rates below 0) may be replaced with default values, or the corresponding record dropped completely. As with data collection, it is important to know the methodology applied to clean the data in order to interpret conclusions correctly.
- **Interpreting Results.** Most data mining tasks do **not** give as their output a set of hypotheses about diseases and their cause. Instead, they merely produce observations about the input data, to some degree of confidence, and it is up to the user to draw their own conclusions. To return to a geographical example, we might plot cancer data across the United States, and observe much higher incidence in some areas, such as Florida. Before forming hypotheses about possible carcinogens prevalent in these areas, we need to consider to what extent this can be explained by already known factors. In this case, if we had not adjusted the data for demographic factors, then the observation may be explained by the fact that many senior citizens retire to Florida, and incidence of cancers increase with age. Great care must be taken to adjust for all relevant factors before claiming that observed results are significant, and frequently subsequent work is needed to verify initial findings, and ensure that the input data was not anomalous.

We continue our discussion of clustering as follows. In the next subsection we will give a mathematical formalism to clustering, and define it as an optimization problem over input data. Then we consider three popular clustering methods: hierarchical clustering, the k-means algorithm, and Expectation Maximization (EM).

2. The Clustering Problem

In order to cluster the input into sets of similar points, we need to be able to define a distance between any pair of points to gauge their similarity. Formally, we assume that the input is a set of points from a *metric space*, with an associated metric, or distance, function. We will denote this distance as d, so the distance between two points x and y is given by $d(x, y)$. If the points are in a metric space, then this gives three requirements on d:

(1) **Identity:** $d(x, x) = 0$ — the distance from any point to itself is zero.
(2) **Symmetry:** $d(x, y) = d(y, x) \geq 0$ — the distance between any two points is the same in both directions, and is non-negative.
(3) **Triangle Inequality:** $d(x, z) \leq d(x, y) + d(y, z)$ — this means that it is never quicker to get from one point to another by going via a different point.

In extensions of clustering applications, it is possible to drop some or all of these conditions, but we will focus on the metric space setting.

Defining an appropriate distance function can be challenging. If all the data is numeric, then we can use the Euclidean distance function (straight line distance) or L_∞ distance (maximum distance in any co-ordinate). However, real data is rarely like this. We could map our data onto numerical values, although the choice of scale can affect the result dramatically. Suppose we had a categorical attribute which takes two values: malign, and benign. We could map benign to 0, and malign to 1, or to 0 and 100, respectively. The choice of this difference effectively determines the extent to which we are emphasizing that attribute relative to the others. One can attempt to normalize the data, by rescaling all values into the range $[0 \ldots 1]$, but this still does not solve the problem completely. Once the distance function has been chosen, we can go on to define the general clustering problem.

DEFINITION 1 (Clustering Algorithm). *A clustering algorithm takes as input a set of points from a metric space, and outputs a set of clusters,* $\mathcal{C} = \{C_1 \ldots C_k\}$.

Note that this definition is very broad—it does not describe how the clusters are described or what criteria they fulfil. This is because there are many ways to define the desired clustering. We give two commonly used formalisms:

DEFINITION 2 (k-center). *A k-center clustering algorithm outputs a set of k points* $\mathcal{C} = \{C_1 \ldots C_k\}$ *("centers") from the metric space to define the clusters: each input data point is associated with the point from* $\mathcal{C}$ *that is closest to it (ties can be broken arbitrarily). The quality of the clustering is determined by the maximum distance of a point to its closest center, ie* $\max_x \min_i d(x, C_i)$.

DEFINITION 3 (k-median). *A k-median clustering algorithm outputs a set of k points* $\mathcal{C}$ *("medians") from the metric space to define the clusters: each input data point is associated with the point from* $\mathcal{C}$ *that is closest to it (ties can be broken arbitrarily). The quality of the clustering is determined by the average distance of points to their closest median, ie for n points this is* $\frac{1}{n} \sum_x \min_i d(x, C_i)$.

Note that in both cases, the way points are allocated to clusters is the same, but it is the *objective function* that varies—that is, the function that we wish to minimize to get the best clustering. To give a good clustering we want to find centers/medians so that the generated clusters give a good covering of the points. This definition also puts each point in exactly one cluster; more general definitions allow a point to belong to multiple clusters, perhaps with some degree of certainty/probability.

Formally speaking, both these objectives are *NP-Hard* to optimize. That is, all known algorithms to find the optimal solution take time exponential in the size of the input. In theoretical computer science, researchers look for algorithms with guaranteed approximation factors, that come provably close to the optimal solution. However, these tend to be complicated and are often slow in practice. Instead, we will focus on describing some clustering algorithms that give few strong guarantees about their output, but which have been observed to work well and efficiently in practice.

3. Hierarchical Clustering

We begin our discussion of clustering algorithms with a simple to describe method [**7**]. The idea of hierarchical (also known as agglomerative) clustering is

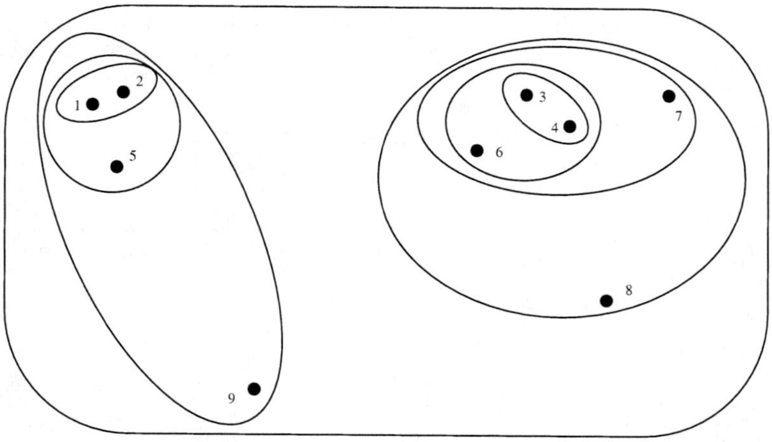

FIGURE 1. Hierarchical clustering of nine points. Ellipses around sets of points illustrate the hierarchy of containment. Initially, points 1 and 2 are closest, so they are merged; then points 3 and 4, and so on. Suppose we wanted to extract three clusters. Then, from this hierarchical clustering we would find the groupings $\{1,2,5\},\{3,4,6,7,8\},\{9\}$, since these are the last three sets to remain in the order of merging.

to begin with each point from the input as a separate cluster. We then build clusters by merging clusters that are close to each other: repeatedly merge the two clusters that are closest to each other out of all pairs. This gives a hierarchy of containment, as each point in the input belongs to a succession of larger clusters. If we keep merging, we end up with a single cluster that contains all points, and the structure of the hierarchy can be represented as a (binary) tree. From this tree we can extract a set of k clusters by, for example, stopping the merging when only k clusters remain, or when the closest pair of clusters are at a distance exceeding some threshold. An example hierarchical clustering is illustrated in Figure 1.

The crucial part of this algorithm is to define the distance between two clusters of multiple points. Several natural definitions suggest themselves: it could be the smallest distance between a point in one cluster and a point in another; the greatest distance between such points; or the average distance. Each definition has its own advantages and disadvantages. For example, taking the minimum cross-cluster distance (also known as *single-link* clustering) can lead to building clusters that are "snakes": long and thin clusters, where each point is close to its closest neighbor, but the whole cluster spreads out very far. Taking the maximum distance (*complete link* clustering) favors clusters that are circular in preference to other shapes that might better capture the nature of the data. And computing the average (*average link* clustering) can considerably slow down the computation of the clustering, which can already be somewhat slow. This is seen as one of the principal disadvantages of the hierarchical approach: even on fairly small data sets, the running time can be quite significant. We need to maintain the distance between each cluster and every other cluster. Initially, there are $\Omega(n^2)$ such inter-cluster distances, since everyone of the n input points is in its own cluster. Every time we merge a pair of clusters, we have to update the distance between the new cluster and all other clusters. Since there are up to n merges of clusters, the total cost of this algorithm is $\Omega(n^3)$ distance computations. This cost can grow to $\Omega(n^4)$ for the average link case.

4. The k-means method

Algorithm 1 The k-means algorithm [8]

Require: set of input *items*, x, in Euclidean space; desired number of clusters, k.

```
for 1 ≤ i ≤ k do
    kmeans[i] ← random item from data
    centroid[i] ← 0
    count[i] ← 0
repeat
    for all x ∈ items do
        mindist ← 1
        for 1 ≤ i ≤ k do
            if ||x − kmeans[i]||_2 < ||x − kmeans[mindist]||_2 then
                mindist ← i
        cluster[x] ← mindist
        centroid[mindist] ← centroid[mindist] + x
        count[mindist] ← count[mindist] + 1
    for 1 ≤ i ≤ k do
        kmeans[i] ← centroid[i]/count[i]
        centroid[i] ← 0
        count[i] ← 0;
until no items reclassified or repetition count exceeded
each x ∈ items is now classified by cluster[x]
```

The k-means algorithm [8] is very widely used to produce clusterings of data, due to its simplicity and speed. The idea is based around clustering items using *centroids*. These are points in the metric space that define the clusters. Each centroid defines a single cluster, and each point from the data is associated with the cluster defined by its closest centroid (ties being broken arbitrarily as usual). The algorithm proceeds in rounds: in each round, every input point is inspected and compared to the k centroid points to find which is closest. At the end of every round, we compute a new set of centroids based on the points in each cluster. For each cluster, we compute the centroid of that cluster, as the "center of mass" of the points. The center of mass can be found efficiently by finding the mean value of each co-ordinate. This leads to an efficient algorithm to compute the new centroids with a single scan of the data: for each of the k clusters, compute the sum of each co-ordinate value of all points that are associated with that cluster, and the count of the number of points in the cluster. The new centroids can then be easily computed after all points have been allocated to clusters. The process terminates either when the clusters do not change (no points are placed in different clusters), or after a set number of iterations. The algorithm is given in pseudocode in Algorithm 1.

From this description, two factors emerge. Firstly, the process relies on the data being numerical in all attributes. The distances measured are implicitly Euclidean distance. So, in the presences of non-numeric data, then k-means cannot be

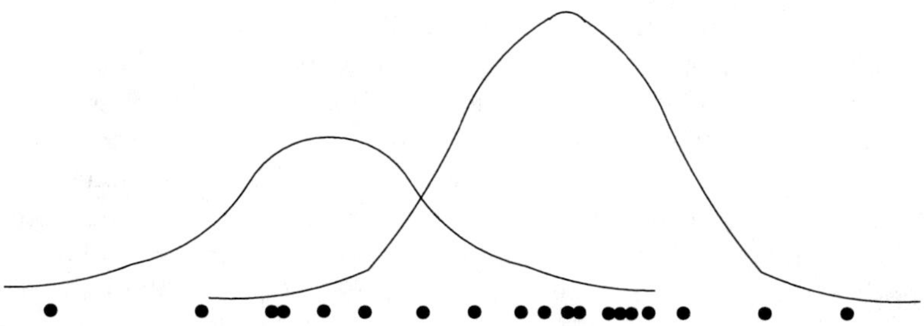

FIGURE 2. Expectation Maximization seeks to find the mixture of distributions that best explains the input set of points.

applied unless some pre-processing of the data is done to convert it to a numerical format. Secondly, the results depend on the choice of the initial setting of the cluster centroids. Typically these are chosen as random points from the input, but other heuristics can be applied. It is observed that the algorithm can be very sensitive to the initial centroids. Different choices can give very different clusterings. Certain bad cases can occur: sometimes, if two centroids are very close to one another, then one tends to dominate the other, so the number of points in one shrinks to almost zero, effectively "wasting" a centroid. Also, outlier points can distort the results, either by stretching the shape of the clusters, or by taking a centroid away from the bulk of the data. Various heuristics can be applied to avoid bad cases, such as repeating the clustering a few times and picking the one with the best score, based on the k-center or k-median criterion.

A more general complaint is that the method requires k to be specified up front, and typically it is not clear in advance how many clusters there are within the data. This applies to several clustering methods, not just k-means. The response of practitioners seems to be to try various values of k until an appropriate value is found. Here at least the speed of the k-means method is an advantage: each round requires each input point to be compared to the current k centroids, and so it can completed in time $O(kn)$. Typically, a relatively small number of rounds are required before a good clustering is found.

5. Expectation Maximization (EM)

In some ways, the Expectation Maximization (EM) [**2**] approach to clustering can be seen as an extension of k-means, with a more solid theoretical underpinning. What is the model that k-means is applying to the data? It is that the each data point belongs to one of k clusters that are defined by a set of k points. The division of space induced by these points can be represented by a Voronoi diagram [**14**]. EM relaxes the assumption that every point comes from a single cluster, and instead models the data as the result of some generative process. For example, typically EM uses a model that says that the data is being generated by a mixture of Gaussian (Normal) distributions. Each distribution gives a probability density over the whole of the space for generating points. If there are k such distributions, then the probability density function comes from taking the scaled union of these individual densities. Each of the distributions can have different parameters—in the case of Gaussians, these need only be the mean and standard deviation for one dimension; for higher dimensions, then there are more parameters to describe the shape of the distribution. This is illustrated in Figure 2. If we accept this model for the data, then the clustering process can be thought of as a search for the parameters of the generating distributions. The Expectation Maximization stage is, given the model and the data, to find the settings of the parameters of the model that best explain the data. That is, they are the most likely settings of the parameters given the data. The result of this means that we do not allocate points to clusters but rather for each data point we can evaluate the produced model at that point and see the relative probabilities that this point came from each of the k different distributions. It is this model which represents the clustering, and which can be used to predict future outcomes.

In order to generate the maximum likelihood settings of the parameters, various algorithms can be employed which, at a high level, resemble k-means. From an initial guess of the settings of the parameters, successive passes over the data refine these guess and improve the fit of the data to the current model. The details depend on the distributions used in the model (Gaussian, Log-Normal, Poisson, Discrete). For a model with a single Gaussian distribution, the sample mean is the maximum likelihood estimator. For two or more Gaussians, one can write out the expression for the mixture of these distributions, and, based on the current estimates of the parameters, compute the likelihood that each input point was generated by each of the distributions. Based on these likelihoods, we can create new settings of the parameters, and iterate. Each step increases the likelihood of the observed data given the current parameters, until a maximum is reached. Note that this maximum may be a local maximum, rather than the global maximum. The maximum that is reached depends on the initial setting of parameters. Hence we see the connection to k-means, the principal differences being the greater emphasis on an underlying model, and the way that each point has a probability or likelihood of belonging to each cluster, rather than a unique parent cluster.

A further advantage of EM is that non-numerical data can more easily be fitted into the models: for categorical data, for example, we can have a discrete probability distribution giving the probability of being in each category for each point. However, the additional cost of evaluating the model and computing the new likelihoods means that it can be slower than k-means. It also requires the user to provide a global hypothesis in advance on the model: not only do they have to give k, the number of distributions, but also describe these: are they k Gaussians, or j Poisson distributions and $k - j$ Gaussians, etc. Compared to the crispness of other so-called "hard clustering" methods, the "fuzzy clustering" produced by EM can disquiet some users.

6. Conclusion

Clustering remains a popular method for extracting hypotheses from large amounts of data. One particular advantage is that, unlike some other data mining methods, it does not require any of the input data to be "labeled", that is, inspected by an expert and tagged with a prognostication. Instead, clustering merely tries to identify groups of similar items within the data and report these back to the user. This falls into the class of "unsupervised learning" techniques, in contrast to "supervised learning", which requires a training set of data to be made available which is tagged with the appropriate class identifier. Understanding the mechanism of the clustering method is important for the user, so that they may evaluate the significance and meaning of the results of clustering. We have only discussed a few of the clustering methods that have been proposed, and mentioned a few of the factors in their use. There have been many variations and alternative methods defined in the database literature on clustering: methods such as CLARANS [**12**], DBSCAN [**3**], CURE [**4**], BIRCH [**17**], and many others.

Many software packages are commercially available that implement such clustering methods. For example, Mathematica [**9**] and Matlab [**10**] both contain routines to perform various clustering operations on input data. XLMiner is a plug-in for Excel that implements k-means clustering and hierarchical clustering [**16**]. Clustan (`http://www.clustan.com/`) is a software package devoted to cluster analysis. In addition to these and many other commercial solutions, one can also find free implementations of a variety of languages: Fortran, C++ and Java being the most popular. For more details on clustering approaches, see one of the several good quality textbooks on data mining [**6, 5, 1**], or tutorials available on the web [**15, 11, 13**].

B. Association Rules

James Abello

1. Association Rules Confidence and Support

Association rules play a central role in the process of identifying valid, novel, potentially useful, and ultimately understandable patterns or models in data [**19**]. Association rules were first introduced by [**79**]. It is useful to think of transactional data as providing information about which items co-occur in a transaction. Using this data one can create a co-occurrence table indicating the number of times that any pair occurs together in the set of transactions. This co-occurrence table allows the establishment of rules of the form: "item i and item j appear together in 35 percent of the transactions". This percentage of co-occurrence is called the *support* of the rule. The ratio of the support of a rule over the frequency of item i in the overall set of transactions is called the *confidence* of the rule "if item i is present then item j is also present". More formally, for the purpose of this write up, let O and A denote sets of objects and attributes respectively and consider data that can be represented as a subset E of object-attribute pairs , i.e. $E \subset O \times A$. A set of pairs (usually referred as an *itemset*) with the first component fixed can be interpreted as the set of items that co-occur in a fixed transaction. If X is a subset of A, let X' denote the set of objects in O which satisfy every property in the set X. An *association rule* is a pair (X, Y) (often written $X \to Y$) with X, Y subsets of A, interpreted to say "in (some) cases where X holds, Y also holds" (near implication), or "in the event of X, event Y also occurs" (conditional event). For an association rule $X \to Y$, Y is called the consequent. *Confidence* and *support* are two functions used to formulate evaluation criteria for association rules, and to control the size of sets of association rules that are created during data mining activity based on a context $\mathbb{K}$. $conf_{\mathbb{K}}(-)$ (confidence) and $supp_{\mathbb{K}}(-)$ (support), are given by

$$conf_{\mathbb{K}}(\ (X,Y)\ ) = \frac{|X' \cap Y'|}{|X'|} \qquad and \qquad supp_{\mathbb{K}}(\ (X,Y)\ ) = \frac{|X' \cap Y'|}{|O|}$$

Confidence outputs the percent of those instances in the data where the hypothesis holds for which the conclusion also holds. This is what statisticians refer to as the conditional probability of Y given X. In the context of association rules this term is observational rather than predictive. *Support* outputs the percent of overall evidence over the entire set of objects O for which the rule is positively witnessed. Even though the most *confident* rules appear to be the best it is in general necessary to measure how much better is a rule at predicting the outcome than just assuming the result. This measure is called an improvement measure and it is defined as the ratio of $p(condition \wedge outcome)/(p(condition)p(outcome))$. When this ratio is greater than one the corresponding rule is better than random chance.

As an example, consider the context of looking for associations between patient symptoms $\mathbb{G}$, where O is the set of patients observed at one practice and A is the set of symptoms presented by each patient (e.g., patient #141 may have complained of tiredness, nausea, vomiting and neck ache). If we consider the rule "nausea → vomiting" and find that

$$supp_{\mathbb{G}}(nausea \to vomiting) = 0.22 \qquad and \qquad conf_{\mathbb{G}}(nausea \to vomiting) = 0.84$$

then of all the observed patients, 22% complained of both nausea and vomiting, and of those patients that had nausea, 84% of them also complained of vomiting.

A theoretical framework for the study of association rules is the so called concept lattice that is discussed in another chapter in this volume [**18**]. There, an intimate connection between the computation of concepts, the derivation of association rules and some fundamental graph decompositions is explored. Some of these connections have been observed by several authors, e.g. [**21, 23**].

2. Generating Association Rules

The most fundamental computational question in this area consists of generating all the association rules whose confidence and support are above certain minimum pre-specified thresholds. Those itemsets with support above the minimum support are called frequent itemsets. The standard method to generate association rules computes first all frequent item sets (this is the expensive part) and uses then the frequent sets to generate all the desired association rules. A version of this process was introduced by [**20**] and it is referred in the literature as the A Priori method. Essentially, the key computational challenge in generating association rules is finding the frequent itemsets. A Priori limits the search space by observing that any frequent itemset must have all its subsets also being frequent. Therefore, it begins by finding all frequent sets of size one (the frequent items), then looks for pairs of these items that are frequent, then triple, quartets, and so on. Thus the algorithm makes multiple passes over the input, collecting information so that after the kth pass, all frequent itemsets of size k and below have been found.

One drawback of the A Priori method is that it can be very costly in terms of the number of possible candidates that must be considered at each step as potential frequent itemsets. This can result in large time and memory requirements. Various other approaches have been proposed to find other tradeoffs between running time and memory cost, and number of scans of the data set. For example, the FP Tree algorithm [**24**] builds a tree structure encoding all potential frequent itemsets, from which the itemsets can be extracted without explicitly generating candidate itemsets, hence reducing the run time cost. However, since a lot of information from the input is represented explicitly within the data structure, the overall memory cost can be higher than the original A Priori algorithm. Many other algorithms for frequent itemset mining have been given in the data mining and knowledge discovery literature.

In addition, during the last decade a host of variations on the method have been introduced some of them addressing some form of optimization required by the application at hand. These include mining of generalized, multi-level, quantitative, weighted and fuzzy association rules. The so-called inter-transaction association rules constituted the first step towards temporal data mining. Maximal association rule mining reduces the number of rules output by insisting that each frequent itemset used is maximal: that is, if any other item is added to the set, then the itemset is no longer frequent. This results in a more concise description of the data, but it can be much more costly to apply the pruning to generated rules to ensure that they are maximal. Sequential pattern mining is a different restriction: here, the transactions are specified as ordered lists, and the patterns sought are ordered subsequences of the list that are frequent. The addition of the order requirement adds further complexity to the task.

The easy conceptual basis for association rules, in addition to the wealth of algorithms to generate them, has led to a variety of work on applying them to all manner of problems. Successful applications of association rules generation and mining include predictive and risk assessment models for the financial services industry; tools for the analysis of genetic sequence data; integration and analysis of customer information to improve customer acquisition and retention; analysis of online shopping behavior; fraud detection, tracking and monitoring; creation of individualized health care plans; optimization of trading strategies; and email spam detectors.

3. Conclusion

Association Rules have become one of the central tools in transactional data mining. We have introduced what they are and briefly mentioned some of their central applications. Some of their uses within epidemiology are addressed by the papers in this volume on concept lattices.

C. Support Vector Machines

Dmitriy Fradkin and Ilya Muchnik

1. Introduction

In many real-life situations we want to be able to assign an object to one of several categories based on some of its characteristics. For example, based on the results of several medical tests we want to be able to say whether a patient has a particular disease or should be recommended a specific treatment.

In computer science such situations are described as classification problems. A binary (two-class) classification problem can be described as follows: given a set of labeled points (x_i, y_i), $i = \overline{1, l}$, where $x_i \in \Re^d$ are vectors of features and $y_i \in \{-1, +1\}$ are class labels, construct a rule that correctly assigns a new point x to one of the classes.

The vectors x_i in this formulation correspond to objects, and the dimensions of the space are the features or characteristics of these objects. For example, a vector may represent a person, with individual features corresponding to the measurements given by some medical tests — blood pressure, cholesterol level, white cell count and so on.

Using labels $\{0, \ldots, K-1\}$ instead of $\{-1, +1\}$ we can describe a multiclass problem with K classes. A classification method or algorithm is a particular way of constructing a rule, also called a classifier, from the labeled data and applying it to the new data.

Support Vector Machines (SVM) recently became one of the most popular classification methods. They have been used in a wide variety of applications such as text classification [**32**], facial expression recognition [**33**], gene analysis[**30**] and many others.

Support Vector Machines can be thought of as a method for constructing a special kind of rule, called a linear classifier, in a way that produces classifiers with theoretical guarantees of good predictive performance (the quality of classification on unseen data). The theoretical foundation of this method is given by statistical learning theory [**39**].

While no general method for producing non-linear rules with such properties is known, the so-called "kernel trick" can be used to construct special kinds of non-linear rules using the SVM methodology.

2. Linear Classifiers

A classifier can frequently be represented as a function $f(x) : \Re^d \rightarrow \Re$. In a two-class case, a point is assigned to the positive class if $f(x) \geq 0$, and to the negative class otherwise.

A classifier function $f(x)$ is linear if it can be expressed as:

(1) $$f(x; w, b) = < w, x > +b$$

where w, b are parameters of the function and $<,>$ denotes the inner product of two vectors.

A set of points (x_i, y_i), $i = \overline{1, l}$, where $y_i \in \{-1, +1\}$ are class labels, is called *linearly separable* if a linear classifier can be found so that $y_i f(x_i) > 0$, $\forall i = 1, \dots, l$.

The use of linear classifiers in machine learning can be traced back to Rosenblatt's work on the perceptron [**38**], though they have been used before that in statistics. The perceptron algorithm works by taking one instance at a time and predicting its class. If the prediction is correct, no adjustments are made. If the prediction is wrong, the parameters, describing a hyperplane, are moved in the direction of the point where the mistake occurred. A scalar value, η, called the *learning rate* determines how the how far the parameters are moved. The choice of a learning rate can significantly affect the number of iterations until convergence on a linearly-separable set. The pseudocode for the perceptron learning, taken from [**28**], is given as Algorithm 2.

Algorithm 2 Online Perceptron Learning Algorithm [**28**]

Require: A linearly separable set S, learning rate $\eta \in \Re^+$

$w_0 = 0; b_0 = 0; k = 0;$

$R = \max\limits_{1 \le i \le l} ||x_i||$

while at least one mistake is made in the **for** loop **do**

    for $i = 1, \dots, l$ **do**

        if $y_i(< w_k, x_i > +b_k) \le 0$ **then**

            $w_{k+1} = w_k + \eta y_i x_i$

            $b_{k+1} = b_k + \eta y_i R^2$ (updating bias[1])

            $k = k + 1$

Return w_k, b_k, where k is the number of mistakes

2.1. Margin and VC dimension. The idea of *margin* (Figure 3) has come to play an important role in the theory of statistical learning.

A hyperplane

$$< w^*, x > +b^* = 0, \ ||w^*|| = 1 \tag{2}$$

is called a γ-margin separating hyperplane if

$$y_i(< w^*, x > +b^*) \ge \gamma \tag{3}$$

for all (x_i, y_i) in set S. Here γ (clearly $\gamma > 0$) is the margin.

Any separating hyperplane can be converted into this form. Suppose

$$y(< w, x > +b) \ge 1. \tag{4}$$

Then, by setting $w^* = \frac{w}{||w||}$ and $b^* = \frac{b}{||w||}$, we obtain a γ-margin separating hyperplane with $\gamma = \frac{1}{||w||}$.

The first result suggesting a relation between the margin and predictive ability of a classifier was Novikov's theorem.

[1]Usually this update is given as $b_{k+1} = b_k + \eta y_i$. However, such formulation makes the result of Novikov's theorem, given below, dependent on the exact value of the bias, b^*, of the separating hyperplane. This reflects the fact that R can be increased simply by moving all points away from the origin. The update used in the Algorithm 2 (suggested in [**28**]) compensates for that.

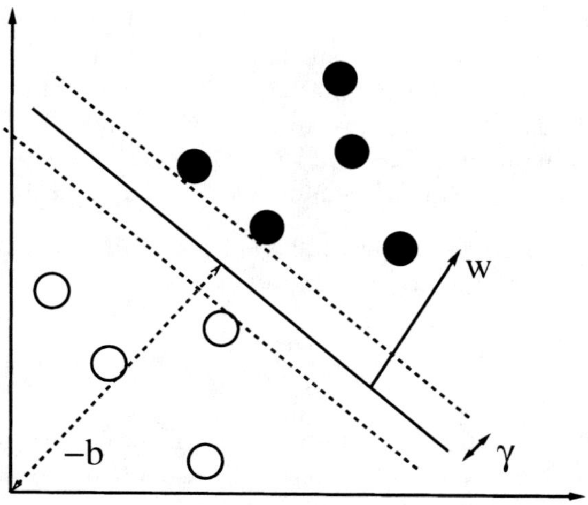

FIGURE 3. Here $(w, -b)$ define the separating hyperplane and γ is the size of the margin. The relation between w and γ is discussed in the text.

THEOREM 2.1. *Novikov's Theorem* [**35**] *Let* S, $|S| = l$ *be a training set, i.e. a set of points with class labels, and let*

$$R = \max_{1 \le i \le l} ||x_i|| \tag{5}$$

Suppose that there exists a γ*-margin separating hyperplane* (w, b) *such that* $y_i(< w, x_i > +b) \ge \gamma$, $\forall\ 1 \le i \le l$. *Then the number of mistakes made by the on-line perceptron algorithm on* S *is at most*

$$\left(\frac{2R}{\gamma}\right)^2 \tag{6}$$

This theorem effectively proves that for a linearly separable set of points the perceptron algorithm finds a separating hyperplane after making a finite number of mistakes. The number of mistakes is directly proportional to the ratio of the volume of the data to the measure of separation of the classes, γ.

Note that Novikov's theorem shows convergence on a periodic training sequence. This result has been extended to an arbitrary infinite sequence of points (each belonging to one of two region that can be linearly separated) by Aizerman et. al. [**25**].

Novikov's theorem bounds the number of errors in the training stage. But in classification we are interested in the accuracy of a classifier on unseen data. Such a number clearly cannot be computed exactly, but it turns out it can be bounded.

Before proceeding let us define the notion of Vapnik-Chevronenkis dimension.

DEFINITION 4. *The* Vapnik-Chervonenkis (VC) dimension *of a set of classifiers is the maximum number* h *of points that can be separated into all possible* 2^h *ways using classifiers in this set. If for any* n *there exists a set of* n *points that can be separated into two classes in all possible ways, the VC dimension of this set of functions is said to be infinite.*

Intuitively, VC dimension measures the complexity of the classifiers in the set. If the classifiers are simple, they have small VC dimension. If they are complicated, the VC dimension is large. For example, the VC dimension of hyperplanes in R^d is known to be $d+1$. The following two results bound the VC dimension of the set of γ-margin separating hyperplanes and the probability of misclassifying an unseen instance with such a hyperplane chosen on the training data.

THEOREM 2.2. **Theorem 5.1 in [39]** *Let $x \in X$ belong to sphere of radius R. The the set of γ-margin separating hyperplanes has VC dimension h bounded by:*

$$h \leq \min\left(\left(\frac{R}{\gamma}\right)^2, d\right) + 1 \tag{7}$$

THEOREM 2.3. **Corollary to Theorem 5.1 in [39]** *With probability $1-\eta$ the probability of a test example not being separated correctly by a γ-margin hyperplane has the bound*

$$P_{error} \leq \frac{m}{l} + \frac{E}{2}\left(1 + \sqrt{1 + \frac{4m}{lE}}\right) \tag{8}$$

where

$$E = 4\frac{h(\ln\frac{2l}{h} + 1) - \ln\frac{\eta}{4}}{l}, \tag{9}$$

m is the number of training examples not separated correctly by γ-margin hyperplane, and h is the bound of the VC dimension given in theorem 2.3.

The bound on the probability of making a mistake on unseen data is proportional to the VC dimension of the set of classifiers. In other words, everything else being equal, a classifier with a lower VC dimension is likely to be a better predictor. Notice that this result does not depend on any assumptions about the distribution of the test data — it is a "distribution-free" bound.

Since the upper bound on VC dimension is inversely proportional to the margin, the strategy for building a good classifier is to have as large a margin as possible while keeping the number of errors on the training set low.

This is somewhat similar to the idea regularization but is motivated from the perspective of the statistical learning theory. It can also be seen as a version of Occam's razor: we want to use the simplest classifier that makes no (or fewest) mistakes on the training set.

2.2. The Maximal Margin in Separable Case. We have seen in the previous section that the probability of making a mistake is inversely proportional to the size of the margin. Thus we would like to find a classifier with the largest margin that still correctly separates the training points.

The maximal-margin separating hyperplane can be found by solving the following optimization problem:

$$\text{minimize}_{w,b} < w, w > \tag{10}$$

subject to:

$$y_i(< w, x_i > +b) \geq 1, \ \forall i = 1, \ldots, l \tag{11}$$

One method for solving optimization problems involves introducing Lagrange multipliers,α_i, for the constraints [**26**]. In this case, the so-called Lagrangian function is given by:

$$L(w, b, \alpha) = \frac{1}{2} < w, w > - \sum_{i=1}^{l} \alpha_i [y_i (< w, x_i > + b) - 1] \tag{12}$$

Taking derivatives with respect to w and b gives:

$$w = \sum_{i=1}^{l} y_i \alpha_i x_i \tag{13}$$

and

$$0 = \sum_{i=1}^{l} y_i \alpha_i \tag{14}$$

Note that w is given by a linear combination of the training points. We will return to this observation later on.

Re-substituting these into the primal problem (12) gives a dual formulation:

$$\text{maximize } W(\alpha) = \sum_{i=1}^{l} \alpha_i - \sum_{i,j=1}^{l} y_i y_j \alpha_i \alpha_j < x_i, x_j > \tag{15}$$

subject to:

$$\sum_{i=1}^{l} y_i \alpha_i = 0, \ \alpha_i \geq 0, \ \forall i = 1, \ldots, l \tag{16}$$

Let α^* be a vector of parameters optimizing $W(\alpha)$. The the weight vector $w^* = \sum_{i=1}^{l} y_i \alpha_i^* x_i$ is a maximal margin hyperplane, with margin

$$\gamma = \frac{1}{||w^*||_2}. \tag{17}$$

The parameter b is not present in the dual problem and has to be computed from the primal constraints (11).

Notice that, because of (13), the classifier $f(x)$ can be expressed as:

$$f(x) =< w, x > +b = \sum_{i=1}^{l} y_i \alpha_i < x_i, x > +b \tag{18}$$

If $\alpha_i = 0$, then x_i is not used in decision rule and can be discarded. Points x_i such that $\alpha_i \neq 0$ lie on the margin and are called support vectors. They determine the decision boundary.

2.3. Extension for the non-separable case. Until now we have discussed only the linearly-separable case. However, similar machinery can be used to handle the non-separable case. The main idea is that those points that lie on the wrong side of the hyperplane are explicitly penalized by introducing *slack* variables, ξ, that control how far on the wrong side of a hyperplane a point lies.

The optimization problem becomes:

$$\text{minimize}_{w,b}\frac{1}{2} < w, w > +C\sum_{i=1}^{l}\xi_i \tag{19}$$

subject to:

$$y_i(< w, x_i > +b) \geq 1 - \xi_i,\ \xi_i \geq 0,\ \forall i = 1, \dots, l \tag{20}$$

where the parameter C, controlling the trade-off between the size of the margin and the training errors, is chosen by the user.

The dual then becomes:

$$\text{maximize} \sum_{i=1}^{l}\alpha_i - \sum_{i,j=1}^{l} y_i y_j \alpha_i \alpha_j < x_i, x_j > \tag{21}$$

subject to:

$$\sum_{i=1}^{l} y_i\alpha_i = 0,\ C \geq \alpha_i \geq 0,\ \forall i = 1, \dots, l \tag{22}$$

Once again the solution is given by a linear combination of inner products with support vectors: $w = \sum_{i=1}^{l} y_i\alpha_i x_i$. There are no general methods for choosing parameters b in a non-separable case - it is usually set to optimize some performance measure on a training or a validation set. The same approach is often taken for choosing a value of C.

2.4. Multi-class classification. Many methods exist for building a multi-class classifier system from binary classifiers (one-vs-all, one-vs-one, error-correcting output codes (ECOC) [**29**], Directed Acyclic Graph (DAG) [**37**]). In all of these approaches multiple binary classifiers are trained separately and their predictions are then combined. For example, in one-vs-all classification, with K classes, K classifiers are constructed. Each recognizes points of one of the classes as positive and those of all others as negative. A new point is assigned to the class h if the corresponding classifier gives this point the highest score among all K classifiers. In one-vs-one, a classifier is trained for each pair of classes. Classification usually proceeds as follows: each of $\frac{K(K-1)}{2}$ classifiers makes a prediction and the number of votes for each class is counted. The point is assigned to the class that has received most votes. DAG and ECOC are more sophisticated in how classifiers are trained and how their predictions are combined.

Special multiclass methods have been developed for SVM. They usually involve solving a single optimization problem. In [**40**] the optimization problem to be solved (over K separating hyperplanes and lK slack variables) is:

$$\text{minimize}_{w^j,b^j,\xi^j}\frac{1}{2}\sum_{j=1}^{K} < w^j, w^j > +C\sum_{i=1}^{l}\sum_{j\neq y_i}\xi_i^j \tag{23}$$

subject to:

$$\begin{aligned}(< w^{y_i}, x_i > +b^{y_i}) \geq (< w^j, x_i > +b^j + 2 - \xi_i^j),\ \forall j \neq y_i \\ \xi_i^j \geq 0,\ \forall i = 1, \dots, l\end{aligned} \tag{24}$$

A new point x is classified as follows:

$$f(x) = \text{argmax}_{j=1,\dots,K}(< w^j, x > + b^j) \tag{25}$$

Cramer and Singer [**27**] suggested a somewhat different formulation, requiring only l slack variables:

$$\text{minimize}_{w^j,\xi} \frac{1}{2} \sum_{j=1}^{K} < w^j, w^j > + C \sum_{i=1}^{l} \xi_i, \tag{26}$$

subject to:

$$\begin{gathered}(< w^{y_i}, x_i > - < w^j, x_i >) \geq 1 - \xi_i \\ \forall i = \overline{1,l},\ j = \overline{1,K} : \xi_i \geq 0,\ j \neq y_i.\end{gathered} \tag{27}$$

The resulting decision function is:

$$f(x) = \text{argmax}_{j=1,\dots,K} < w^j, x > \tag{28}$$

2.5. Computational Issues. We have shown that the problem of finding a maximal margin hyperplane can be formulated as a particular quadratic optimization problem. Many numerical methods for solving general quadratic optimization problems are known. For the special kind of optimization needed for SVM there exist particularly efficient algorithms such as Platt's sequential minimal optimization (SMO) [**36**] capable of handling thousands of vectors in thousand-dimensional spaces.

3. The "Kernel Trick"

The main idea behind the "kernel trick" is to map the data into a different space, called *feature space*, and to construct a linear classifier in this space. It can also be seen as a way to construct non-linear classifiers in the original space. Below we explain what the kernel trick is and how these two views are reconciled.

Notice that in the the dual problem (15) the training points are included only via their inner products. Also, as can be seen in (18), the classifier function $f(x)$ can be expressed as a sum of inner products with support vectors.

An important result, called Mercer's theorem, states that any symmetric positive semi-definite function $K(x,z)$ is an inner product in some space (and vice-versa). In other words, any such function $K(x,z)$ implicitly defines a mapping into so-called feature space $\phi : x \to \phi(x)$ such that $K(x,z) =< \phi(x), \phi(z) >$. Such functions K are called kernels.

The feature space can be high-dimensional or even have infinite dimension. However we don't need to know the actual mapping since we can use kernel function to compute similarity in the feature space.

Some examples of kernels include polynomial kernels

$$K(x,z) = (< x, z > + 1)^p \tag{29}$$

and gaussian kernels

$$K(x,z) = e^{-\frac{||x-z||^2}{2\sigma^2}}. \tag{30}$$

Many kernels have been developed for special applications such as sequence matching in bioinformatics [**31**]. General properties of kernels are described in many publications, including [**28**].

By replacing the inner product in the formulation of SVM by a kernel and solving for Lagrange multipliers α_i, we can obtain via (18) a maximal margin separating hyperplane in the feature space defined by this kernel. Thus choosing non-linear kernels allows us to construct classifiers that are linear in the feature space, even though they are non-linear in the original space.

The dual problem in the kernel form is:

$$\text{maximize } W(\alpha) = \sum_{i=1}^{l} \alpha_i - \sum_{i,j=1}^{l} y_i y_j \alpha_i \alpha_j K(x_i, x_j) \tag{31}$$

$$\text{subject to } 0 = \sum_{i=1}^{l} y_i \alpha_i, \ \alpha_i \geq 0, \ \forall i = 1, \dots, l \tag{32}$$

and the classifier is given by:

$$f(x) = \sum_{i=1}^{l} y_i \alpha_i K(x_i, x). \tag{33}$$

The idea of viewing kernels as implicit maps into a feature space was first suggested in [**25**]. However this approach was not widely used until the emergence of SVM. Many algorithms other than SVM have now been "kernelized" — reformulated in terms of kernels rather than inner products. A survey of kernel-based methods is given by [**34**].

4. Conclusion

In this note we attempted to highlight the main ideas underlying the SVM method. For a detailed explanation of these, and many other ideas in statistical learning and kernel methods an interested reader is referred to [**28, 39**]. While [**28**] provides a clear and broad introduction to the area, [**39**] goes into much greater depth. Both of these books provide many references to relevant literature. Another valuable resource is kernel-machines website (`http://www.kernel-machines.org/`) which contains information on books, articles and software related to SVM and other kernel-based methods.

D. Statistics and Data Mining

David Madigan

The field of Statistics develops methodology for data analysis. Key statistical activities include experimental design, sampling, exploratory data analysis, stochastic modeling, testing, and prediction. Traditionally Statistics has closely aligned itself with Mathematics, and much statistical research has focused on often-arcane mathematical properties of statistical artifacts. Increasingly however, major developments in Statistics draw as much from Computer Science as from Mathematics. The emergence of massive data sets and ever more sophisticated modeling requirements are having a profound effect on the cutting edge of statistical research and practice.

1. The Big Ideas

All of the "big ideas" in Statistics apply to data mining. These include:

- Sampling: A random sample of 1,500 from a population of millions or even billions can estimate the percentage of the entire population who have a certain trait or opinion to within 3%. That is, the difference between the sample-based estimate and the correct answer is no more than 3% for 95% of such random samples, at least when the true percentage is not very close to either 0% or 100%.
- Experimentation: Advances in experimental design have revolutionized fields as diverse as medicine and manufacturing. Standard methods allow us to routinely and reliably infer causation from practically-sized experiments.
- Prediction: A staggering array of statistical techniques is now available to facilitate well-calibrated predictions about future observables. No forecaster has a crystal ball, but intelligently chosen statistical approaches can properly account for uncertainty and dramatically improve the quality of decision making under uncertainty.
- Visualization: Developments in statistical graphics now enable viewing of up to 100,000 data points in 20 or more dimensions - see, for example, `http://www.ggobi.org`.
- Bayesian Inference: Until quite recently, Bayesian inference occupied a quirky and somewhat annoying Statistical backwater. "Bayesians" were long on talk but short on action. Developments in Monte Carlo methods combined with raw computing power have changed all that, and the front-line statistical journals are packed with elaborate Bayesian applications.

Real-world application of these ideas requires some care. To quote Deming [**41**]:

> "So-called modern 'theories of estimation' are not theories of estimation at all, but are rather theories of distribution and are a disappointment to one who is faced with the necessity of making a

> prediction from his data, i.e., of basing some critical course of action on them, The conviction that such devices as confidence limits and Student's t provide a basis for action regardless of the size of the sample whence they were computed, even under conditions of statistical control, is too common a fallacy."

Nowhere is this concern more prescient than in arenas such as medical research where "P-values" have unfortunately emerged as the key analytical outputs from clinical trials . The P-value is the probability associated with the event that the test statistic was as extreme as the value observed, or more so. However, the event that actually happened was that a specific value of the test statistic was observed. Consequently, the relationship between the P-value and the veracity of the target hypothesis is subtle at best. Jeffreys [**44**] puts it this way:

> "I have always considered the arguments for the use of P absurd. They amount to saying that a hypothesis that may or may not be true is rejected because a greater departure from the trial value was improbable; that is, that it has not predicted something that has not happened."

The fully-fleshed out Bayesian decision theoretic framework does address these concerns, but routine Bayesian analyses rarely go all the way.

2. The Bayesian Perspective

The standard "classical" or "frequentist" approach to statistics revolves around the idea that we are trying to estimate fixed unknowns (or "parameters") and it regards the data values before us as only one possible outcome of the supposedly random process of data-generation. Thus with this approach the data are viewed as random and the unknowns as fixed.

With the Bayesian approach, we hold constant things we know, including the data values, and we use the machinery of probability to quantify our uncertainty about the unknowns. That is, with this approach the data are fixed and the unknowns are random. As a result, Bayesian inferential statements tend to be easier to interpret, and it is often easier with the Bayesian approach to build highly complex models when such complexity makes sense. The Bayesian approach also provides a natural framework for sequential learning. Before the data arrive, a prior distribution over the unknowns represents the available prior knowledge (often a very flat distribution). The arriving data then update this prior distribution to create the posterior distribution. This posterior distribution in turn plays the role of a prior distribution awaiting more data.

As an example of the interpretability of Bayesian outputs, consider the interpretation of interval estimates. A Bayesian 90% probability interval for a mean, for instance, has a 90% probability of containing the unknown mean. A classical 90% confidence interval, on the other hand, can only be interpreted in relation to a sequence of similar inferences that might be made with other data sets.

The Bayesian approach to hierarchical modeling is exquisitely straightforward. Consider the following fictitious example. Columbo Inc., a large healthcare corporation, owns say 50 major hospitals. Total hip replacements (THR) are performed at each of these hospitals although the frequency with which the hospitals performed the procedure in 2003 varies from a minimum of 18 at one hospital to a maximum of 650 at another hospital. Columbo wishes to compare THR outcomes across the hospitals. One common outcome measure for THR is length of stay. A naive comparison of length-of-stay measures across the hospitals clearly could be quite misleading since it could well be the case that some hospitals handle more "risky" patients than others. A standard approach in these situations [**43**] is to adjust for risk using a regression model. So, here we have:

$$\text{Length-of-stay} = B_0 + (B_1 * \text{Risk}) + \text{error}$$

(Customized risk scores exist for a large number of procedures and disease—see [**43**]). How should we estimate the parameters of this model? One possibility would be to lump all the patients together and ignore the fact that they attended different hospitals. This will almost certainly lead to tricky heterogeneity issues in modeling the error however, and affords no way to incorporate known hospital covariates such as hospital size or location. Another possibility would be fit a single model for each hospital, and then compare the risk-adjusted lengths of stay across the hospitals. However, it is clear that the model for the hospital with 18 procedures will be considerably less reliable than the model for the hospital with 650 procedures. Furthermore, the B_1's for the different hospitals will presumably be somewhat similar, as will the B_0's and the error distributions—fitting separate models ignores this fact. The Bayesian hierarchical approach allows us to bridge the gap between these two extremes. On the one hand it does use all the data. On the other hand, it allows for heterogeneity amongst the hospitals. How does it do this? The basic idea is to fit a separate model for each hospital, but to assume that the parameters of the 50 models represent a sample from a population of parameters. For instance, we might assume that the B_1's for the 50 hospitals arise from a normal distribution with some mean and variance *a priori*. In this way the different hospitals can "borrow strength" from each other - what we learn from the hospital with 650 procedures will sharpen our inferences about the hospital with 18 procedures, and to a lesser extent, vice versa. Incorporation of hospital-level data is also straightforward.

The predictive benefits of the Bayesian approach can be significant. [**45**] describe a Bayesian approach to locating users in wireless networks. In a standard Wi-Fi setup, for example, one or more access points serve end-users. Wi-Fi location estimation can then use the received signal strength (RSS). The standard approach uses supervised learning techniques. The training data comprise vectors of signal strengths, one for each of a collection of known locations. The dimension of each vector equals the number of access points. Collection of the location data is labor intensive requiring physical distance measurements with respect to a reference object such as a wall. Consequently, minimizing the number of training observations needed to adequately profile a particular site is an important objective. The key finding in [**45**] is that a hierarchical Bayesian approach, incorporating prior physical knowledge about the nature of Wi-Fi signals, can provide accurate location estimates without *any* location information in the training data. Specifically the training data comprise signal strength vectors alone. Cheap sniffing devices can gather such vectors repeatedly and without cost from whatever wireless devices are available. In the context of an infrastructure-based deployment, the Bayesian model can thus eliminate profiling entirely.

In practice, Bayesian data analyses typically begin with a simple model that aims to capture some of the coarse level structure in the data generating mechanism.

A battery of model assessment tools exists to assist with subsequent model elaboration (see, for example, [**42**]). Such elaborations justify themselves primarily in terms of their ability to improve the preditive accuracy of the model. Since all but the most trival Bayesian analyses require numerical methods to compute the requisite posterior distributions, tools such as BUGS provide excellent model building environments. BUGS[2] allows the user to specify models visually using the language of probabilistic graphical models and frees the user from the details of the underlying Markov chain Monte Carlo numerical methods. BUGS is intended for complex models in which there may be many unknown quantities but for which substantial conditional independence assumptions are appropriate. Particular structures include generalised linear models with hierarchical or crossed random effects, latent variable or frailty models, measurement errors in responses and covariates, informative censoring, constrained estimation, and missing data. The two volumes of examples that are included in BUGS provide an excellent starting point for many Bayesian analyses. BUGS does have its limitations however, and truly large-scale models are still off-limits to general purpose tools.

3. Conclusion

The diversity of activity within Statistics is striking and no two statisticians would agree on what constitutes the core of the field. Furthermore, the statistical process, like the data mining process, is complex and spans a range of activities from gathering data to looking at data to making inferences about quantities that are not observed. Statistics and Data Mining overlap almost completely and it seems self-evident to us that both fields could benefit from more interaction.

[2]`http://www.mrc-bsu.cam.ac.uk/bugs/`

E. Boosting

Ofer Melnik

Making accurate predictions based on past observations is a main direction of Machine Learning techniques. One form of prediction is classification, where items are assigned labels using measurements. For example, a classification task might be to give a medical diagnosis using lab results and symptom information. Classical approaches for this task might involve building diagnostic models in the form of "***if** we observe these A symptoms **then** diagnose B*" (expert systems [**56**]) or building probabilistic models that capture the relationships between symptoms and diagnoses (probabilistic networks [**47**]). Unlike these approaches that require direct expert knowledge for constructing classification rules (classifiers), Machine Learning approaches attempt to gather much of this knowledge automatically and implicitly by observing examples of correct classification.

One successful Machine Learning method for building classifiers is called Boosting. It is based on the idea that while it may be difficult to take examples and build a highly accurate prediction rule in one shot, it may be possible to do so incrementally by gradually constructing and combining weak prediction rules. A weak prediction rule in this case can be thought of as a rough rule of thumb that has some basis but does not capture the data completely. For example, in diagnosis a high temperature might indicate an infection but not conclusively and consistently. Boosting approaches are general in the sense that they do not require weak rules of a particular type, rather they assume that they are given a weak learning algorithm that for different distributions of training examples can return a weak rule that is slightly better than random.

A boosting algorithm receives a training dataset of preclassified examples and a weak learning algorithm. At each iteration the boosting algorithm assigns an importance to each training example (a distribution) and builds a weak prediction rule over this distribution. At its termination the boosting algorithm returns a prediction rule that is a combination of the weak prediction rules. Assuming the weak learning algorithm works, the resulting combined prediction rule minimizes the misclassification error on the training examples.

Intuitively boosting works by adjusting the example distribution to focus on the "harder" examples. That is, the importance of examples that are already covered by existing rules is diminished while the misclassified examples are emphasized to motivate the formation of weak prediction rules to address them. The weak rules are combined using a weighted majority vote, where the weights are selected to maximize classification accuracy.

1. Adaboost

Adaboost [**53**] was the first practical Boosting algorithm. It was the catalyst that sparked much of the practical and theoretical interest in boosting as a method for building predictive models. Algorithm 3 shows the Adaboost algorithm for binary classification.

1.1. Training error reduction. Assuming the weak learners are consistently better than random, the Adaboost algorithm reduces the training error and converges exponentially in the number of iterations. If the error of each weak learner, h_t, is better than random by γ_t then since it can be proven that the training error (left) is bounded by the exponential (right)

$$\frac{1}{m}\left|\{i : H(x_i) \neq y_i\}\right| \leq \exp\left(-\sum_t \gamma_t/2\right)$$

— the training error is minimized exponentially fast. Thus the Adaboost algorithm combines the weak learning rules to build a combined prediction rule with an arbitrarily low training error rate.

1.2. Generalization. While achieving low training error is a prerequisite for building accurate predictive models, low training error does not necessarily mean good generalization to unseen data. A typical pitfall in building predictive models is called over-fitting. Over fitting takes place when the model matches the training data too closely rather than generalizing from it. One of the fears with procedures like boosting that incrementally build more and more complex models is that they would tend to over-fit. However, one of the initial conundrums of the Adaboost algorithm was that it apparently avoided over-fitting even when run for thousands of iterations [**49, 63**]. In fact it appeared that iterating actually continued to improve generalization on test data even after achieving convergence on the training data. While later experiments showed that over-fitting does occur if the algorithm is run long enough and that this phenomenon is particular to relatively noise free datasets, it is still one of the strengths of Boosting. One explanation for this phenomena is that Adaboost acts to increase the margins of the prediction on the training data, where the margin, $margin(x, y) = y \sum \alpha_t h_t(x) / \sum |\alpha_t|$, can be interpreted as the confidence in the prediction [**65**]. The principle of margin maximization is also a motivating factor of another successful Machine Learning technique, Support Vector Machines (SVMs) [**69**]. Note that there are other interpretations of what the Adaboost algorithm is doing, including paradigms from entropy minimization[**58**], game theory [**54**] and optimization [**60**].

2. Extensions and other Algorithms

The core Adaboost algorithm is designed for two-class problems. Various multi-class variations of Boosting exist. Some of these require variations in the weak learning algorithm to achieve provable results [**53**]. Other methods using error-correcting codes allow regular binary weak learners to be used [**57, 66**].

Another prediction task is regression, where a measurement is assigned a numeric value rather than a label (classification). Different boosting algorithms for regression exist [**50, 55**]. Most of these algorithms work in ways similar to the classification case, where a distribution is modified to emphasize the examples with large residuals. As such, similar convergence proofs for regression can also be demonstrated.

Boosting algorithms also exist for the task of generating and combining ranks [**52**], for example, in applications of collaborative filtering and meta search.

Algorithm 3 The Adaboost algorithm

Require: $(x_1, y_1), \ldots, (x_n, y_n)$, the training examples, where $x_i \in X$ is a measurement and $y_i \in \{-1, 1\}$ is a classification label.

1: Initialize the example distribution $D_1(i) = 1/n$
2: **for** $t = 1 \ldots T$ **do**
3: Train a weak prediction rule, h_t, using distribution D_t.
4: Choose $\alpha_t = \frac{1}{2} \ln \left(\frac{1-\epsilon_t}{\epsilon_t} \right)$ where $\epsilon_t = \Pr_{i \sim D_t} \left[h_t(x_i) \neq y_i \right]$ is the classification error of the rule.
5: Update:
$D_{t+1}(i) = \frac{D_t(i) \exp(-\alpha_t y_t h_t(x_t))}{Z_t}$
where Z_t is chosen to make D_{t+1} a distribution.
6: Output the combined classification rule: $H(x) = sign \left(\sum_{t=1}^{T} \alpha_t h_t(x) \right)$

The issue of noisy data has been addressed in different ways for boosting. One of the first approaches is the *LogitBoost* algorithm which applies a different error bound to the data that does not emphasize misclassified examples as much. More explicitly, algorithms like $Adaboost_{Reg}$ [**64**], *BrownBoost* [**51**] and *SmoothBoost* [**68**] impose limitations on the training distributions and the impact individual examples can have. Other approaches [**59**] look at margins over the whole distribution rather than individual examples.

3. Conclusion

Boosting is an effective approach for building predictive models from example data. Medical applications of Boosting include Melanoma diagnosis [**61**], Lung Cancer identification [**70**] and tumor classification from gene expression data [**48**]. It has also been successfully applied to other fields, including engineering [**62**] , text classification [**67**] and finance [**46**]. Boosting is based on the idea of constructing highly accurate models by incrementally combining weak prediction rules. Extensions of Boosting exist to cover different problem types, including binary classification, multi-class classification and regression. In recent years Boosting and related algorithms have been extensively studied and refined. A valuable resource for the interested practitioner is `http://boosting.org`, which contains links to papers, software and information about the boosting community.

F. External Memory Algorithms (A Digest)

James Abello

ABSTRACT. The Input-Output communication (or simply, IO) between the different levels of storage devices is often a significant bottleneck in applications that process massive amounts of data. Explicit management of the contents of each storage level helps to incorporate locality directly into the algorithms. This results in many instances in substantial performance gains. This section contains a brief sample of some of the major existing techniques for the design and analysis of external memory algorithms and data structures. It is intended for non-specialists and it is modeled after the survey articles [**81, 110**].

1. Introduction

When data is too large to fit entirely in the computer's fast internal memory it is usually stored in slower external storage devices such as magnetic disks. Essentially, internal memory is fast because it provides random access to its contents. On the other hand, external storage devices are substantially cheaper but provide only sequential access to the data. The transfer of data between internal memory and external storage has been recognized as a major bottleneck. It is termed the *IO* bottleneck. Modern systems employ several types of caching and prefetching mechanisms to alleviate the *IO* bottleneck. However, for certain class of computations substantial performance gains are achieved by incorporating locality directly into the algorithms [**77, 111, 75**]. In other words, bypassing the virtual memory system and devising algorithms that manage explicitly the transfer of data between fast internal memory and slower external storage is in many instances a sound way to approach the solution to problems that deal with massive data. These algorithms are called *External Memory Algorithms* or *out of core* algorithms.

Such techniques are of interest in the study of epidemiology for several reasons. Firstly, as the ability to capture and store data continues to increase rapidly, it is outpacing our ability to hold complete data sets within computer memory. For example, as patient records are increasingly stored electronically, there is the potential (once privacy and anonymity issues are resolved) to search for patterns and connections within vast collections of electronic records. As the complete genomes of different species are sequenced, we want to search, index and compare such sequences, which in totality are many times larger than available memory. In order to make the searching and analysis of such data sets tractable, and hence to allow interactive exploration of the data for researchers with even modest computational resources, one needs carefully designed storage and processing structures. Secondly, many emerging monitoring applications inherently generate massive amounts of data. Later in this volume there is discussion of the EpiSims project, which stores data on movements of many individuals across time. Currently, such data is stretching the resources available to track interaction patterns. Similarly, other monitoring applications, based on widely distributed sensor deployments, also generate many millions of readings every hour, or even every second. All these collections of data require appropriate techniques and algorithms so that analysis can keep pace with the generation of new readings. Lastly, External Memory Algorithms are of interest for conceptual reasons. The approaches used, of taking multiple linear passes through the data, of carefully arranging the data into trees or grids force us to separate *how* the algorithm is computing a solution from *what* the algorithm is computing. Further, the techniques of passing over the data, or following graph edges within the data, have conceptual connections to the spread of disease through a population, and the waves of infection.

This write up constitutes a biased and very brief sample of some of the major existing techniques on external memory algorithms and data structures. First we present the *parallel disk model*which incorporate the three more relevant measures for analyzing the performance of external memory algorithms. These measures are the *number of IO operations, the disk space usage* and *the internal CPU time.* Second we discuss some canonical external memory problems that include sorting, matrix multiplication, typical combinatorial problems on graphs and also point out some computational geometry related problems.

2. A Basic Computational Model

Modeling accurately disk and memory systems is a very complex task. Differentiation of sequential data access from random access is at the heart of this modeling process. The fundamental quantity of interest is the number of IO's necessary and sufficient to solve a given problem as a function of the available random access memory (M), the number of items transferred per IO (B) and the amount of disk space. Some models consider the effects of disk buffer caches and shared buses to reduce the time per IO operation and others consider asynchronous data transfers from multiple disks [**105, 84, 108, 95**]. We limit ourselves here to the *Parallel Disk Model* [**77, 111, 103**] since it facilitates the design of efficient IO algorithms and exemplifies the main issues we want to address.

2.1. The Parallel Disk Model. The number of data items in the input (assumed to be of fixed length) is denoted by N. M denotes the number of data items that fit in internal memory and $M < N$. The fundamental unit of transfer between fast internal memory and slower external storage is called a **block**. This is just a large collection of B contiguous data items. In a single IO each disk can simultaneously transfer a block of B data items.

Often B is between 512 bytes and 8 Kilobytes for online applications and a little larger than the track size for batch applications (about 100 Kilobytes). However, these values are not theoretically essential since they are strictly technology driven. Different applications may need adjustment of the block size to optimize performance. The measures of performance in this model are the number of IO's used to solve a problem, as well as the number of disk **blocks** used and the internal memory computation time. Computation can only be performed on objects residing in internal memory. These measures of performance are functions of N, M and B.

To account for multiprocessor systems let D and P denote the number of independent disks and processors respectively. It is assumed that the processors are linked by an interconnection network and that the D block transfers in one IO are synchronous. With these conventions it makes sense to assume that $2 \leq 2DB \leq M$. It is possible that $P > D$ or that $D > P$. The essential parameter is the aggregated memory M, i.e. each processor has internal memory equal to M/P.

2.2. Fundamental Operations. *Scanning, sorting and blocked output* are three fundamental operations in terms of which one can express the IO performance of a variety of external memory algorithms. One of the reasons is the standard assumption that the input and output data is organized in the D disks in such a way that a file with N data items can be read or written in $O(N/(DB))$ IO's. This quantity is called **a scan**. It corresponds to one pass over the data. In the case of one disk and one processor, the IO complexity of externally sorting a file of N data items is $O((N/B)\log_{(M/B)}(N/B))$ [**77**] . This corresponds to the fact that external sorting can be achieved with a logarithmic number of **scans** over the data. It is worth to notice here that the base of the logarithm is M/B which is precisely the number of data blocks that fit in internal memory and N/B is the number of disk blocks used to hold the data. In the case of multiple independent disks, this last quantity becomes $N/(DB)$. Contrast this with the complexity of sorting in internal memory which is $O(n\log_2(n))$, i.e. n plays the role of $N/(DB)$ and the base of the logarithm is 2.

2.3. Problem Classification. The problems considered are broadly divided into batch and online problems:

- **Batched Problems**. In this case the entire file of data items must be processed with one or more passes over the data. Typical examples include external sorting, permutation problems, fast Fourier transform, grid and linear algebra computations and some problems in graph theory and computational geometry. The corresponding basic algorithmic techniques include distribution and merging. For several graph problems, IO efficient algorithms can be obtained by using sorting to simulate some known parallel algorithms. For computational geometry problems, distribution sweep, persistent B-Trees, batched filtering and randomized incremental constructions with gradations have become prominent. As a guide to detecting if a problem has an efficient IO algorithm it helps to recall a result of [**93**] which basically states that the existence of an efficient parallel algorithm (even theoretically) guarantees the existence of an efficient IO algorithmic solution. The reverse direction has not been formulated in a satisfactory manner yet and it is still an interesting question to ponder.
- **On Line Problems**. These are problems for which computation is done to answer a series of queries. When the data is **static** it can be preprocessed for efficient query answers. However, in the more general **dynamic** setting data updates are allowed making the problems substantially more challenging.

3. Fundamental Algorithmic Techniques

3.1. Data locality and Load Balancing. Naive deployment of an internal memory algorithm that does not exploit data locality, into an external memory setting, can result in embarrassing performance even in the case that the system posses only one disk. The essential reason is that virtual memory is used to handle page management. In the case of multiple disks, *disk striping* [**102, 106**] is an important technique to transform a class of single disk algorithms into algorithms for multiple disks. However, optimal sorting on multiple disks requires more sophisticated load balancing techniques than disk striping. These techniques are fundamental versions of the recursive distribution and merging paradigms [**103**]. These paradigms are very useful beyond the sorting context as will be exemplified later in the graph algorithms section.

3.2. Sorting and Related Computations. In *Distribution sorting* the data is ordered into a collection of buckets by a set of partitioning elements. Each bucket is then recursively sorted. This fundamental process is coupled with online load balancing to guarantee that each IO operation accesses data items that are evenly distributed on the D disks. When external sorting is done via *merging*, N/M sorted runs are striped across the disks and they are subsequently merged in an online manner(at most M runs at a time) resulting in $O(\log_M(N))$ passes over the data. As in distribution sort, this process has to be coupled with clever load balancing techniques to guarantee even items distribution. These techniques include Greed Sort [**104**], Sharesort [**78**], Randomized Striping [**85, 103**] and a block duplicating technique of [**107**]. It is worth to notice here that the mentioned methods operate on passes over the data and do not rely on the use of specialized data structures. The situation is quite different if we want to externally sort K strings of total length N. In this case, efficient external memory algorithms have been developed that make use of the *String B-tree* [**96**] and the *Buffer Tree* [**81**] data structures (see Section 4). Since *matrix transposition* is a special case of *permuting* which is in turn a special case of *sorting* specialized methods have been developed for them [**91, 77**]. The algorithms for the *Fast Fourier Transform* are simpler and faster than sorting because their communication patterns are fixed in advance [**92**].

3.3. Matrix Computations. A fundamental operation on a matrix **A** is to decompose it into a product of a lower triangular matrix **L** and an upper triangular matrix **U** (referred to as an **LU** decomposition). The computation of an **LU** decomposition of a $K \times K$ matrix can be done in external memory optimally with the same number of IO's as those required to multiply two $K \times K$ matrices [**112**]. Both of these fundamental problems benefit from decomposing the input matrix into $\sqrt{B} \times \sqrt{B}$ submatrices. For computations which can be expressed in tensor form there are automatic ways to derive efficient IO algorithms [**98**]. A good discussion of external memory algorithms for numerical problems can be found in [**109**].

3.4. Graph Problems. A (loopless) *directed graph* $\mathfrak{G}$ is a pair (V, E) where V is a nonempty set and E is a subset of $V \times V$, the set of ordered pairs of V. Elements of V are called *vertices*, while elements of E are called *edges*. $\mathfrak{G}$ is called *undirected* if instead of ordered pairs of vertices we consider two subsets of V. A graph G is called *semi-external* if only its vertex set fits in RAM . If neither the vertex set nor the edge set fits in RAM , G is called *fully external.* Several standard problems like finding connected and biconnected components and minimum spanning forests of a semi-external undirected graph can be solved in an optimal number of IO's [**72**]. However, for fully external graphs their IO complexities remain open [**93**]. This is the case also for shortest paths, depth first search and transitive closure. There seems to be an inherent connection between problems which are parallelizable and problems that can be solved efficiently in external storage. The reason is that if each step of an efficient parallel algorithm can be simulated by few sorting steps then it can be converted into a linear data scan [**93**]. On the other hand, those problems which are theoretically proven to be hard to parallelize (i.e. P-complete problems) are natural candidates not to have efficient external memory solutions (i.e. lexicographically first depth first search). However, this line of research has proven elusive.

3.4.1. *Fundamental External Memory Graph Techniques.* The most successful fundamental operations to deal with fully external memory graphs without the use of data structures include sorting, permuting, transposition, randomization and edge contractions. As a guiding principle, it is advantageous to check if the problem in question can be decomposed recursively in terms of one of several of these fundamental operations. [**72**] exploit this idea in their functional approach to external memory algorithms. As an illustration, consider the computation of a minimum spanning forest of a weighted fully external memory graph. A very elegant deterministic algorithmic idea consists of first externally sorting the edges in non-decreasing weight order; solving next an internal memory version of the problem for the subgraph formed with the first M weighted edges, contracting the obtained solution over the entire data set and recursing (A version of this idea was originally proposed by Borůvka in 1926 [**89**], about two decades before models of computation were even formalized by Turing). Better IO bounds can be obtained by incorporating randomization during the selection of the M edges on which to operate in internal memory. This is a standard approach used in several parallel graph connectivity algorithms [**72**].

An orthogonal and substantially more complicated approach consists of using amortized data structures for binary heaps, tournament trees [**100**] and cross trees [**97**]. In the next section we will discuss some fundamental external memory data structures.

4. Fundamental External Memory Data Structures

Space efficient data structures on external storage devices are used to store dynamically changing data sets in order to answer queries efficiently. The database community main concern has traditionally focused on the development of efficient indexes. Relatively recently there has been a renewed interest on the worst case efficiency of external memory data structures. We review briefly some of the most popular external data structures used in practice and point out some of the most prominent structures used for geometric data.

4.1. B-Trees and Variants. The most fundamental one dimensional external data structure is the **B-Tree** [**86, 90, 103**]. B+ and B* trees are popular variants of the basic B-Tree. A B-tree is essentially a $\Theta(B)$-ary tree build on top of same level $\Theta(N/B)$ leaves where each tree node is stored in one disc block. In the simplest version, the N data elements are stored in the leaves and the internal nodes hold $\Theta(B)$ "splitting" elements used to guide searches. With a fan out of $\Theta(B^c)$ for some constant c between 0 and 1 and keeping $\Theta(N/B)$ leaves produces a tree with $O(N/B)$ space and height $O(\log_B N)$. Range queries, insertions and deletions can be handled in a logarithmic number of IO's. A B-Tree can be built with the same number of IO's as sorting by first sorting the elements and then building the tree bottom-up level by level.

Weight balanced B-Trees are obtained from a normal B-Tree by requiring the number of elements stored in the leaves of each subtree of height h to be $\Theta(B^{ch})$ [**82**].

Level balanced B-Trees [**76**] constitute another variation that use a global balance condition instead of the local degree or weight conditions explained above. This is done by imposing a constraint on the number of nodes on each level of the tree and by rebuilding the entire subtrees at that level and above when the constraint is violated. Level balanced B-Trees support efficient divide and merge operations and traversals of leaves to root paths.

In evolving or temporal data base applications it is sometimes necessary to query different versions of the data base. In these cases one needs some form of *persistent* data structure. B-Trees can be made persistent by augmenting each data element with a time interval indicating its insertion and possible deletion times. An element is called *alive* in its time interval. By making sure that a node contains $\Theta(B)$ alive elements in its time interval one guarantees that the nodes whose time intervals contain a given time t form a B-Tree on the elements alive at that time. If N is the number of performed updates, the obtained structure still uses $O(N/B)$ space and can handle insertions and deletions in $O(\log_B(N))$ IO's.

String B-Trees offer an elegant solution to the sorting of elements with different lengths [**96**]. It is basically a B-Tree built on N pointers to the N suffixes of a given set of K strings, in lexicographic order. Each internal node contains what is called a compacted trie structure which fits in one disk block [**103**]. A good entry point to results on string B-Trees processing can be found in [**94**].

4.2. The Logarithmic Method. Transforming a static external memory data structure into an efficient dynamic structure is possible via an external version of the so called *logarithmic method* [**87**]. The basic idea is to partition a set of N elements into $\log_B(N)$ sets such that the ith set S_i has size less than $B^i + 1$ and to construct an efficient static external memory structure for each set S_i. By this choice, the sets $S_1, S_2, \ldots, S_j$ do not contain enough elements to build a set S_{j+1} of size B^{j+1}. Assuming we have an static data structure that can be constructed in $O(N/B\log_B(N))$ IO's and that answers queries in $O(\log_B(N))$ IO's, one can answer a global query over all the $\log_B(N)$ sets, by simply querying each S_i and combining the results using $O(\log_B^2(N))$ IO's. Insertions and deletions can be handled efficiently by rebuilding selected substructures, [**83**].

4.3. Higher Dimensional Structures. B-Trees are external memory data structures which are suitable to answer queries on one dimensional data. The analogous queries for higher dimensional data are well captured by what is called *Range Search* queries. In particular the *stabbing query* problem in two dimensions consists of maintaining a dynamically changing set of intervals such that one can report efficiently all the intervals containing a given query point. A clever use of a persistent B-tree together with an elegant technique called *sweeping* provides an IO efficient solution for the static version. The dynamic version solution is obtained by building, on the endpoints of the intervals, a weight balanced B-Tree with fan out $\Theta(\sqrt{B})$ and using some auxiliary secondary structures to store the intervals associated with the internal nodes of the tree [**82**].

Planar Range Searching is the problem of finding among a given point set all the points contained within a query rectangle. External memory versions of interval trees and priority search trees have been used to find efficient solutions.

An elegant and optimal linear space cross-tree data structure was developed by Grossi and Italiano [**97**] for this problem. The essential idea is to divide the plane into $\Theta(\sqrt{N/B})$ vertical slabs and $\Theta(\sqrt{N/B})$ horizontal slabs each containing $\Theta(\sqrt{NB})$ points. These slabs determine an irregular grid of $\Theta(N/B)$ basic squares each of them containing between 0 and $\sqrt{N/B}$ points. Points in vertically adjacent basic squares containing less than B points are placed together to form groups of $\Theta(B)$ points and stored in blocks together. Those points in a basic square containing more than B points are stored in a B-Tree. Altogether this structure uses $O(N/B)$ space. An upper level search structure is built on top to determine the basic square containing a given point. This upper level structure consists basically of two B-Trees, one for the horizontal slabs and another for the vertical slabs. Each of these trees has fan out $\sqrt{B}$.

For dimensions greater than or equal to 3 the reader is referred to the papers by Agarwal *et al* [**76**].

4.4. The Buffer Tree and the R-Tree: Two general purpose data structures. It is very often the case that we want to answer a diverse set of queries on a single data structure rather than having specialized data structures for each query. This together with the fact that in massive data set applications we are constrained to having linear space suggest the development of heuristics that perform well in most practical instances rather than striving for worst case performance guarantees. In a nutshell, in linear space scenarios fundamental lower bounds often prevent logarithmic worst case search even for relatively simple problems.

4.4.1. *R-Trees.* In data bases that manage information on objects with a spatial extent, it pays off not to store the objects themselves but instead to store some minimal axes parallel rectangle enclosing the object together with a pointer to the object itself [**99**]. *R-Trees* are specially suited for efficient storage and querying of minimal bounding rectangles. An R-Tree is a multiway tree very similar to a B-Tree. All leaf nodes are at the same level and each leaf contains $\Theta(B)$ data rectangles. Each internal node with the possible exception of the root has $\Theta(B)$ children. It contains for each of its children a minimal bounding rectangle of all the rectangles on each child subtree. An R-Tree has height $O(\log_B(N))$ and uses $O(N/B)$ space. Insertions can be performed with $O(\log_B(N))$ IO's in a B-Tree. Deletions can not be done in general with the same logarithmic number of IO's. Constructing an R-Tree by repeated insertions may result in a suboptimal structure for query performance. Specialized construction methods have been proposed by [**88**] and the structure can be efficiently maintained in a dynamic setting.

4.4.2. *Buffer Trees.* [**80**] The buffer tree is a B-Tree with fan out $\Theta(M/B)$ where each internal node has a buffer of size $\Theta(M)$. It has height $O(\log_{(M/B)}(N/B))$ The essential idea is to collect operations until we have a block of insertions that we then insert into the root of the tree. When a buffer gets full its elements are pushed down to buffers in the next level. Inserting N elements requires $O((N/B)\log_{(M/B)}(N/B))$ IO's in total. Deletions and one dimensional range queries can also be supported efficiently using buffers. Arge has used Buffer Trees for solving a general class of high dimensional problems. Buffer trees have been applied successfully to certain graph problems.

5. Conclusions

We have provided a bird's eye view of some of the main techniques in external memory algorithms and data structures. The intention was to provide quick entry points to the literature in this research area since we believe that conceptually several problems in epidemiology may benefit from an algorithmic perspective.

References

1. T. Dasu and T. Johnson. *Exploratory Data Mining and Data Cleaning.* John Wiley, 2003.
2. A. Dempster, N. Laird, and D. Rubin. Maximum likelihood from incomplete data via the EM algorithm. *Journal of the Royal Statistical Society, Series B*, 39(1):1–38, 1977.
3. M. Ester, H-P. Kriegel, J. Sander, and X. Xu. A density-based algorithm for discovering clusters in large spatial databases with noise. In *Proceedings of the Second International Conference on Knowledge Discovery and Data Mining*, page 226, 1996.
4. S. Guha, R. Rastogi, and K. Shim. CURE: An efficient clustering algorithm for large databases. In *Proceedings of ACM SIGMOD International Conference on Management of Data*, pages 73–84, 1998.
5. J. Han and M. Kamber. *Data Mining: Concepts and Techniques.* Morgan Kaufmann, 2001.
6. A. K. Jain and R. C. Dubes. *Algorithms for Clustering Data.* Prentice-Hall, 1988.
7. S. C. Johnson. Hierarchical clustering schemes. *Psychometrika*, 2:241–254, 1967.
8. J. B. MacQueen. Some method for the classification and analysis of multivariate observations. In *Proceedings of the 5th Berkeley Symposium on Mathematical Structures*, pages 281–297, 1967.
9. Mathematica. `http://www.wolfram.com/`.
10. Matlab. `http://www.mathworks.com/`.
11. A. Moore. k-means and hierarchical clustering. `http://www-2.cs.cmu.edu/~awm/tutorials/kmeans.html`.
12. R. T. Ng and J. Han. Efficient and effective clustering methods for spatial data mining. In *Proceedings of the International Conference on Very Large Data Bases*, pages 144–155. Morgan Kaufmann, 1994.
13. A tutorial on clustering algorithms. `http://www.elet.polimi.it/upload/matteucc/Clustering/tutorial_html/`.
14. J-R Sack and J. Urrutia, editors. *Handbook on Computational Geometry.* Elsevier Science, 1998.
15. J. Ullman. Lecture notes on clustering. `http://www-db.stanford.edu/~ullman/mining/cluster1.pdf`.
16. XLMiner. `http://www.xlminer.net/`.
17. T. Zhang, R. Ramakrishnan, and M. Livny. BIRCH: an efficient data clustering method for very large databases. In *Proceedings of ACM SIGMOD International Conference on Management of Data*, pages 103–114, 1996.
18. J. Abello and A. Pogel. Graph Partitions and Concept Lattices. This volume.
19. U. Fayyad, G. Piatetsky-Shapiro and P. Smyth. From Data Mining to Knowledge Discovery: An Overview. In *Fayyad et al, 1996.*
20. R. Agrawal and R. Srikant. Fast Algorithms for Mining Association Rules In *Proceedings of the 20th International Conference on Very Large Databases*, 1994
21. Gerd Stumme, Rafik Taouil, Yves Bastide, Nicolas Pasquier, and Lotfi Lakhal. Computing iceberg concept lattices with TITANIC. *Data and Knowledge Engineering*, 42(2):189-222, 2002.
22. J. Abello, M. Resende, and S. Sudarsky. Massive Quasi-Clique Detection. In *Proceedings of Latinamerican Informatics*, Springer Verlag LNCS, 2002.
23. M. Zaki and M. Ogihara. Theoretical Foundations of Associations Rules. In *Proceedings of 3rd SIGMOD'98 Workshop on Research Issues in Data Mining and Knowledge Discovery (DMKD'98)*, Seattle, Washington, 1998.
24. J. Han, J. Pei and Y. Yin Mining Frequent Patterns without Candidate Generation In *ACM SIGMOD International Conference on Management of Data*, 2000.
25. M. Aizerman, E. M. Braverman, and L. I. Rozenoer. Theoretical foundations of the potential function method in pattern recognition learning. *Automation and Remote Control*, 25(6):821–837, June 1964.
26. S. Boyd and L. Vandenberghe. *Convex Optimization.* Cambridge University Press, 2004.
27. K. Crammer and Y. Singer. On the learnability and design of output codes for multiclass problems. In *Computational Learning Theory*, pages 35–46, 2000.
28. N. Cristianini and J. Shawe-Taylor. *An Introduction to support vector machines and other kernelbased learning methods.* Cambridge University Press, 2000.

29. T. G. Dietterich and G. Bakiri. Solving multiclass learning problems via error-correcting output codes. *Journal of Artificial Intelligence Research*, 2:263–286, 1995.
30. I. Guyon, J. Weston, S. Barnhill, and V. Vapnik. Gene selection for cancer classification using support vector machines. *Machine Learning*, 46(1-3):389–422, 2002.
31. T. Jaakkola, M. Diekhaus, and D. Haussler. Using the fisher kernel method to detect remote protein homologies. pages 149–158, 1999.
32. T. Joachims. Text categorization with support vector machines: Learning with many relevant features. In *Proceedings of the European Conference on Machine Learning*. Springer, 1998.
33. P. Michel and R. E. Kaliouby. Real time facial expresion recognition in video using support vector machines. In *Proceedings of ICMI'03*, pages 258–264, 2003.
34. K.-R. Muller, S. Mika, G. Ratsch, K. Tsuda, and B. B. Schölkopf. An introduction to kernel-based learning algorithms. *IEEE Transactions on Neural Networks*, 12(2):181–202, March 2001.
35. A. Novikov. On convergence proofs for perceptrons. In *Proceedings of the Symposium of the Mathematical Theory of Automata*, volume 12, pages 615–622, 1962.
36. J. Platt. Fast training of support vector machines using sequential minimal optimization. In C. B. B. Schölkopf and A. Smola, editors, *Advances in Kernel Methods — Support Vector Learning*, pages 185–208. MIT Press, 1999.
37. J. Platt, N. Cristianini, and J. Shawe-Taylor. Large margin DAGs for multiclass classification. *Advances in Neural Information Processing Systems*, 12:547–553, 2000.
38. F. Rosenblatt. The perceptron: a probabilistic model for information storage and organization of the brain. *Psychological Review*, 65:386–408, 1959.
39. V. Vapnik. *The Nature of Statistical Learning Theory*. Springer-Verlag, 2nd edition, 1998.
40. J. Weston and C. Watkins. Multi-class support vector machines. Technical Report CSD-TR-98-04, Department of Computer Science, Royal Holloway, University of London, 1998.
41. W.E. Deming. Comments on Professor Hoteling's paper. *Annals of Mathematical Statistics*, **11**, 470–1, 1940.
42. A. Gelman, J.B. Carlin, H. Stern, and D.R. Rubin. *Bayesian Data Analysis (second edition)*, Chapman and Hall, 2003.
43. L.I. Iezzoni. *Risk Adjustment for Measuring Health Care Outcomes*. Health Administration Press, 1994.
44. H. Jeffreys. *Theory of Probability*, Oxford University Press, 1980.
45. D. Madigan, E. Elnahrawy, R.P. Martin, W. Ju, P. Krishnan, and A.S. Krishnakumar. Bayesian Indoor Positioning Systems. *Proceedings of IEEE Infocom*, 2005.
46. F. Audrino and P. Bühlmann. Volatility estimation with functional gradient descent for very high-dimensional financial time series. *Journal of Computational Finance.*, 2002. To appear. See `http://stat.ethz.ch/~buhlmann/bibliog.html`.
47. R.G. Cowell, A.P. Dawid, S.L. Lauritzen, and D.J. Spiegehalter. *Probabilistic Networks and Expert Systems*. Springer-Verlag, 1999.
48. M. Dettling and P. Bühlmann. How to use boosting for tumor classification with gene expression data. Preprint. See `http://stat.ethz.ch/~dettling/boosting`, 2002.
49. H. Drucker and C. Cortes. Boosting decision trees. In *Advances in Neural Information Processing Systems 8*, pages 479–485, 1996.
50. N. Duffy and D. Helmbold. Boosting methods for regression. *Machine Learning*, 2/3, 2002.
51. Y. Freund. An adaptive version of the boost by majority algorithm. *Machine Learning*, 43(3):293–318, June 2001.
52. Y. Freund, R. Iyer, R.E. Schapire, and Y. Singer. An efficient boosting algorithm for combining preferences. *Journal of Machine Learning Research*, 4:933–969, 2003.
53. Y. Freund and R.E. Schapire. A decision-theoretic generalization of on-line learning and an application to boosting. *Journal of Computer and System Sciences*, 55(1):119–139, August 1997.
54. Y. Freund and R.E. Schapire. Adaptive game playing using multiplicative weights. *Games and Economic Behaviour*, 29:79–103, 1999.
55. J.H. Friedman. Greedy function approximation: A gradient boosting machine. *The Annals of Statistics*, 5, 2001.
56. J.C. Giarratano and G.D. Riley. *Expert Systems: Principles and Programming*. Course Technology, 1998.

57. V. Guruswami and A. Sahai. Multiclass learning, boosting, and error-correcting codes. In *Proc. COLT'99*, 1999.
58. J. Kivinen and M. Warmuth. Boosting as entropy projection. In *Proc. 12th Annual Conference on Computational Learning Theory*, pages 134–144. ACM Press, 1999.
59. L. Mason, P.L. Bartlett, and J. Baxter. Improved generalization through explicit optimization of margins. Technical report, Dept. of Systems Engineering, Australian National University, 1998.
60. R. Meir and G. Rätsch. An introduction to boosting and leveraging. In S. Mendelson and A. Smola, editors, *Advanced Lectures on Machine Learning*, LNCS, pages 119–184. Springer, 2003. In press. Copyright by Springer Verlag.
61. S. Merler, C. Furlanello, B. Larcher, and A. Sboner. Tuning cost-sensitive boosting and its application to melanoma diagnosis. In J. Kittler and F. Roli, editors, *Proceedings of the 2nd Internationa Workshop on Multiple Classifier Systems MCS2001*, volume 2096 of *LNCS*, pages 32–42. Springer, 2001.
62. T. Onoda, G. Ratsch, and K.-R. Muller. A non-intrusive monitoring system for household electric appliances with inverters. In *Proc. of NC'2000*, 2000.
63. J.R. Quinlan. Bagging, boosting and c4.5. In *Proceedings of the Thirteenth National Conference on Artificial Intelligence*, pages 725–730, 1996.
64. G. Ratsch, T. Onoda, and K.-R. Muller. Soft margins for adaboost. *Machine Learning*, 3:287–320, 2001.
65. R.E. Schapire, Y. Freund, P. Bartlett, and W. S. Lee. Boosting the margin: A new explanation for the effectiveness of voting methods. *The Annals of Statistics*, 26(5):1651–1686, October 1998.
66. R.E. Schapire and Y. Singer. Improved boosting algorithms using confidence-rated predictions. *Machine Learning*, 3:297–336, 1999.
67. R.E. Schapire and Y. Singer. Boostexter: A boosting-based system for text categorization. *Machine Learning*, 2/3:135–168, 2000.
68. R.A. Servedio. Smooth boosting and learning with malicious noise. In *Proceedings of the 14th Ann. Conf. on Computational Learning Theory*, pages 473–489, 2001.
69. V. Vapnik. *The Nature of Statistical Learning Theory*. Springer, N.Y., 1995.
70. Z.-H. Zhou, Y. Jiang, Y.-B. Yang, and S.-F. Chen. Lung cancer cell identification based on artificial neural network ensembles. *Artificial Intelligence in Medicine*, 24(1):25–36, 2002.
71. J. Abello, A. Buschbaum, and J. Westbrook. A Functional Approach to External Memory Algorithms. *In Proceedings of the 6th Annual European Symposium on Algorithms*, Vol 1461, LNCS, pages 332-343, Springer Verlag, 1998.
72. J. Abello, A. Buschbaum, and J. Westbrook. A Functional Approach to External Graph Algorithms. *Algorithmica* 32(3): 437-458, 2002.
73. J. Abello and J. Korn. MGV: A System for Visualizing Massive Multidigraphs. *IEEE Transactions on Visualization and Computer Graphics* **8** No. 1, January-March 2002.
74. J. Abello, A. Pogel and L. Miller: Breadth First Search Partitions and Concept Lattices. *Journal of Universal Computer Science*, Vol. 10, No. 8, 2004.
75. J. Abello and J. S. Vitter (eds): External Memory Algorithms. Vol 50 of the AMS-DIMACS Series in Discrete Mathematics and Theorethical Computer Science, 1999.
76. P.K. Agarwal, L. Arge, G.S. Brodal, and J.S. Vitter. IO Efficient Dynamic Point Location in Monotone Planar Subdivisions. *In Proceedings of the ACM-SIAM Symposium on Discrete Algorithms*, pages 1116-1127, 1999.
77. A. Aggarwal and J.S. Vitter. The IO Complexity of Sorting and Related Problems. *Communications of the ACM* **31** No. 9, 1116-1127, 1988.
78. A. Aggarwal and C.G. Plaxton. Optimal Parallel Sorting in Multi Level Storage. *In Proceedings of the Fifth Annual ACM-SIAM Symposium on Discrete Algorithms*, pages 659-668, 1994.
79. R. Agrawal, T. Imielinski and A. Swami. Mining association rules between sets of items in large databases. In *ACM SIGMOD Intl. Conf. Management of Data*, May 1993.
80. L. Arge. The Buffer Tree: A New Technique for Optimal IO Algorithms. *In Proceedings of the Workshop on Algorithms and Data Structures*, LNCS 955, pages 334-345, 1995.
81. L. Arge. External Memory Data Structures. *In Handbook of Massive Data Sets*, J. Abello, P. Pardalos and M. Resende(editors), Kluwer Publishers, North Holland, pages 313-357, 2002.

82. L. Arge and J. S. Vitter. Optimal Dynamic Interval Management in External Memory. *In Proceedings of the IEEE Symposium on the Foundations of Computer Science*, pages 560-569, 1996.
83. L. Arge and J. Vahrenhold. I/O Efficient dynamic planar point location. In *Proceedings of the ACM Symposium on Computational Geometry*, pages 191–200, 2000.
84. R.D. Barve, A. M. Shriver, P.B. Gibbons, B. K. Hillyer, Y. Matias,and J. S. Vitter. Modeling and Optimizing IO Throughput of Multiple Disks on a Bus. *In SIGMETRICS Joint Internatinal Conference on Measurement and Modeling of Computer Systems*, pages 83-92, 1999.
85. R.D. Barve and J.S. Vitter. A Simple and Efficient Parallel Disk Merge Sort. *In Proceedings of the 11th Annual ACM Symposium on Parallel Algorithms and Architectures*, pages 232-241, 1999.
86. R. Bayer and E. McCreight. Organization and Maintenance of Large Ordered Indexes. *Acta Informatica*, 1:173-189, 1972.
87. J.L. Bentley. Decomposable searching problems. *Information Processing Letters*, 8(5):244–251, 1979.
88. M. de Berg, J. Gudmundson, M. Hammar and M. Overmars. On R-Trees with Low Stabbing Number. *In Proceedings of the Annual European Symposium on Algorithms*, pages 167-178, 2000.
89. O. Borůvka. O jistém problému minimálním *Moravské Přírodověd. Spol v Brně 3*, pages 37–58, 1926.
90. D. Comer. The Ubiquitous B-Tree. *ACM Computing Surveys*, 11(2):121-137.
91. T. H. Cormen, C.E. Leiserson and R.L. Rivest, Introduction to Algorithns, M.I.T. Press, 1990.
92. T.H. Cormen and D.M. Nicol. Performing out-of-core FFTs on parallel disk systems. *Parallel Computing*, 24:5–20, 1998.
93. Y.J. Chiang, M.T. Goodrich, E.F. Grove, R. Tamassia, D.E. Vengroff. and J.S. Vitter. External Memory Graph Algorithms. *In Proceedings of the ACM-SIAM Symposium on Discrete Algorithms*, pages 139-149, 1995.
94. A. Crauser, P. Ferragina and K. Mehlhorn, U. Meyer and E. A. Ramos. I/O-optimal computation of segment intersections. In *External Memory Algorithms*, DIMACS Series on Discrete Mathematic and Theoretical Computer Science, pages 131–138. American Mathematical Society, 1999.
95. M. Farach, P. Ferragina, and S. Muthukrishnan. Overcoming the Memory Bottleneck in Suffix Tree Construction. *In Proceedings of the IEEE Symposium on Foundations of Computer Science*, pages 174-183, 1998.
96. P. Ferragina and R. Grossi. The String B-Tree: A New Data Structure for String Search in External Memory and its Applications. *In Proceedings of the 27th Annual Annual ACM Symposium on Theory on Computing*, pages 693-702, 1995.
97. R. Grossi, and G. F. Italiano. Efficient Cross-Trees for External Memory. *In J. Abello and J. S. Vitter, External Memory Algorithms*, Volume 50 of the AMS-DIMACS Series, American Mathematical Society, pages 87-106, 1998.
98. S.K.S. Gupta, Z. Li, and J. H. Reif. Generating Efficient Programs for Two Level Memories from Tensor Products. *In Proceedings of the Seventeenth IASTED/ISMM International Conference on Parallel and Distributed Computing and Systems*, pages 510-513, 1995.
99. A. Guttman. R-trees: A dynamic index structure for spatial searching. In *Proceedings of the SIGMOD International Conference on Management of Data*, pages 47–57, 1984.
100. V. Kumar and E. Schwabe. Improved Algorithms and Data Structures for solving Graph Problems in external memory. In *Proceeedings of the 8th IEEE Symposium on Parallel and Distrtributed Processing*, pages 169–176, 1996.
101. K. Mehlhorn. Data Structures and Algorithms 1: Sorting and Searching. Springer Verlag, EACTS Monographs on Theoretical Computer Science, 1984.
102. M.Y. Kim. Synchronized Disk Interleaving. *IEEE Transactions on Computers*, Vol 35, 978-988, 1986.
103. D. Knuth. Sorting and Searching, Volume 3 of the Art of Computer Programming. Addison Wesley, Reading MA, second edition, 1998.
104. M.H. Nodine and J.S. Vitter. Greed Sort: An Optimal Sorting Algorithm for Multiple Disks. *Journal of the ACM*, Volume 42, pages 919-933, 1995.

105. C. Ruemmler and J. Wilkes. An Introduction to Disk Drive Modeling. *IEEE Computer*, pages 17-28, 1994.
106. K. Salem and H. Garcia Molina. Disk Striping. *In Proceedings of the 2nd IEEE Data Engineering Conference*, pages 332-342, 1986.
107. P. Sanders, S. Egner, and J. Korst. Fast Concurrent Access to Parallel Disks. *In Proceedings of the 11th Annual ACM-SIAM Symposium on Discrete Algorithms*, pages 849-858, 2000.
108. E. Shriver, A. Merchant and J. Wilkes. An Analytic Behaviour Model for Disk Drives with Read Ahead Caches and Request Ordering. *In Joint International Conference on Measurement and Modeling of Computer Systems*, pages 182-191, 1998.
109. S. Toledo. A Survey of Out of Core Algorithms in Numerical Linear Algebra. *In J. Abello and J.S. Vitter (Editors), External Memory Algorithms*, AMS-DIMACS Series, Volume 50, pages 161-179, American Mathematical Society, 1999.
110. J.S. Vitter. External Memory Algorithms. *In Handbook of Massive Data Sets*, J. Abello, P. Pardalos and M. Resende(editors), Kluwer Publishers, North Holland, pages 359-416, 2002.
111. J.S. Vitter and E.A.M. Shriver. Algorithms for Parallel Memory I and II. *Algorithmica*, Vol 12:pages 110-169, 1994.
112. D. Womble, D. Greenberg, S. Wheat, and R. Riesen. Beyond Core: Making Parallel Computers IO Practical. *In Proceedings of the 1993 DAGS-PC Symposium*, pages 56-63, 1993.

DIMACS Research Institute, Rutgers University, Piscataway, NJ 08854, USA
E-mail address: abello@dimacs.rutgers.edu

DIMACS Research Institute, Rutgers University, Piscataway, NJ 08854, USA
Current address: Bell Laboratories, 600 Mountain Avenue, Murray Hill, NJ 07974, USA
E-mail address: cormode@lucent.com

Department of Computer Science, Rutgers University, Piscataway, NJ 08854, USA
E-mail address: dfradkin@cs.rutgers.edu

Department of Statistics, Rutgers University, Piscataway, NJ 08855, USA
E-mail address: dmadigan@rutgers.edu

DIMACS Research Institute, Rutgers University, Piscataway, NJ 08854, USA
E-mail address: melnik@dimacs.rutgers.edu

DIMACS Research Institute, Rutgers University, Piscataway, NJ 08854, USA
E-mail address: muchnik@dimacs.rutgers.edu

DIMACS Series in Discrete Mathematics
and Theoretical Computer Science
Volume **70**, 2006

Descriptive Epidemiology: A Brief Introduction

Dona Schneider

ABSTRACT. Epidemiologists are trained to be wary of data dredging as the process of making multiple comparisons may yield spurious results. Today, with large health-related and biological data sets readily available, and with powerful computers and sophisticated software widely accessible, data mining has become the newest recast tool for examining data sets for underlying patterns. Yet the ability to utilize data mining techniques is more likely to be found among computer scientists or mathematicians than among epidemiologists and the two fields are not openly communicating. The following brief review of descriptive epidemiology is designed especially for data miners, to make them aware of some of the pitfalls epidemiologists have long recognized in the most commonly used health-related data sets and the most commonly used statistical tools of the trade. Readers should also come away with an understanding of why those trained exclusively in epidemiology have difficulty in overcoming skepticism about data mining.

1. Introduction

The goals of descriptive epidemiology are to evaluate trends in health and disease and to compare these trends among countries or population subgroups. Simply put, descriptive epidemiology studies:

- Who gets sick and who does not (person variables)
- Where rates are highest and lowest (place or space variables)
- Temporal patterns of disease (time variables)

Good epidemiologic training includes learning about data limitations as well as learning to examine data sets for bias and confounding. Typical topics that the student of epidemiology must master include the uses of population-based data sets, especially census and vital statistics data. All final exams in introductory epidemiology require students to know two points, that 1) descriptive epidemiology cannot test hypotheses and 2) finding a statistical association does not constitute cause. Why these points are so important may not be immediately obvious to the data miner, but they are at the foundation of epidemiology and a recurrent theme of this chapter.

2000 *Mathematics Subject Classification.* Primary 92-01 Instructional exposition; 92D30 Epidemiology.

The rapid reporting of results based on statistical associations from a single study has caused repeated and distressing problems for epidemiologists. Those lacking an understanding about what constitutes cause in epidemiology have further tainted the field, producing widespread feeling that the discipline generates "meaningless findings" that yield "the scare of the week." Much of the fault for epidemiology's bad publicity can be ascribed to the process of data dredging in biased and confounded data sets [**1**]. Indeed, medical journalist James Le Fanu became so frustrated with this practice that he proposed that "The simple expedient of closing down most university departments of epidemiology could both extinguish the endlessly fertile source of anxiety mongering while simultaneously releasing funds for serious research" [**2**]. In other words, epidemiologists and pretenders to the craft have been burned by data dredging. They harbor the fear that data mining simply provides more techniques that will lead to spurious associations. In order to combat this fear, novices to epidemiology need to understand limitations of the health-related data sets they choose to mine. They also need to understand what constitutes cause in epidemiology, as it is not simply statistical association. If they master these two areas, perhaps data miners can contribute to epidemiology by providing new insights into data sets and by helping to formulate new hypotheses from their data mining results. Such efforts should open new avenues for discussion with those trained exclusively in epidemiology.

2. Showing Cause in Epidemiology

A bit of history may help the data miner understand how epidemiologists think about cause, a matter more reflective of good judgment than mathematical proof. In the late 19th century, most disease was infectious and average life expectancy at birth was about 20 years shorter than it is today. Showing cause, i.e., that a particular agent caused a particular disease, was done in the laboratory under experimental conditions. If you met the criteria of the Henle-Koch postulates (one agent, one disease), you could conclude that Agent A caused Disease A, Agent B caused Disease B, etc. As we entered the 20th century, improvements in sanitation, vaccines, food storage, transportation and medical care all helped to increase life expectancy. The causes of death shifted to chronic conditions such as cancer and heart disease, conditions with complex causes that did not lend themselves to microbiologic confirmation. Showing cause became problematic, not only because diseases became more complex, but because epidemiology is an observational science and most of the health-related data sets available to study disease outcomes have data limitations, including bias and confounding.

Epidemiologists consider bias "any systematic error in the design, conduct or analysis of a study that results in a mistaken estimate of an exposure's effect on the risk of disease" [**3**]. Gordis provides a lengthy discussion of the types of bias inherent in data sets [**4**]. In contrast to bias is confounding, a condition that occurs when there is an association between disease and exposure caused by a third factor not taken into consideration. A confounder, then, is a variable that is associated with the exposure and, independent of that exposure, is a risk factor for the disease. For example, cirrhosis of the liver is statistically associated with cigarette smoking. No matter how strong that association, we cannot conclude that smoking causes cirrhosis because we know that the most likely biologic cause remains excessive alcohol consumption. As heavy drinkers also tend to be heavy smokers, smoking is a confounding rather than causal variable in studies of cirrhosis. A good epidemiologist, then, seeks to understand the biology of the disease, the human behavior related to that disease, and the problems with bias and confounding inherent in the data set before seeking to find a statistical association.

The best example of why statistical association is not sufficient to show cause is perhaps the furor about the link between smoking and lung cancer that emerged in the 1940s and 50s. Arguments about how to establish the causal link abounded, with Sir Austin Bradford-Hill finally setting forth "viewpoints" that would allow epidemiologists to judge whether an association that could not be proven in the microbiology laboratory was likely to be causal [**5**]. These nine are still important for epidemiology and remain useful for making judgments about cause related to non-infectious agents today:

- *Strength of Association* — The stronger the association, the less likely the relationship is due to chance or a confounding variable.
- *Consistency of the Observed Association* — If the association is observed in different populations and if it is found using different methods, it is unlikely to be due to chance.
- *Specificity* — If an association is limited to specific persons, sites and types of disease, and if there is no association between the exposure and other outcomes, then the relationship supports causation.
- *Temporality* — The exposure of interest must precede the outcome by a period consistent with any proposed biologic mechanism.
- *Biologic Gradient* — There is a gradient of risk associated with the degree of exposure (dose-response relationship).
- *Biologic Plausibility* — The exposure might reasonably alter the risk of developing the disease by a known or postulated mechanism.
- *Coherence* — The observed data must not conflict with known facts about the natural history and biology of the disease.
- *Experiment* — The strongest support for causation may be obtained through controlled experiments (clinical trials, intervention studies, and animal experiments).
- *Analogy* — In some cases, it is fair to judge cause-effect relationships by analogy, especially when the outcome may be devastating (the experience with thalidomide makes it fair to accept less but similar evidence to conclude that another drug with the same qualities might produce the same effects).

The above postulates are sound, but it is rare for the epidemiologist to be able to meet all of them. Failing to try, however, has put many in poor standing with both the public and the scientific community. It is the prudent epidemiologist, therefore, that remains wary of those seeking to show cause by statistical association alone. Indeed, drawing conclusions about causal relationships is beyond the scope of descriptive epidemiology, a field focused on identifying patterns among person, place and time variables, not on statistical inference.

3. Understanding Epidemiologic Data

Finding interesting patterns for types of diseases in a variety of subpopulations located in different places over time can be exciting. Indeed, there may be valid reasons for some trends, such as changes in the age distribution of a population, changes in survivorship, or the number of new cases of disease because of environmental exposures or other factors. It is also possible, however, that trends emerge simply because of data artifacts. For example, the number of cases of disease may vary in place and time simply because there are changes in disease recognition, changes in disease reporting, and/or changes in the rules and procedures for classifying disease or the cause of death. Variations in estimating the population-at-risk may result from migration or from changing the way the population is enumerated. Some of the best-understood data artifacts in population-based data sets are presented below.

3.1. Person Variables.

3.1.1. *Vital Statistics Data.* Birth and death (vital statistics) registration in North America began with the earliest settlers, but the information was used for legal purposes, not for statistical reporting. Vital statistics reporting in the United States began in Massachusetts around 1850. By 1933, all states reported their birth and death certificate data to the federal government. Hetzel [**6**] describes the history of the national vital statistics system, as well as providing tables listing the variables included in birth and death certificates by year. The National Center for Health Statistics (NCHS), located in the Centers for Disease Control and Prevention within the Department of Health and Human Services in Hyattsville, MD, gathers and aggregates the vital statistics from the states. It also issues annual reports on vital statistics data and provides case-level data sets for researchers to download from the Internet [**7**].

Coding Issues for Mortality Data. International comparisons of mortality or death statistics are possible using the International Classification of Diseases (ICD) promulgated through the World Health Organization (WHO). The coding rules for the ICD have changed over time, with new diseases entering the system and others disappearing or undergoing reclassification. Ten revisions of the ICD coding scheme now exist and these provide significant challenges for the researcher doing longitudinal work. For example, the 9th revision (ICD-9) uses a 4-digit numeric system and 4,000 categories of disease. In contrast, the 10th revision (ICD-10) uses a 4-digit alphanumeric system and 8,000 categories of disease. The ICD revisions and the years for which each coding system was in place in the United States appear in Table 1. In addition to using ICD-9 coding from 1979-98, the United States introduced its own classification and coding rules for Human Immunodeficiency Virus infection (HIV) beginning in 1987 and these data cannot be readily used for international comparisons. Data miners should be wary of discontinuities in mortality data due to ICD changes and they should use appropriate care in examining secular trends for tracking specific diseases, especially across nations. Algorithms are available for transforming the data across revisions, mostly available through third party providers.

A related classification system, the International Classification of Diseases, Clinical Modification (ICD-9-CM) is used in the United States for morbidity (illness or injury) rather than mortality data, primarily to assign diagnostic billing codes associated with inpatient, outpatient, and physician office utilization. Finally, cancer registries such as the Surveillance, Epidemiology and End Results (SEER) and state-based registries utilize the WHO's International Classification of Diseases for Oncology (ICD-O) for classifying information on each cancer case. The ICD-O system has now undergone three revisions. Again, data miners may

TABLE 1. ICD revision and years covered for US data

ICD	Years
1	1900-09
2	1910-20
3	1921-29
4	1930-38
5	1939-48
6	1949-57
7	1958-67
8	1968-78
9	1979-98
10	1999-present

need to use algorithms to translate between ICD coding schemes in order follow disease trends using cancer registry data. Those that exist should be obtained directly from the cancer registry providing the data set being utilized. For instance, a colleague studying cancer mortality trends in the United States between 1950 and 1980 found a remarkable increase in liver cancer deaths. It took more than a dozen phone calls to locate the person (who had retired from government service) who knew that the coding scheme for liver cancer changed and was responsible for the artificial trend. Failure to follow through in finding coding changes over time can cause the researcher to come to invalid conclusions [**8**].

Beyond understanding ICD codes, it is important for investigators to understand how health-related data are gathered and processed. NCHS has public-use documentation and technical appendices for each year of mortality data on its website [**7**]. Before embarking on the use of these mortality data sets, it is important to spend significant time with these resources and to understand the data limitations. For example, missing data are often imputed for fields such as race, while for others such as occupation they intentionally are left blank. In New Jersey during the early 1970s, for instance, no racial or ethnic data were collected. The data were imputed by using data from the previous and following years. In 1972, half the deaths for Alaska and Hawaii remain missing [**9**].

Coding Issues for Natality Data. Natality or birth statistics also present challenges. For instance, the definition of a live birth has historically differed among societies. Both the WHO and the NCHS currently define a live birth as the complete expulsion or extraction from its mother of a product of conception, irrespective of the duration of the pregnancy, which, after such separation, breathes or shows any other evidence of life such as heartbeat, umbilical cord pulsation, or definite movement of voluntary muscles, whether the umbilical cord has been cut or the placenta is attached. This is far from straightforward, as the definition does not incorporate body length, weight or gestational age. Yet WHO puts forth criteria for perinatal mortality statistics that include these data fields and even recommends different criteria for calculating national perinatal statistics vs. international ones (Table 2). The consumer of natality data is warned that "perinatal" is defined in different ways across data sets, from the 20th–28th week of gestation to from 1–4 weeks after birth. Furthermore, perinatal data are biased because women who have

TABLE 2. WHO inclusion criteria for perinatal mortality statistics

Minimum value	National perinatal statistics	International perinatal statistics
Birthweight at least	500 g	1000 g
Gestational age at least	22 wk	28 wk
Body length at least	25 cm	35 cm

access to medical care may be more likely than women without health-care access to have information on their early spontaneous abortions and fetal deaths recorded.

3.1.2. *Demographic Data.* The US Constitution mandates a decennial census (Article 1, Section 2) for determining representation in the House of Representatives. The Census Bureau, located in the Economics and Statistics Administration, Department of Commerce is responsible for gathering this information. All other uses of census data are secondary, which makes the use of census data for determining demographics or populations-at-risk fraught with pitfalls. For example, the first census took place in 1790, at which time the census counted only six categories of persons: free white males $\geq$16 years (to assess the country's industrial, military and tax potential), free white males <16 years, free white females, all other free persons (by sex and color), and slaves. Since that time, the census categories for race and ethnicity have changed significantly, reflecting the social and political concerns of their respective times (See Table 3).

Before 1997, race and ethnicity variables were not standardized across federal data sets because different branches of government gathered data on the population for different purposes. It is important to recognize that race and ethnicity are highly subjective variables, usually obtained through self-report except in cases of unattended deaths. Because they are sensitive data fields, they are sometimes left blank. Algorithms for imputing missing racial and ethnic data exist but they are not standardized across data sets. For example, race and ethnicity are imputed in vital statistics data by assigning the race or ethnicity of the preceding record. Other data sets impute missing racial and ethnic data by using typical surnames. Still others leave the missing data fields blank. To deal with the problem of incompatible data sources, the Office of Management and Budget (OMB) issued a policy directive revision requiring that all federal data sets have at least five categories for race and two for ethnicity beginning with the 2000 census. The minimum categories for race were American Indian or Alaska Native, Asian, Black or African American, Native Hawaiian or Other Pacific Islander, and White. Those for ethnicity were "Hispanic or Latino" and "Not Hispanic or Latino." The OMB further required that respondents be directed to "check all that apply" for racial and ethnic variables [**10**] and that implementation of the directive begin with the 2000 census and be completed for all federal data sets by January 1, 2003.

Researchers often use race and ethnicity as surrogate variables for socioeconomic status (SES), especially in data sets that do not contain other income variables (i.e., vital statistics). This is an important practice, as one of the best predictors of health outcomes, along with age, is SES. Unfortunately, researchers using race and ethnicity in their analyses often misinterpret their results, reinforcing

TABLE 3. Racial categories in the US Census, 1860–2000

1860	1890	1900	1970	2000[1]
White	White	White	White	White
Black	Black	Black (of Negro descent)	Negro or Black	Black, African American
Mulatto	Mulatto[2] Quadroon Octoroon			
	Chinese	Chinese	Chinese	Chinese
	Indian	Indian	Indian (American)	American Indian or Alaskan Native
	Japanese	Japanese	Japanese	Japanese
			Filipino	Filipino
				Asian Indian
			Korean	Korean
			Hawaiian	Native Hawaiian
				Vietnamese
				Guamanian or Chamorro
				Samoan
				Other Asian
				Other Pacific Islander
			Other	Some other race

Source: 200 Years of US Census Taking: Population and Housing Questions 1790-1990. US Department of Commerce. US Bureau of the Census.
1. Categories printed in the 2000 Census questionnaire.
2. In 1890, mulatto was split into three categories: mulatto was defined as a person who was three-eighths to five-eighths black. A quadroon was one-quarter black and an octoroon one-eighth black.

racial and ethnic stereotypes rather than understanding the surrogacy of the variables [**11**]. As the population becomes more diverse, and as data sources increasingly reflect respondents use of the "check all that apply" option, our ability to use race and ethnicity as surrogates for SES will diminish. How that will affect our ability to draw conclusions about patterns of disease remains to be seen [**12**].

3.2. Place (Spatial) Variables and Methods. Place is a geographic area that we usually define according to political boundaries (country, state, county, city, etc.) although it could be defined by functional area (such as zip code or watershed district). Place variables lend themselves to mapping, i.e., to defining spatial distributions. The classic example of disease mapping comes from John Snow's map of a cholera outbreak in London more than a century and a half ago (Figure 1). Snow was a physician with an avid interest in cholera. Using a dot map, he plotted all cases of cholera during the summer epidemic of 1854 in the Golden Square neighborhood of London. The pattern of dots indicated that the Broad Street pump (Pump A) was the probable source of the epidemic [**13**]. Snow's work was seminal in understanding that cholera transmission can occur through a public water supply.

Dot mapping is still widely used today in local health departments, by using a simple street map and colored pins to "pinpoint" locations of contaminated wells, the locations of dead birds (indicating probable infection with West Nile Virus), hot

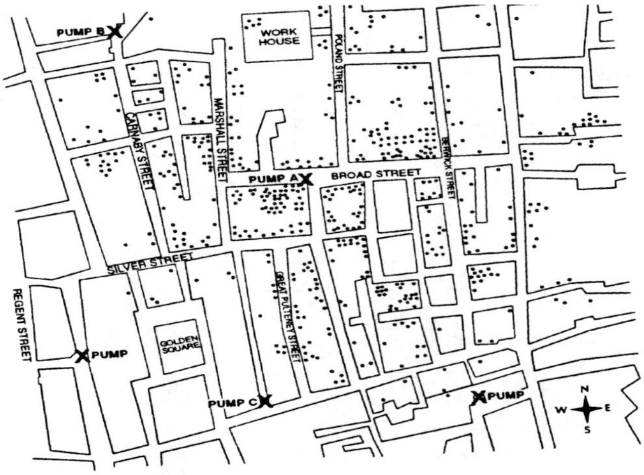

Source: Snow 1860 [**13**]

FIGURE 1. John Snow's map of cholera in London, Aug–Sept 1854

spots for deer-vehicle collisions, and other health-related information. For complex data, the pin system is replaced by computer mapping, a system that uses geocoding and a grid that identifies place data with latitude and longitude (lat-long) coordinates. To examine multiple variables, data layers (each representing one variable) are inserted into a geographic information system (GIS) and statistically analyzed. Data miners might best understand this process as computer mapping using a relational database with each point identified by lat-long coordinates.

Computer mapping goes beyond dot mapping and into complex presentations of data using isopleths (or contours that portray harmonic or equal measures) and choropleths (to portray aggregate data at a variety of geographic scales). Typical isopleth maps are the weather maps showing areas of equal barometric pressure (isobars) published in daily newspapers. When medical geographers or epidemiologists use isopleth mapping with health-related data, the diffusion of a disease or population migration patterns can be graphically depicted using isolines (Figure 2). Alternatively, the levels of contamination (exposure) can be portrayed and statistically related to disease outcome (Figure 3). When the amount of exposure is related to disease outcome, epidemiologists term the relationship a dose-response one. Dose-response relationships are one factor in helping determine causality.

Choropleth maps portray rates of disease for aggregate areas, typically using county or state lines to show differences in disease rates. Epidemiologists and medical geographers use political boundaries routinely for choropleth mapping because population-at-risk data are available at those particular aggregations from the census. Disease, of course, does not respect political boundaries and there are limitations to using these boundaries to examine patterns of disease. Figure 4 portrays one of these limitations, the effect of geographic scale on the pattern of adverse outcomes. Note how the pattern of low birth weight shifts dramatically depending upon the level of geographic analysis selected. Data miners are warned that small geographic areas are likely to produce small numbers of cases, thereby creating large confidence intervals and limiting the ability to make comparisons.

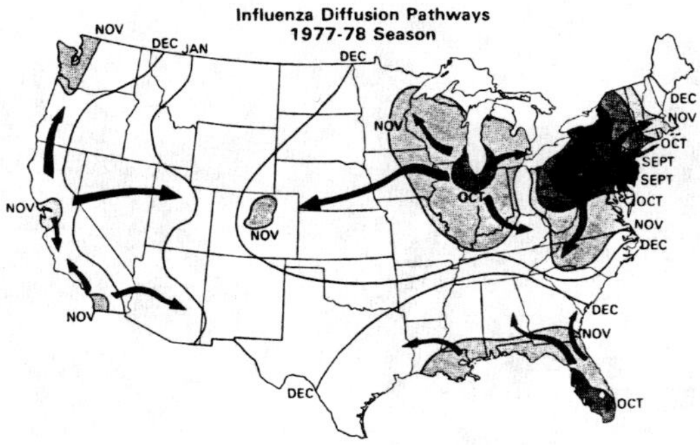

Source: Pyle 1986 [**14**]

FIGURE 2. Influenza diffusion, 1977–78, using harmonic measures

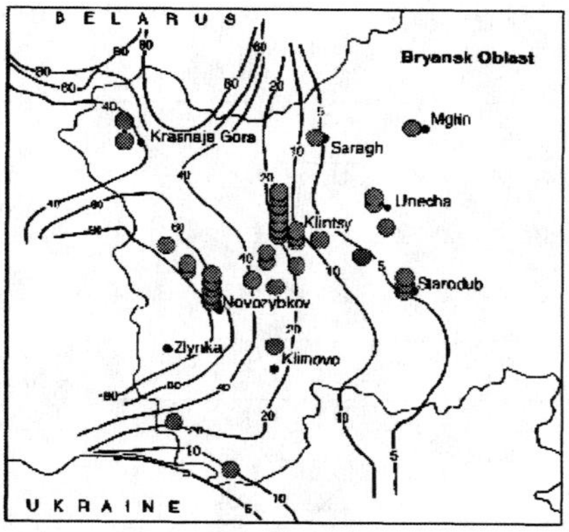

Source: Parshkov et al. 1997 [**15**]

FIGURE 3. Levels of soil contamination and cases of thyroid cancer cases in Russia after the Chernobyl disaster

On the other hand, large areas may not be helpful for locating specific populations to target for interventions. It is important, therefore, to understand the how selecting the geographic scale for analysis affects results. Mapping may generate random variation due to multiple comparisons. Furthermore, large, sparsely-populated areas containing few cases may predominate, yielding a distorted image. For instance, in Canada where data for a relatively small population covers a large geographic area, the image generated from a few cases can present a false impression of results. In these cases, dot maps are preferable to choropleth ones. Researchers not trained in the use of geographic information systems (GIS) should consult a medical geographer about the limitations of various visualization and cartographic techniques before trying to analyze a data set spatially.

3.3. Time Variables (Cross-sectional, Cohort and Longitudinal Data). The epidemiologist might segment time into hours, days, weeks, or even decades, depending on the number of cases examined and the importance of time between exposure and screening, diagnosis, disease progression and ultimate outcome. In

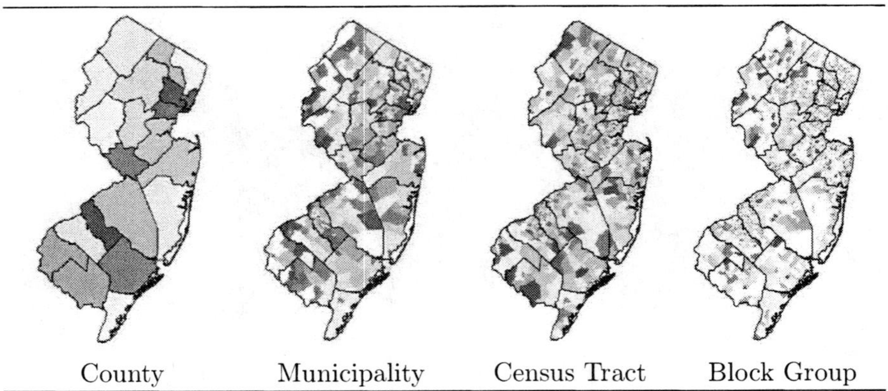

Data Source: New Jersey Vital Statistics, Natality, 1998

FIGURE 4. Percent low birthweight births, New Jersey 1998

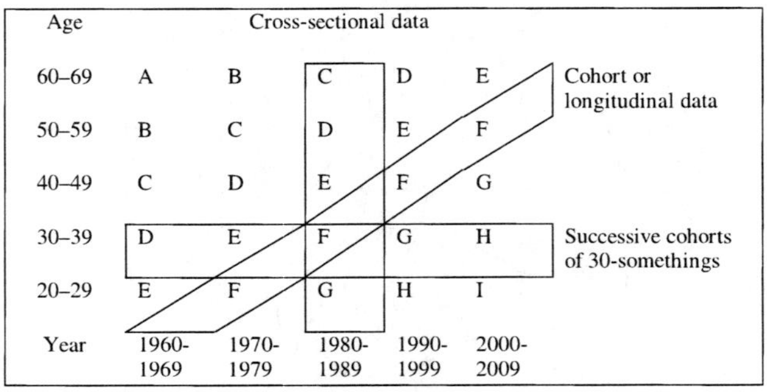

FIGURE 5. Evaluating data sets for cross-sectional and longitudinal studies

addition, the way the research question is posed determines the approach the epidemiologist will take with the time variables in the data set.

For example, Figure 5 portrays a hypothetical data set for staff employed by a major university. Between 1960 and 1969, group E was between 20 and 29 years of age; group D was 30 to 39 years, etc. If the epidemiologist wanted to know the rate of back injuries among university staff over time, he or she would use cross-sectional data to compare rates across decades. Perhaps the occupational health nurse noted that she was seeing quite a few 30-somethings for back injury. The epidemiologist might then examine the data to determine whether 30-somethings really have higher rates. It might even be interesting to examine data on successive cohorts (groups sharing one or more attributes), such as successive groups of 30-somethings, to determine whether the problem of back injury in this population is exacerbating or improving. Perhaps the university is concerned that aging increases the likelihood of back injuries and asks the epidemiologist for guidance about restricting older workers to less strenuous jobs. While an analysis stratified by age group might yield good information, a second approach might be to use or longitudinal data to address the question.

As with place variables, time variables are likely to show different patterns depending on the time scale selected. For example, the author and colleagues examined homicide and suicide data at a variety of time scales, finding that homicides were more likely to happen on Thursdays. Such a finding was new and the researchers searched for potential reasons for the pattern. They found that welfare checks came out on Thursdays and hypothesized that demands for money perhaps led to conflicts that ended in homicide [**16**]. In another instance, the author and colleagues examined pediatric cancer incidence data and found clusters in both time and space emerged and disappeared depending on the cut points selected [**17**]. It is prudent, therefore, to examine data at a variety of time and place scales and to consider carefully whether these make sense in terms of the outcome.

4. Study Designs in Descriptive Epidemiology

Epidemiologists use several types of study designs to look for patterns in person, place and time variables, ranging from the individual case report to sophisticated statistical analyses. These are described below.

4.1. Case Reports and Case Series. Medical journals often publish case reports as teaching examples and to point out the particulars if an individual case. Case reports allow physicians and other medical practitioners to recognize new syndromes or atypical presentations of known diseases in a timely fashion. For example, the first case of bioterrorism-related inhalation anthrax diagnosed in Palm Beach County, Florida found its way into the medical literature within 15 days, alerting the national medical community and increasing the awareness of all citizens of the disease's signs and symptoms [**18**]. If a case series emerges (three or more cases), the information provided can be examined for commonalities, to create diagnostic standards and to predict prognosis. A case series may also provide clues for tracking down likely exposures and preventing future cases [**19**]. The limitation of case series data is that there is no way to test for statistical associations because there is no relevant comparison group.

4.2. Cross-sectional (Prevalence) Studies. Cross-sectional studies measure disease and exposure at the same time. They are equivalent to asking people 1) "Do you have heart disease?" and 2) "Do you smoke?" on the same questionnaire. In data mining terms, the design might be described as summarizing the joint occurrences of the attributes. Because cross-sectional studies are designed to elicit the proportion of disease in the entire population under study, they are also called prevalence studies.

Cross-sectional or prevalence studies use a simple 2×2 table for statistical analysis (Figure 6). Depending on the variable of interest, the proportion of disease in the exposed group (a/a+b) may be compared to that for the not exposed group (c/c+d). Alternatively, the proportion of exposure in the diseased group (a/a+c) may be compared to that for the group without disease (b/b+d). Such comparisons allow the researcher to describe patterns in the data, to identify variables for future analytic studies.

An advantage to the cross-sectional design is that it determines the prevalence of disease in the general population, not simply those cases that seek medical care. For example, the design can pick up mild cases of disease where people might choose to "tough-it-out" or self-medicate (especially for common diseases such as arthritis,

	Disease	No Disease
Exposed	A	B
Not Exposed	C	D

FIGURE 6. Standard 2 × 2 table

high blood pressure, or allergies). This allows the entire spectrum of disease to be addressed.

One disadvantage of cross-sectional studies is that they are more likely to pick up cases of long duration rather than recent ones and this biases the data towards survivors and survival factors. For example, when an individual first becomes symptomatic, they are likely to seek medical care and restrict their activities (such as with Lyme disease or arthritis). As they begin to respond to treatment or recover, they are more likely to participate in cross-sectional surveys. The researcher, then is likely to pick up cases of long duration, those under doctor's care, or those in a stable or recovery phase rather than cases of active illness with restricted activities.

The cross-sectional study design is also plagued by a lack of temporality, i.e., because exposure and outcome are measured at the same time, the researcher cannot determine whether the exposure preceded the disease. This chicken-and-egg problem means that cross-sectional studies cannot be used to make a case for causality. Rather, these studies can and should be used to generate hypotheses about a potential cause.

4.3. Ecologic (Correlational) Studies. Ecologic studies use aggregate data to compare risk factors of interest, such as age, time, utilization of services, or exposures. The study design is useful for generating hypotheses about disease-exposure relationships or for identifying high- or low-risk populations, geographic regions, or time periods for future analytic studies. On the other hand, ecologic studies are limited by the lack of case-level data. Only with case-level data can the researcher control for potential confounders and relate exposure directly to outcome (including examining the data for a dose-response relationship), thereby helping to build a case for cause.

The epidemiologist is also trained to avoid drawing inappropriate conclusions from ecologic studies, i.e., to avoid committing "ecological fallacy." This blunder arises when the researcher attributes group characteristics to individuals, characteristics they may not possess. For example, the author and colleagues used an ecological analysis that uncovered high rates of childhood cancer in several locations [**20**]. Rather than assume that places with increased rates likely had increased risk, they identified places to examine the case-level data. In at least one instance, in-migrants were responsible for the increased rate. Specifically, a family moved to a northern New Jersey community from Puerto Rico. After they arrived, their child was diagnosed with leukemia and successfully treated at a regional hospital. Word got back to Puerto Rico that the hospital provided good medical care and several additional families with children with leukemia moved to that community in order to receive the same services. In other words, the patterns found in the ecological analysis did not imply individual risk for developing childhood leukemia, only that an increased number of cases existed at that location. It is important to remember that only individual-level factors can indicate risk, not aggregate-level ones.

Because individual-level variables cannot be controlled in an ecological analysis, individual risk cannot be estimated.

5. Rates and Measures

5.1. Crude Rates. Crude rates are simple to calculate by using the number of diagnosed cases and assuming the whole population is at risk. This tactic is useful for examining the general burden of disease in a population; thus, crude rates are widely used for health planning and administrative purposes. Yet any comparison of crude rates must be done with extreme care and with an understanding of the disease process so that the researcher does not draw inappropriate conclusions.

For instance, one state's Cancer Registry calculates crude rates for breast cancer incidence by county to determine where rates are highest and where they are lowest. It would be irresponsible to conclude that places with high rates have a higher risk for breast cancer than places with lower rates or that places with lower rates are healthier places to live based on crude rates alone. Rather, the Cancer Registry targets places with low crude rates in order to increase access to breast cancer screening services, especially for underserved populations. This use of crude rates allows an administrative use of cancer registry data that is novel, to say the least.

It is important to understand that age differences alone drive crude mortality rates. Florida, for example, has a large proportion of retirees whereas Alaska has a high proportion of young workers that in-migrate to take advantage of high salary offers. The result is that Florida has a high crude mortality rate and Alaska has a relatively low one. Again, this does not mean that Florida is an unhealthy place to live nor that Alaska is a healthy one. Rather, their respective crude rates reflect the age distributions of their populations.

5.2. Specific Rates. Age is the best predictor of disease and death. Because crude rates do not take the age structure of populations into account, places with larger proportions of elderly are more likely to have high crude rates than places with younger populations. In order to control for age or other factors that are likely to influence outcomes, epidemiologists calculate specific rates (or stratum-specific rates) for subgroups. Specific rates provide the detail that allows comparison between and among subpopulations. In Figure 5, for instance, it is possible to compare age-specific rates for 20-somethings with those for 30-somethings. Groups can be further stratified by gender, race and ethnicity, income and other factors that might influence disease status. Such detail is useful in comparing specific groups, such as 0–4 year old white males with 0–4 year old white females, or with 0–4 year old black males, or with 5–9 year old white males, etc., but it sorely limits the ability of comparing whole populations. The data become cumbersome with no summary figure to facilitate population-wide comparisons.

5.3. Adjusted Rates. To make comparisons between or among whole populations while controlling for potential confounders (especially age), epidemiologists use adjusted or standardized rates. Data miners might recognize adjusted rates as linear combinations of component rates where the determination of weighting coefficients is fixed by various conventions. Adjusted rates come in two forms, directly and indirectly adjusted. Directly adjusted rates involve the calculation of a weighted mean using a standard population, and the most commonly reported outcome measure of direct adjustment is the age-adjusted rate (AAR). By convention,

TABLE 4. Advantages and disadvantages of rates

Type	Advantages	Disadvantages
Crude	Actual rates Easy to calculate	Difficult to interpret due to underlying differences in population structure
Specific	Controls for subgroups Provides detail	Cumbersome if there are many subgroups No summary figure
Adjusted	Provides summary figure Controls for confounders Permits population comparisons	Fictional rate Magnitude of differences depend on the standard selected Hides subgroup differences

US mortality statistics before the year 2000 are directly standardized to the 1940 US population (the first census after US vital statistics become available for all the states). Beginning with the year 2000, mortality data are standardized to the 2000 US population. The exception to this rule is that US cancer mortality has been and continues to be standardized to the 1970 US population (the census closest to the inception of the SEER program). Data miners are warned that the WHO and the US government use different age standards, which means that their rates are not directly comparable. The United States has chosen to continue to use a national standard, whereas many other nations and the WHO have selected a world standard. Failure to standardize using the conventional population standards will probably get submissions to refereed journals rejected.

Epidemiologists sometimes calculate indirectly standardized rates by using a standard disease rate rather than a standard population. The summary figure for indirectly standardized rates is called a standardized mortality or morbidity ratio (SMR), calculated by dividing the observed cases by the expected cases (calculated from the standard disease rate) and multiplying by 100. Selection of the disease standard for indirect standardization is dependent upon the disease and population being studied rather than the conventions in the literature. These rates are widely used in occupational epidemiology and allow a specific occupational cohort to be compared to other working cohorts as well as to the local non-occupational population.

Adjusted rates are fictional rates and the public does not relate to them well, making them difficult to use for risk communication purposes. Adjusted rates hide subpopulation differences and the magnitude of the differences between and among populations depends on the standard selected for the adjustment. Adjusted rates do however allow comparisons between and among populations as long as the researcher uses the same standard. This makes adjusted rates an invaluable tool for the epidemiologist's tool chest (Table 4).

5.4. Incidence and Prevalence. Incidence and prevalence are epidemiologic concepts that are easily confused. Incidence is a rate, or the proportion of those susceptible (the population-at-risk) that develop a disease or outcome over a given period of time. Incidence rates are usually multiplied by a constant (in this case 1000) so they are readily grasped by the public. An attack rate is a type of incidence rate, reflecting the proportion of new cases that develop in a population-at-risk, usually for a short time period during an epidemic.

TABLE 5. Examples of the relationship of prevalence with incidence and the time duration of disease

Pancreatic cancer	**Common cold**
Prevalence low	Prevalence low
Incidence low	Incidence high
Duration short	Duration short
Type I diabetes	**Essential hypertension**
Prevalence high	Prevalence high
Incidence low	Incidence high
Duration long	Duration long

$$\text{Incidence Rate} = \frac{\text{Number of new cases}}{\text{Population-at-risk}} \times 1000$$

In contrast to incidence, prevalence is not reported as a rate (an exception is for HIV/AIDS data) as it does not reflect newly developed cases over time. Rather, prevalence reflects the proportion of existing cases (old and new) in a population at a point or period in time (point prevalence or period prevalence). Prevalence is the most effective way to describe the burden of disease in a population.

$$\text{Prevalence} = \frac{\text{Number of existing cases (old and new)}}{\text{Population-at-risk}} \times 1000$$

The relationship between incidence and prevalence is dependent upon the time duration of disease, written as $P \cong ID$ (i.e., prevalence is about equal to incidence times duration). Table 5 shows examples of this relationship. On the left we have two diseases where the incidence is low, pancreatic cancer and type I (juvenile or insulin-dependent) diabetes. On the right we have two diseases where the population-based incidence of disease is high, the common cold and essential hypertension. The top row shows that both diseases have a low prevalence because their duration is short. Conversely, the bottom row indicates a high prevalence for both diseases because their duration is long. The duration of disease may be long because the disease entity causes debilitation rather than death (as for arthritis) or when there is adequate treatment to maintain survival (as for some chemotherapies). Duration may be short when there is either rapid recovery (as for most single headaches) or when the disease progression is rapidly fatal (as for Ebola virus).

Beyond the simple $P \cong ID$ formula, epidemiologists recognize that prevalence in a geographic area is increased by an in-migration of cases, an out-migration of healthy people, an in-migration of susceptible persons, and improved diagnostic facilities (or better reporting) [**21**]. Prevalence decreases by an in-migration of healthy people, an out-migration of cases and improved cure rates. These concepts were of particular importance when the AIDS epidemic was in its early stages and cases migrated to centers most prepared to treat the new disease. Understanding population change and human behavior, then, is important for interpreting many disease trends.

We understand a great deal about how a disease impacts a population by considering its incidence and prevalence. Table 6 below lists two of the three variables

TABLE 6. Incident cases, prevalence and mortality for select diseases, United States 2000

Disease	Incident cases	Prevalence	Mortality
Lung cancer	170,400	—	160,288
Asthma	—	31 million	4,487
SARS	192	—	0

(incident number of cases, prevalence, or mortality) for three diseases. The table shows that 170,400 new cases of lung cancer were diagnosed in the year 2000. In that same year, 160,288 people died of the disease. Given the large annual number of deaths from lung cancer relative to the new cases diagnosed, it is logical to conclude that the prevalence of lung cancer in the general population is not very high. On the other hand, asthma accounted for 4,487 deaths in 2000, but the table shows that 31 million people are currently living with the disease. Given that people with asthma generally live a long time with the disease, it is logical to conclude that the incidence rate for asthma is high, but nowhere nearly as high as its prevalence. For SARS, the incident number of cases was low (192) in the year 2000, with mortality at 0. We can conclude that the prevalence of SARS was also low as the duration of the disease is short (weeks).

5.5. Proportionate Mortality. Proportionate mortality is simply that proportion of all mortality ascribed to a particular cause for a given population. It is sometimes written as the proportionate mortality rate as it exemplifies the mortality experience of a population for a given time period, usually one year. Some epidemiologists take issue with the term rate in relation to proportionate mortality as the measure does not measure risk. Use of the term is, therefore, not standard across the epidemiologic literature.

Proportionate mortality should not be confused with cause-specific death rates, as the denominator used for the calculation of proportionate mortality is all deaths, not the population-at-risk. For example, Table 7 shows the leading causes of death in the United States for 1991, by number, proportionate mortality rate and cause-specific death rate. The proportions must always add to unity, whereas rates are relative to population size and characteristics.

5.6. Proportionate Mortality Ratio (PMR). Epidemiologists often compare the proportionate mortality experience in one subpopulation to that of the population as a whole, either for deaths from all causes or from a specific cause. That particular calculation is termed a proportionate mortality ratio and it is directly comparable to an SMR, using proportions instead of rates. As with proportionate mortality, a PMR does not directly measure the risk or probability that a person in a population will die from a specific disease, but it does measure the differences in mortality from other causes of death. PMRs are used to examine the relative importance of specific causes of death in the total mortality picture of a given population. The formula is written:

$$\text{PMR} = \frac{\text{observed proportionate mortality}}{\text{expected deaths (based on proportion in a standard population)}} \times 100$$

TABLE 7. Leading causes of death, 25–44 year olds, United States, 1991

Rank	Cause of Death	Number	Proportionate Mortality Rate (%)	Cause-specific Death Rate per 100,000
1	Accidents and adverse effects	26,526	18.0	32.2
2	Malignant neoplasms	22,228	15.0	27.0
3	HIV/AIDS infection	21,747	14.7	36.4
4	Diseases of the heart	15,822	10.7	19.2
5	Homicide and legal intervention	12,372	8.4	15.0
6	Suicide	12,281	8.3	14.9
7	Chronic liver diseases and cirrhosis	4,449	3.0	5.4
8	Cardiovascular diseases	3,343	2.3	4.1
9	Diabetes mellitus	2,211	1.5	2.7
10	Pneumonia and influenza	2,203	1.5	2.7
	All cases	147,750	100	

Note: Population = 82,438,000
Source: `http://wonder.cdc.gov/`

5.7. Case Fatality Rates. Case fatality rates are not to be confused with mortality rates. Mortality rates are based on the total population-at-risk and indicate risk, whereas case fatality rates are based on the total number of cases of a particular disease and imply risk only for those who already have a given disease entity. Data miners might better recognize a case fatality rate as a conditional probability (the risk of dying given you have contracted the disease). For example, assume that in Lexington, KY (with a 2001 population of 100,000) there were 20 cases of Disease X. Of those cases, 18 individuals died from the disease, one remains stricken and one recovered. The mortality and case fatality rates for Disease X in Lexington, KY in 2001 would then be:

$$\text{Mortality rate from Disease X} = \frac{18}{100,000} = 0.00018 = 0.018\% \text{ in 2001}$$

$$\text{Case fatality rate from Disease X} = \frac{18}{20} = 0.9 = 90\% \text{ in 2001}$$

If mentioned on the nightly news, the mortality rate from Disease X would not likely cause a panic among the city's population, but the case fatality rate might easily do so, especially if it was not explained in detail. Indeed, as the case fatality rate does not imply risk to the general population, it is not usually used by health educators/risk communicators to explain risk to the public.

5.8. Years of Potential Life Lost. Years of Potential Life Lost (YPLL) is becoming a popular mortality measure because it recognizes that the death of an individual at an early age results in a greater loss of productivity than if that same individual lived to an average life span, by convention equal to 75 years. YPLL (or PYLL in some of the epidemiologic literature) can be calculated for either an individual or for group data. Suppose, for instance, that an individual died at age 20. That individual would contribute 55 potential years of life lost to a YPLL calculation ($75 - 20 = 55$ YPLL). For group data, individuals 75 years or older are excluded from the analysis. The group rate is obtained by dividing the total potential years of life lost by the total population less than 75 years of age.

6. Understanding Survival Measures

The convention for calculating survival measures, particularly for cancer, is 5 years. Five, however, may not be the appropriate choice of survival time for all cases because survival is subject to lead-time bias. Lead time bias reflects the fact that people screened for disease enter a data set earlier and may appear to survive longer than people who enter a data set at the usual time of diagnosis, i.e., when symptoms occur. When many people enter a data set through screening, they shift survival curves so that screening programs appear, perhaps inaccurately, to improve survival from a given disease.

Related to lead time bias is length bias. Length bias refers to the fact that screening programs are more likely to identify the lesser aggressive forms of disease. Since aggressive disease has a short asymptomatic period, cases with aggressive disease are less likely to be identified through the screening process. Data obtained from screening programs, then, are almost always biased in terms of cases with lesser aggressive forms of a disease.

A case in point is the recent debate over whether PSA screening and aggressive treatment of newly diagnosed prostate cancer makes sense [**22**]. Some experts argue that aggressive treatment of early disease is always desirable as the goal of screening is to identify cases early when they have the best chance for cure. Others argue that since PSA screening is biased towards finding less aggressive forms of the disease, watchful waiting for disease progression may be a better choice than aggressive treatments that carry a risk of serious side effects such as incontinence and impotence [**23**]. The research results to answer this question are not yet available and may not be for several more years.

6.1. Life Tables. Epidemiologists, demographers and actuaries use mortality tables or life tables to measure longevity, fertility, migration, population growth, and both length of working life and length of disability-free life. Life tables describe the process of population extinction and they end with the death of the last individual. Simple life tables are calculated from the age-specific mortality rates for whole populations or their subgroups. Complex life tables are calculated by using mortality rates and other demographic data to build complex models. One significant advantage of life tables is that they are not impacted by the age distribution of a population and do not require the use of a standard population for comparative analyses. The tables yield information on the probability of surviving fixed segments of time (weeks, months, or years). Their drawback is that they assume that no changes in conditions occur over the time period of observation. Life tables also require a minimal loss to follow-up of the individuals in the population under study. Where individuals are lost to follow-up, or if they enter the cohort after the beginning of a time segment, they are termed "withdrawls" and by convention are calculated as contributing half their numbers to the mortality for their respective time periods. Small populations do not lend themselves to life table analysis as migration drastically affects the population structure and small numbers of deaths yield imprecise results. For an in-depth discussion of risk estimation from life table analysis see Rothman and Greenland [**24**].

6.2. Kaplan-Meier Method. The Kaplan-Meier method is a better choice for analyzing data on small populations than is the life table method. In international epidemiology circles, the Kaplan-Meier method is sometimes called the crude survival method or the observed survival method. Kaplan-Meier analyses do not use fixed segments of time but set the time periods for analysis by the time of death or diagnosis of each case. Where withdrawls in life table analysis partially contribute to the mortality experience of the population under study, they are removed from the analysis in the Kaplan-Meier method.

Historically, Kaplan-Meier was reserved for small data sets and standard life tables were used for larger ones. With the advent of new computer programs, the method is now being used on large data sets and the epidemiology literature reflects an increasing number of studies utilizing the Kaplan-Meier method for describing survival. In 2001, the United Kingdom Association of Cancer Registries held a workshop and determined that SAS, SPSS, SPlus, and Stata are adequate for running Kaplan-Meier analyses, producing comparable results [**25**]. For the mathematics of the Kaplan-Meier method and examples of how to use it, see Kelsey and colleagues [**26**] or Koepsell and Weiss [**27**].

6.3. Median and Relative Survival. Median survival is the time that half the population survives, either from a given diagnosis or from an exposure. Median survival is not affected by outliers and is quite useful as it can be reported when half, rather than the entire population succumbs to an outcome. It is estimated by linear interpolation within the interval containing the survival probability equal to 0.50. A limitation of using median survival is that it is not yet available as part of standard statistical packages. In addition, algorithms have not yet been standardized for the measure and different algorithms yield different results [**25**].

Relative survival compares the survival of a group with a particular disease to a comparable group who do not have the disease (Table 8). Changes in relative survival are sensitive to changes in technology (e.g., finding early cases of disease that may be more responsive to treatment) or to improvements in treatments that lengthen life. The outcome measure is calculated as:

$$\text{Relative survival (\%)} = \frac{\text{Observed cases}}{\text{Expected cases (based on disease-free population)}} \times 100$$

New software has become available to calculate relative survival (i.e., the stand-alone program SURV3 or the Stata macro *strel*). Relative survival commands are also available in SPlus [**25**].

7. Summary

If data miners and epidemiologists are to make progress in working together to find patterns in person, place and time variables related to health outcomes in large data sets, they must speak a common vocabulary and bridge the gap in mindset between their professions. While the former have new and different statistical tools for examining large data sets, the latter remain skeptical and worry that these tools are simply another form of data dredging. To begin the mindset bridging process, data miners must bring more than originality and enthusiasm to the table. They must understand and be willing to discuss data limitations and the way in which epidemiologists think about cause [**28**]. They must recognize that while finding and rapidly reporting statistical associations can get you in the newspaper, it has the potential of disparaging the good work epidemiology can do [**1**]. On the other hand, epidemiologists must embrace the possibility that using

TABLE 8. Relative survival* (%) during three time periods by cancer site

Cancer	1974-1976	1983-1985	1992-1998
All sites	50	52	62
Breast (female)	75	78	86
Colon and rectum	50	57	62
Leukemia	34	41	46
Lung and bronchus	12	14	15
Melanoma	80	85	89
Non-Hodgkin's lymphoma	47	54	55
Ovary	37	41	53
Pancreas	3	3	4
Prostate	67	75	97
Urinary bladder	73	78	82

Source: Surveillance, Epidemiology, and End Results Program, 1973-1999.
Division of Cancer Control and Population Sciences, National Cancer Institute, 2002.
* 5-year relative survival rates based on follow up of patients through 1999.

novel approaches to explore health-related data sets might bring new insights that standard epidemiologic techniques have not yet uncovered. They must take the initiative to educate data miners about data limitations and be the conscience for those drawing conclusions about results. If data mining can become yet another tool in the descriptive epidemiology toolbox, it may lead to new insights about health risks and outcomes not yet considered in existing data sets. That, indeed, is what descriptive epidemiology is all about.

References

1. Smith GD and Ebrahim S. Data dredging, bias, or confounding. They can all get you into the BMJ and the Friday papers. *BMJ* 2002(2128 Dec);325:1437–8.
2. Le Fanu, J The Rise and Fall of Modern Medicine. New York: Carroll and Graf Pubs, 2000.
3. Schlesselman JJ. Case-Control Studies: Design, Conduct, and Analysis. New York: Oxford University Press, 1982.
4. Gordis L. More on causal inferences: Bias, confounding, and interaction (Chapter 14). In: Epidemiology (2nd ed.). New York: WB Saunders, 2000.
5. Bradford-Hill, A. The Environment and Disease: Association or Causation? President's Address. *Proc Royal Soc Med* 1965;9:295–300.
6. Hertzel AM. History and organization of the vital statistics system. National Center for Health Statistics. 1977. See `http://www.cdc.gov/nchs/data/misc/usvss.pdf`.
7. National Center for Health Statistics. See `http://www.cdc.gov/nchs/nvss.htm`.
8. Greenberg MR. Urbanization and Cancer Mortality: The United States Experience 1950–1975. New York: Oxford University Press, 1983.
9. Personal communication with MR Greenberg, Edward J Bloustein School of Planning and Public Policy, Rutgers University, New Brunswick, NJ. July 25, 2004.
10. Office of Management and Budget. Revision of Statistical Policy Directive No. 15, Race and Ethnic Standards for Federal Statistics and Administrative Reporting. Federal Register 1997 (Oct 30). See `http://www.whitehouse.gov/omb/fedreg/1997standards.html`.
11. Williams DR. Race and health: basic questions, emerging directions. *Ann Epidemiol* 1997 Jul;7(5):322–33.
12. Sondik EJ, Lucas JW, Madans JH, Smith SS. Race/ethnicity and the 2000 census: implications for public health. *Am J Public Health* 2000 Nov;90(11):1709-13.
13. Snow J. On the Mode of Communication of Cholera (2nd ed.). London: John Churchill, 1860. Available online at `http://www.deltaomega.org/snowfin.pdf`.

14. Pyle GF. The Diffusion of Influenza: Patterns and Paradigms. Totowa, NJ: Rowman & Littlefield, 1986.
15. Parshkov EM, Chebotareva IV, Sokolov VA, et al. Additional thyroid dose factor from transportation sources in Russia after the Chernobyl disaster. *Environ Health Perspect* 1997 Dec;105 Suppl 6:1491-6.
16. Greenberg MR and Schneider D. Blue Thursday? Homicide and suicide among urban 15–24 year old black male Americans. *Public Health Rep* 1992; 107(3): 264–68.
17. Schneider D, Greenberg MR, Donaldson MH, and Choi D. Cancer clusters: Investigating multiple geographic scales. *Soc Sci Med* 1993; 37(6): 753–59.
18. Notice to readers: Ongoing investigation of anthrax—Florida, October 2001. *Morb Mortal Wkly Rep* 2001 Oct 19;50(41):889–93. See `http://www.cdc.gov/mmwr/preview/mmwrhtml/mm5040a5.htm`.
19. Jerrigan JA, Stephens DS, Ashford DA, et al. Bioterrorism-related inhalational anthrax: The first 10 cases reported in the United States. *Emerg Infect Dis* 2001 Nov-Dec;7(6): 933–44.
20. Schneider D, Greenberg M R, Donaldson M H, Abe T, and Choi D. Childhood and young adult cancer in New Jersey and four SEER states. *NJ Med* 1992; 89(12): 929–34.
21. Polissar L. The effect of migration on comparison of disease rates in geographic studies in the United States. *Am J Epidemiol* 1980; 111: 175–82.
22. Dennis LK and Resnick MI. Analysis of recent trends in prostate cancer incidence and mortality. *Prostate* 2000 Mar 1;42(4):247–52.
23. D'Amico AV, Chen MH, Roehl KA, Catalona WJ. Preoperative PSA velocity and the risk of death from prostate cancer after radical prostatectomy. *N Engl J Med* 2004 Jul 8;351(2):125–35.
24. Rothman KJ and Greenland S. Modern Epidemiology (2nd ed.). Philadelphia: Lippincott-Raven Publishers, 1998. pp. 287–294.
25. See `http://www.ukacr.org.uk/survival/survivalreport.htm`.
26. Kelsey JL, Whittemore AS, Evans AS and Thompson WD. Methods in Observational Epidemiology (2nd ed.). New York: Oxford University Press, 1996.
27. Koepsell TD and Weiss NS. Epidemiologic Methods: Studying the Occurrence of Illness. New York: Oxford University Press 2003.
28. Gori GB. Considerations on guidelines of epidemiologic practice. *AEP* 2002;12(2):73–78.

E. J. Bloustein School of Planning and Public Policy, Rutgers University
E-mail address: `donas@rci.rutgers.edu`

DIMACS Series in Discrete Mathematics
and Theoretical Computer Science
Volume **70**, 2006

Biostatistical Challenges in Molecular Data Analysis

William D. Shannon

ABSTRACT. Epidemiology is the study of the distribution and size of disease problems in human populations, in particular to identify etiological factors in the pathogenesis of diseases and to provide the data essential for the management, evaluation and planning of services for the prevention, control and treatment of disease [**4**]. Molecular epidemiology uses molecular biology to identify the etiological factors, and is a growing and important area of biomedical research.

Molecular epidemiology presents new challenges to data analysts. Modern molecular biology can measure tens of thousands of molecular variables rapidly and cheaply (e.g., gene chips measure the activity of tens of thousands of genes, genotyping is routinely done at hundreds or thousands of markers, and proteomics has the potential of characterizing the entire protein content of tissues). The limiting step in molecular epidemiology is the small number of human subjects these measurements are made on relative to the large number of variables (the large P, small N problem).

In this paper I address three statistical problems faced when analyzing molecular epidemiology data. The first problem is the proper identification of patient subgroups within which statistical tests of genotype-phenotype association should be applied. The second problem is the testing of clinical covariates against a large number of molecular variables. The third problem is the selection of important molecular factors related to disease. While these problems can be defined in the language of classical statistics (i.e., population stratification, over-determined systems, and variable selection, respectively), I believe their solution will require combining statistics with discrete mathematics and computer science.

1. Epidemiology

Epidemiology has been defined as the "study of the *distribution and size of disease* problems in human populations, in particular to *identify etiological factors* in the pathogenesis of diseases and to provide the data essential for the management, evaluation and planning of *services for the prevention, control and treatment of disease*" [**4**]. By quantifying disease occurrence and location, and using this information to identify etiological causes of the diseases by observing differences in exposures among areas with different distributions and size of the disease problem, modern epidemiologists have successfully identified serious risk factors associated

2000 *Mathematics Subject Classification.* Primary 65C60 Computational problems in statistics; Secondary 62P10 Applications to biology and medical sciences.

TABLE 1. A contingency table of exposure by disease for calculating an odds ratio.

		Exposure	
		Yes	No
Disease	Yes	N_{YY}	N_{YN}
	No	N_{NY}	N_{NN}

with many diseases. For example, heart disease, skin cancer, and lung cancer have very clear etiological risk factors obesity, sun, smoking contributing to their occurrence. These were all identified through modern epidemiological studies.

The quantitative statistical tools of modern epidemiology have been well worked out both theoretically and for applied data analysis. Consider the simple case of trying to decide whether a particular exposure increases the odds of having a disease. Under a suitable controlled (and defined) experiment a set of cases (those with the disease) and controls (those without the disease but in all other senses similar to the cases) are obtained and the frequency of the exposure in the two groups is compared. This is displayed in Table 1 where N_{YY} is the number of people with the disease and with the exposure, N_{YN} is the number of people with the disease and without the exposure, etc. From this we calculate the odds ratio (OR) which is a statistical measure of the association of exposure with disease by the simple formula:

$$OR = \frac{N_{YY} \times N_{NN}}{N_{YN} \times N_{NY}}$$

This has many well established theoretical advantages of which the most important is the clear interpretation of its value. If the $OR = 1$ (signified by a P value greater than 0.05) then we conclude the exposure is unrelated to the disease. On the other hand, if the $OR > 1$ or $OR < 1$ (signified by a P value less than or equal to 0.05) then we conclude the exposure is related to the disease. The odds ratio and many other classical statistical (e.g., vital statistics, life tables, logistic regression) and observational studies (e.g., cohort studies, case-control) methods have become part of the epidemiologists toolbox and are applied daily with great success in discovering etiological causes of disease. However, the complexity of data in molecular epidemiology, whose goal is the same as classical epidemiology of relating etiological exposures to disease, often will not fall into the same framework where the existing tools of epidemiology apply.

2. Molecular Biology

The term molecular biology was first described as "...an approach from the viewpoint of the so-called basic sciences with the leading idea of *searching below the large-scale manifestations of classical biology* for the corresponding molecular plan. It is concerned particularly with the *forms of biological molecules* and... is predominantly three-dimensional and structural and... it must at the same time inquire into genesis and function" [**1**]. In the intervening 40 years we have successfully gone below classical biology and amazingly unraveled the forms and structures of these biological molecules. Only now are we able to begin to uncover their genesis

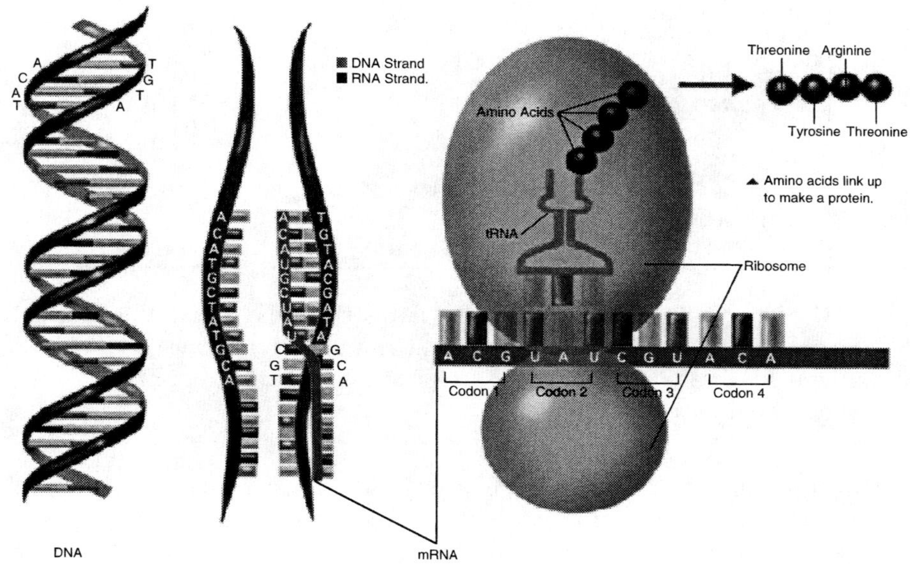

FIGURE 1. Schematic of the storage, transmission and expression of genetic information. The 'type' of information relates to the specific DNA sequences and the 'rate' of information exchange is the amount of mRNA and protein produced.

and function, and more excitingly, begin to apply this knowledge as biotechnology to benefit mankind in terms of advances in pharmaceuticals, medicine, and agriculture.

That genes encode information for cell functioning and proteins process information for cellular functioning is well established and defined in the central dogma of molecular biology: DNA makes RNA makes Protein. Figure 1 (taken from "How Genes Work", `http://www.nigms.nih.gov`) shows how DNA unravels to transcribe RNA, which moves to the ribosome, and is subsequently translated into protein. What has become evident in the last few years is that for biotechnology it is more important to know the *Type* and *Rate* of information transfer from gene to protein which defines the cell's phenotype, and therefore have a direct impact on the biotechnology product. For simplicity we view the "Type" of information as the organisms genotype and the "Rate" of information transferred as the activity of the gene.

The "Type" of information being stored in genes is often measured as single nucleotide polymorphisms, or SNPs, which indicate where in a gene a base shows variation across individuals. (Other aspects of 'type' might include alternative slice sites or methylation, but we will not be concerned with those factors in this paper.) In In Figure 2, the box to the left shows a short segment of the ABCB1 gene which is involved in transporting chemotherapeutic drug (irinotecan for colon cancer) into and out of the cancer cell. A SNP at position 3435 shows some individuals with the C nucleotide and some with the T nucleotide at this position in the gene. The differences in this nucleotide is being investigated as possibly effecting patient response to irinotecan. The "Rate" of information transferred is routinely measured

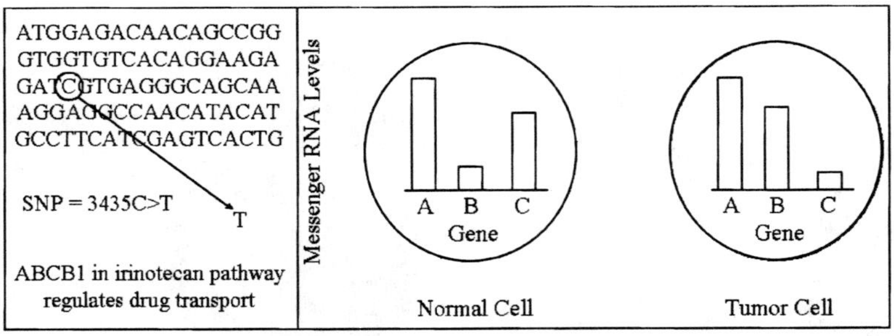

FIGURE 2. The figure on the left shows the 'type' of information stored in DNA as a SNP single-nucleotide polymorphism. The figure to the right shows the 'rate' of information transferred as captured in microarray data.

by RNA levels in cells using techniques such as microarrays. The histograms in the box to the right in Figure 2 shows how mRNA levels vary in genes across tissue types (or any other tissue samples). In this illustration Gene A has high expression in both tissues, B is low in normal and high in tumor tissue, etc. The challenge for microarrays is that there will be upwards of 40,000 genes to analyze in a single experiment and not just three as Figure 2 suggests.

Analyzing the effect of the Type and Rate of information transfer on biotechnology products present novel biostatistical challenges which this paper addresses.

3. Epidemiology and Molecular Biology: Statistical Challenges

The molecular epidemiology questions are similar in nature to classical epidemiology questions:

- How do different SNPs (type of information transferred) effect drug metabolism?
- How do different SNPs (type of information transferred) effect patient outcome?
- How do we select genes with similar expression profiles (rate of information transferred)?
- How do we select genes whose expression profiles (rate of information transferred) distinguish tissue subgroups?

However, the nature and complexity of the data pose serious problems to the analyst that cannot be overlooked, and that provide methodologists with exciting new problems to tackle. In this section I present three problems related to the data analysis of this data, and present (in brief outline) strategies my lab has taken to overcome them. The inclusion of this chapter in the book is hopefully to introduce the reader to a broad range of open problems in data analysis whose solutions might eventually be most efficiently solved by combining statistics, discrete mathematics, and computer science.

For the reader with little or no background in molecular biology I recommend two things. First, read "How Genes Work" which is online and free at `http://www.nigms.nih.gov`, and "DNA: The Secret of Life" by James Watson and Andrew Berry (Knopf, 2003) as good simple introductions to the complexities of molecular biology. Second, find a biologist working on molecular epidemiology problems and work closely with them - attend their weekly lab meetings, provide service support for their standard data analyses to show you are a good citizen, and help solve 'their' problems. From these interactions you will begin to find the open data analysis problems that should be solved and therefore identify methodology that you can develop and will drive your research agenda. But before the non-epidemiologist reader knows what tools need to be developed (and I guarantee they are not the tools we think are needed or probably the tools we have developed thinking the world of molecular epidemiology will flock to our door) we need to know what the real problems being faced by the molecular biologist are.

3.1. Subgroup Identification. Under ideal conditions many statistical genetic methods have good power to detect phenotype-genotype relationships. However, the power decreases significantly in less than ideal situations. When possible we compensate for loss of power due to heterogeneous genetic etiology in the dataset (e.g., genotypic variation at locus A contributes to trait variation in some samples but not in others) by identifying subgroups within which statistical analyses are performed separately. In the following 2 x 2 table we see a statistically nonsignificant result indicating no relation between the genotype (SNP) and outcome:

		SNP		
		T	*C*	
Outcome	*Live*	60	50	*P*=0.22
	Die	50	60	

However, a well known problem in epidemiology is the subgroup analysis and if a covariate is able to partition the population into say 2 subgroups, the analysis within each subgroup may increase power to detect an effect:

Subgroup 1		*SNP*		
		T	*C*	
Outcome	*Live*	20	5	*P*=0.0001
	Die	5	20	

Subgroup 2		*SNP*		
		T	*C*	
Outcome	*Live*	40	45	*P*=0.54
	Die	45	40	

This is a reasonable scenario in molecular epidemiology where the effect of a gene may be dependent on other genes not measured. Technically this is known as epistasis, or gene-gene interaction, and is becoming an important area of research in genetics [**3**] and new methods to solve the computational complexity are very much needed. Analogous to the gene-gene interaction is gene-environment interaction, though the term epistasis does not apply to this.

We developed an approach for automatically identifying subgroups in genetic epidemiology data. By modifying the recursive partitioning algorithm for molecular data, we were able to increase the power to locate genes related to phenotype in simulation studies [**7, 8**]. Applications of our methods to real data are also showing promising results. In one application for cardiovascular disease [**2**] using matched data (i.e., sibpairs), a gene was identified related to blood pressure in individuals whose matched sibling was discordant to them in having a high blood pressure diagnosis, younger than 48, and high cholesterol levels. In all other subgroups this gene had no effect on blood pressure, and when all the data was pooled and analyzed together, the gene was not significant. Performing the statistical analyses on subgroups separately resulted in increased signal for identifying disease associated genes.

Nonparametric hierarchical cluster analysis, which plays a prominent role in the statistical analysis of molecular data [**9**], is another powerful data reduction tool used in molecular epidemiology to identify subgroups. The analytical goal of cluster analysis is to find subgroups such that samples (or genes) within a subgroup are more similar to each other than they are to samples (or genes) in different subgroups. Because molecular data often consists of large numbers of predictors, for example genes in a microarray or a large number of measured SNP's, the data must be reduced before the relationship between genes and phenotypes can be assessed. Putative relationships between clusters of samples and phenotypes need to be recognized as nothing more than hypotheses generated by clustering methods. Additional experiments must be done to statistically and biologically validate the relationships.

Unlike standard statistical methods such as the t-test and analysis-of-variance, statistical hierarchical clustering does not have a probabilistic foundation. Because of this, there are no statistical tests or P values to determine how many subgroups are in the data and which subgroups are valid. We take two novel approaches to improve hierarchical cluster analysis in molecular data analysis, and to formally test for the number of clusters in the data. We use consensus methods to combine results from multiple cluster analyses into a final, more stable cluster, and show that these final clusters indicate more clearly how many clusters exist in the data. We will also apply a probability model applicable to graphs to determine the significance level of the consensus model and allow the number of clusters to be statistically tested using a likelihood-ratio test [**6, 10**]. It should be noted that mixture models for finding subgroups are based on mixtures of probability models and have an objective rule for deciding how many clusters are in the data based on a likelihood ratio test. Other approaches such as Bayesian information criteria (BIC) or MCMC to get the posterior distribution on the number of clusters exist which purport to provide more objective measures. However these approaches require major assumptions about how the data are distributed which this author is reluctant to do.

3.2. Testing Covariates Against Molecular Variables. Analyses testing the relationship of covariates with molecular variables generally proceed in two steps. First, a statistical data reduction method such as hierarchical clustering is applied to the molecular variables (without reference to the covariate data) to identify sample subgroups. Second, covariate values are compared across the subgroups found in the first stage of analysis (e.g., if we split the data into subgroups identified by the dendrograms is one phenotype more likely to appear in one subgroup than in another). This "two-stage" analysis is a very powerful paradigm, and has been used successfully in many microarray analyses, but is qualitative and provides no measures of association or statistical tests and P values.

We focus on using methods which directly test the statistical association of molecular data with clinical covariates [**11**]. The two-stage analysis described above is likely to result in a loss of power. A preferred analysis is to analyze the gene expression and covariate data simultaneously, such as through a regression or correlation type analysis. However, standard correlation and regression approaches to analyzing gene chip data are not appropriate since these experiments generate large amounts of data on a small number of samples resulting in an overparameterized (unidentifiable) model. We therefore have been developing and applying Mantel statistics to allow the simultaneous and valid statistical analysis of molecular variables and sample covariates.

The Mantel correlation is simple to describe. Suppose two datasets are available on a set of subjects: a dataset containing genetic variables and a dataset containing standard clinical covariates. Calculate the subject pairwise distance matrices separately for the covariates, D_X, and the genetic information, D_G, unravel the upper triangle of the distance matrices, and correlate the d_{ij} pairwise distances:

$$D_X \overset{Unravel}{\longrightarrow} \begin{bmatrix} d_{12} \\ d_{13} \\ \vdots \\ d_{N-1,N} \end{bmatrix}_{Covariate} \times \begin{bmatrix} d_{12} \\ d_{13} \\ \vdots \\ d_{N-1,N} \end{bmatrix}_{Genetic} \overset{Unravel}{\longleftarrow} D_G$$

Moving the analysis from raw data to pairwise distances we avoid the problem of an over-determined model and can begin to interpret complex genomic data for the epidemiologist. For example, highly correlated distances in the two matrices indicate the genetic and covariate data are related, while zero correlation indicates no relation. We are currently applying genetic algorithms in combination with Mantel correlation to identify subsets of genes that are most likely related to clinically meaningful covariates.

3.3. Selection of Molecular Variables. Perhaps the statistical problem getting the most attention in molecular data analysis is known as multiple testing. This occurs when multiple statistical tests have been performed to select genes from a microarray experiment which distinguishes sample types. In this case a P value is generated for each gene and genes are selected based on their ordering (e.g., 10, 100, or 1000 genes with the smallest P values). It is well known that this results in a significant increase in the number of false positives (i.e., number of genes declared significant when in fact they are not). Attempts to reduce this error are proposed based on Bonferroni, permutation, and false discovery rate adjustments. However, these adjustments simply move the threshold for saying which genes to retain (e.g., 2, 65, 250 with the smallest adjusted P values versus 10, 100, or 1000 genes with the smallest unadjusted P values).

Current multiple adjustment techniques do not allow genes to be selected out of the order of the P values. In other words, genes with small fold changes (differences in the ratio of the mean expression values across two sample groups) can not be selected. This makes sense statistically but not biologically since many cases where a small change in a molecule results in drastic changes in phenotype. Figure 3 shows a Quantile Volcano Plot display of 223 genes from a region on human chromosome 9 identified as possibly related to cytotoxicity in cells treated with a cancer drug [**12**]. The two dashed horizontal lines show arbitrary cutoff points for declaring genes significant depending on if they are above the horizontal line (bottom line is the unadjusted P value and the top line is the Bonferroni adjusted P value). We have developed a novel method [**5**] for gene selection based on fitting nonlinear quantile regression lines (the curved line following the shape of the data) and selecting those

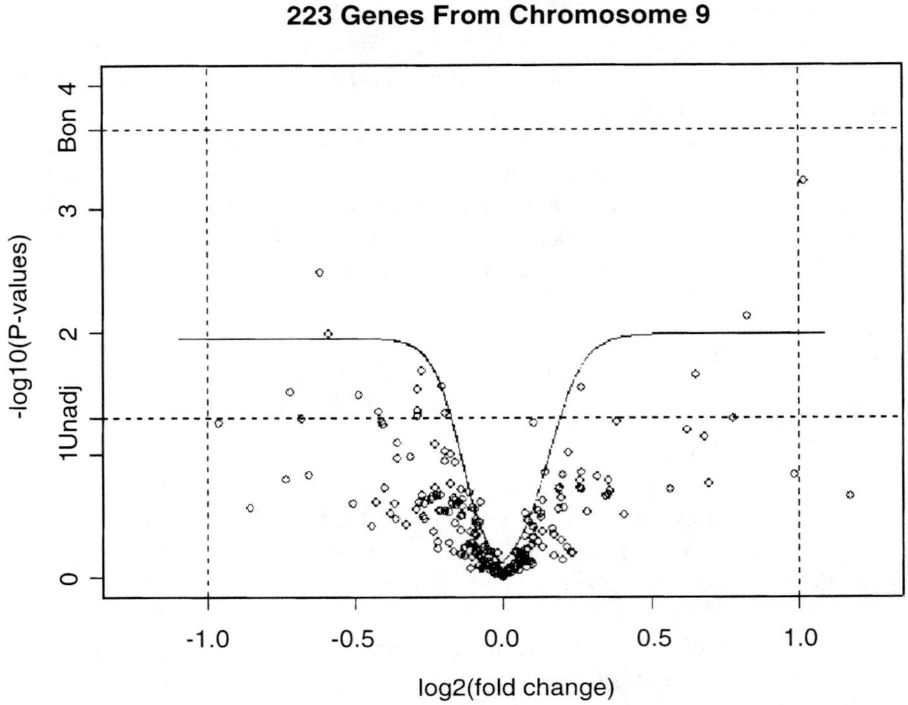

FIGURE 3. A Quantile Volcano Plot with a non-linear decision boundary (curve) with the genes above the curve being declared significant.

genes above this line as significant. The advantage of our approach is that we allow genes with small differences in expression level between groups (x-axis variable) to now be selected which would not be allowed with the adjustments described above.

4. Discussion

We believe that modern molecular data requires new methods of analysis to extract useful and valid information for biotechnology. In this brief paper we have identified three existing challenges of molecular data—subgroup identification, testing covariates against molecular variables, and selecting molecular variables—and discussed the approaches we have developed and routinely apply to overcome these challenges. We believe that researchers with skills in discrete mathematics and computer science, as well as in statistics, if working closely with molecular epidemiologists to solve their problems, can identify and make valuable methodological contributions.

In should be remembered that these models, such as classification and regression trees and hierarchical clustering, often have statistical problems such as biased selection of covariates or no probabilistic framework. However, as a data mining technique these models can provide insight into the molecular biology being studied without having a formal statistical hypothesis testing procedure, and provide ideas and directions for future studies and formal hypotheses that can be tested in a subsequent study.

References

1. Astbury W.T. Editorial *Nature* 1961, 190:1124
2. Costello, Swartz et al. *BioMedCentral Genetics* 2003 Suppl. 4:66
3. Culverhouse R, Klein T, Shannon W. "Detecting epistatic interactions contributing to quantitative traits". *Genetic Epidemiology* , 2004
4. Everitt, B. *The Cambridge Dictionary of Statistics.* Cambridge University Press, 1998.
5. Li X., Culverhouse, R., Watters, J., McLeod, H., Shannon, W. "Quantile Volcano Plots for Identifying Significant Genes in Microarray Data". *The American Statistician* Under Review.
6. Shannon W, Banks D. "Combining classification trees using maximum likelihood estimation". *Statistics in Medicine* 1999, 18(6):727-740.
7. Shannon W, Province M, Rao DC. "Tree-based recursive partitioning methods for subdividing sibpairs into relatively more homogeneous subgroups". *Genetic Epidemiology* Apr 2001; 20(3):293-306.
8. Shannon W, Faifer M, Province M, Rao DC. "Tree-based recursive partitioning methods for fitting stratified linear regression models". *Journal of Classification* 2002; 19:113-130.
9. Shannon W, Culverhouse R, Duncan J. "Analyzing microarray data using cluster analysis". *Pharmacogenomics*, 2003, 4(1):41-51.
10. Shannon W, Klein T, Culverhouse R. "A likelihood approach for determining cluster number". *Computing Science and Statistics* In Press.
11. Shannon W, Watson M, Perry A, Rich K. "Mantel statistics to correlate gene expression levels from microarrays with clinical covariates". *Genetic Epidemiology*, 2002,23:87-96.
12. Watters, J. W., Kraja, A., Meucci, M. A., Province, M. A., and McLeod, H. L. "Genome-wide discovery of loci influencing chemotherapy cytotoxicity". *Proc Natl Acad Sci USA* 2004, 101, 11809-11814.

WASHINGTON UNIV. SCHOOL OF MEDICINE 660 S. EUCLID AVE., CAMPUS BOX 8005 ST. LOUIS, MO 63110

E-mail address: `wshannon@wustl.edu`

DIMACS Series in Discrete Mathematics
and Theoretical Computer Science
Volume **70**, 2006

Mining Online Media for Global Disease Outbreak Monitoring

Lynette Hirschman and Laurie E. Damianos

1. Introduction

This paper discusses text mining applied to medical data and illustrates how text mining is maturing to support selected applications in epidemiology. We describe an operational prototype, MiTAP, that collects open source information, particularly *local* information from news wire sources, to assist public health practitioners in tracking disease outbreaks around the world.

The paper begins with a brief overview describing the need to monitor disease outbreak worldwide. This is followed by a short summary of the kinds of textual information that can be processed today, e.g., syndromic surveillance data, patient record data, and news wire reports of events, with several examples of the organizations and systems that are doing this. We then introduce MiTAP, a system for the capture of multilingual information on disease outbreak, and the next two sections discuss specific natural language technologies in use in MiTAP and applications of MiTAP. The final section discusses research challenges and new directions that text mining will enable.

2. Need for Global Disease Monitoring

With the recent outbreaks of West Nile Virus, SARS, and avian influenza, there is greatly increased awareness of the need for global monitoring of infectious disease. Infectious disease is not only a public health issue, with 15 million of 57 million annual deaths attributable to infectious disease worldwide [**16**], but it is increasingly a political issue — due to the possibility of bioterrorism. It is also a major economic issue: the SARS outbreak is estimated to have resulted in losses of at least $30 billion [**14, 24**]; the current avian influenza outbreak in Southeast Asia has led to the culling of millions of poultry, with serious economic impact on the poultry farmers in the region, not to mention the threat to public health, tourism, and trade for the local and national economies.

There is an urgent need to identify emerging outbreaks quickly, in order to mobilize effective global response. Global connectivity has been greatly expanded by international trade and travel; as a result, there are new "vectors" for disease

2000 *Mathematics Subject Classification.* Primary 68T50 Natural language processing; Secondary 92C60 Medical epidemiology.

outbreak, including airplanes (SARS) and trade: monkey pox was introduced into the US by trade in exotic pets; a Thai man was recently caught smuggling hawks infected with avian influenza into England. In order to prevent the rapid spread of new diseases, it is critical to identify outbreaks in the early stages, before they have a chance to spread unchecked to immunologically naïve populations around the world.

Rapid response requires constant monitoring of disease outbreaks around the world. There are, of course, international mechanisms in place to collect and share data about such global outbreaks. These include the World Health Organization (WHO), which coordinated the successful response to the SARS outbreak, and the US Centers for Disease Control and Prevention (CDC), as well as local and national public health agencies across the world. These agencies publish regular reports, such as the Weekly Epidemiological Reports by WHO (`http://www.who.int/csr/don/archive/country/ind/en/`) and in the US, the Morbidity and Mortality Weekly Report from CDC (`http://www.cdc.gov/mmwr/`). However, both of these are weekly reports based on evidence evaluated by staff at WHO or CDC. As a result, there is often a time lag between the first report of a disease, and its appearance in one of these authoritative reports. Moreover, WHO depends on voluntary contribution of information from participating countries. There are many reasons why such reporting is not always prompt, including inadequate public health infrastructure, or threat of loss of tourism or quarantine of agricultural products. In the case of SARS, there was a 3 month lag between the initial outbreak and the first mentions of the outbreak in the media, allowing the disease to spread to neighboring countries and translocate to North America via air travel. Prompt reporting could perhaps have triggered a more timely containment strategy, limiting its spread and the resulting economic devastation and loss of life.

3. Capture of Timely Outbreak Information

There are additional sources of information on disease outbreak, namely the news media, particularly locally reported news. Two important sources that rely on local media and local contacts are GPHIN (Global Public Health Intelligence Network), from Health Canada, and ProMED (Program for Monitoring Emerging Diseases). GPHIN collects multilingual news sources and organizes these to provide an early warning system for public health events around the world (`http://gphin-rmisp.hc-sc.gc.ca/about.html`). GPHIN is in use at WHO, CDC and at a limited number of public health agencies. ProMED is a program of the International Society for Infectious Diseases that provides an expert-moderated e-mail forum for reporting outbreaks of emerging infectious diseases (`http://www.promedmail.org`). ProMED collects information from participating physicians worldwide, as well as from local news sources. ProMED Mail can be received by no-cost subscription and its web site is openly accessible [**26, 25**].

Figure 1 contains a message that appeared in ProMED on Feb. 10, 2003, relaying a report of hospital closings and people dying in Guangdong. This was the first report on SARS that appeared in Western media[**11**]. The advantage of sources such as ProMED and GPHIN is that they are timely — they capture news as it is reported. The disadvantage, of course, is that the assessment of the outbreak is less authoritative than those assessments published in the official weekly reports of

PNEUMONIA - CHINA (GUANGDONG): RFI
****

A ProMED-mail post
<http://www.promedmail.org>
ProMED-mail is a program of the International
Society for Infectious Diseases
<http://www.isis.org>

Date: 10 Feb 2003
From: Stephen O. Cunnion, MD, PhD, MPH
<cunnion@erols.com>

This morning I received this e-mail and then searched your archives and found nothing that pertained to it. Does anyone know anything about this problem?

"Have you heard of an epidemic in Guangzhou? An acquaintance of mine from a teacher's chat room lives there and reports that the hospitals there have been closed and people are dying."

--
Stephen O. Cunnion, MD, PhD, MPH
International Consultants in Health, Inc
Member ASTM&H, ISTM
<cunnion@erols.com>

FIGURE 1. First ProMED Report Related to SARS (Feb. 10, 2003) [**19**].

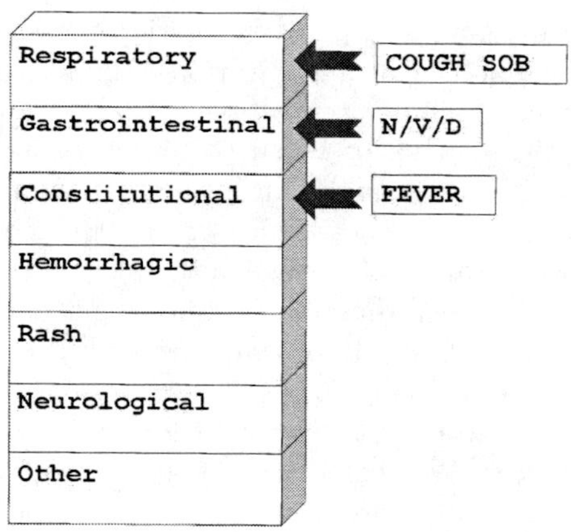

FIGURE 2. Binning of Triage Reports into Syndromes

major public health organizations, which require careful verification of information before reporting it.

Ideally, information about outbreaks could be gathered directly via health care services, such as hotlines, triage reports, or even patient admission data from hospitals and clinics. We are beginning to see the development of such systems in the United States. For example, the Real-time Outbreak and Disease Surveillance (RODS) system from the University of Pittsburgh and Carnegie Mellon University (`http://www.health.pitt.edu/rods/`) collects and analyzes real-time disease surveillance data in Western Pennsylvania and other areas. RODS uses text mining to provide syndromic surveillance, processing Triage Chief Complaint reports to gather timely information on patient symptoms. Triage chief complaints are short (50-character or less) sets of key phrases or abbreviations entered by a triage nurse describing the reason for the patient's emergency room visit. Several examples of triage chief complaints are shown in Figure 2, with their associated syndromic "bins." The text is highly telegraphic, with many abbreviations, e.g., "N/V/D" for *nausea, vomiting, diarrhea*; and "SOB" for *shortness of breath.* The RODS M+ (Medical Probabilistic Language Understanding) system processes the triage reports using a chart parser plus a Bayes network semantic model [**4, 17**]. It obtained good agreement (96-100% AROC accuracy[1]) with the results from a trained physician doing the same syndromic binning task by hand. These results provide an example where text mining can be used to automate a task at an accuracy comparable to humans.[2]

The techniques used in M+ for triage chief complaint may not scale well to more complex patient records, which have a combination of fixed fields and more extensive free text information. There are other systems that can handle complex patient record data, for example, the MEDLEE system[**9, 10**], which has been used at Columbia Presbyterian in a number of applications and studies. MEDLEE can handle complex medical narrative and extract relevant facts. However, there are several limitations. First, MEDLEE must be tailored to each new application, especially if a different type of hospital record is involved, or a different hospital information system. Second, there is a time lag between patient admission and the processing of the record. Moreover, the systematic processing of patient records over a large area (e.g., for public health monitoring) requires a highly interconnected health infrastructure which includes protection of patient confidentiality and also protections related to the sharing of sensitive hospital-specific data. Currently, this kind of information is only available in limited regional settings in developed countries. Thus, at least for now, these kinds of surveillance systems do not solve the problem for global monitoring of disease outbreak.

For these reasons, it is clear that if we want to get early warning of disease outbreak worldwide, we need the kind of timely (if unverified) information that is available on-line in local news media, web sites and mailing lists. This remainder of this article examines the role of text mining for rapid identification of disease outbreaks using such sources. We begin with a description of MiTAP, MITRE's system for capture of multi-lingual information on disease outbreak. We then describe some of the applications of MiTAP to date, and we conclude with a discussion of future directions for text mining for global disease monitoring.

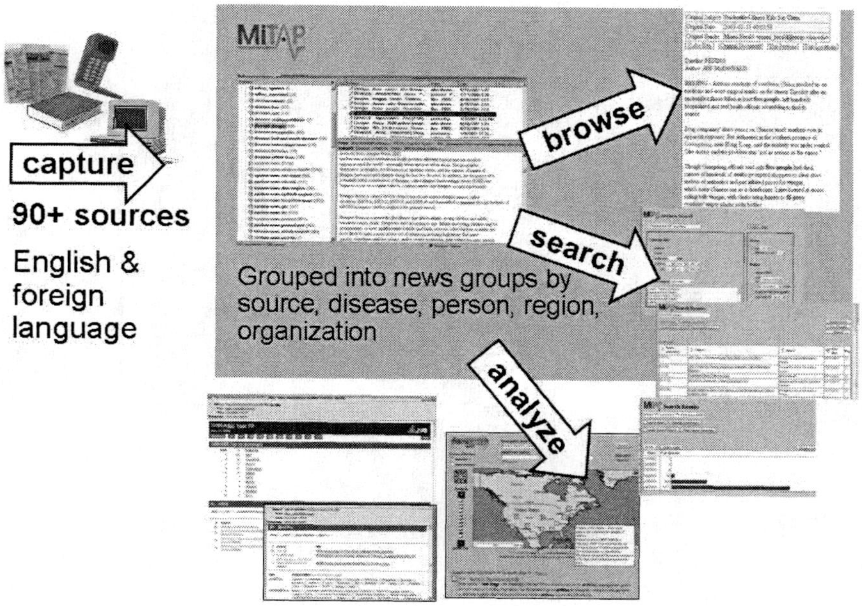

FIGURE 3. Schematic Overview of MiTAP

4. The MiTAP System for Monitoring Disease Outbreak

The MiTAP system[3] [**5, 6, 7**] was developed as an experimental prototype using human language technologies for monitoring infectious disease outbreaks and other global disasters. The goal of MiTAP is to provide timely multi-lingual information access for medical personnel, members of non-governmental organizations, and members of humanitarian assistance/disaster relief organizations. An initial working prototype has been available since June 2001.[4] The system now captures, on a daily basis, between 2000 and 10,000 articles from over ninety on-line sources. These are then filtered, translated, tagged, summarized, categorized by content, and made available to users via a news server and web-based search engine. Text mining technology plays a critical role in many of these processes, allowing information to be presented in ways that facilitate browsing, searching, sorting, and scanning of articles. Machine translation provides users with access to foreign language information that would otherwise be inaccessible to English speakers. By

[1]AROC stands for Area under the Receiver Operating Characteristic curve. This measures trade-off between specificity and sensitivity. A perfectly performing system would cover 100% of the area; the reported measures for M+ in the major syndromic categories of 96-100% show good agreement with expert human judgment.

[2]The claim here is only that text mining can be used to do syndromic binning for triage chief complaints at a level of accuracy comparable to experts. There are no claims about the value of syndromic surveillance or the relative merits of triage chief complaints as compared to other sources of data.

[3]The MiTAP system was funded in part by the Defense Advanced Research Projects Agency (DARPA) Translingual Information Detection Extraction and Summarization (TIDES) program under contract numbers DAAB07-01-C-C201 and W15P7T-04-C-D001.

[4]An English-language-only version is available at `http://mitap.sdsu.edu`; the web site includes an overview of the system and instructions for obtaining an account.

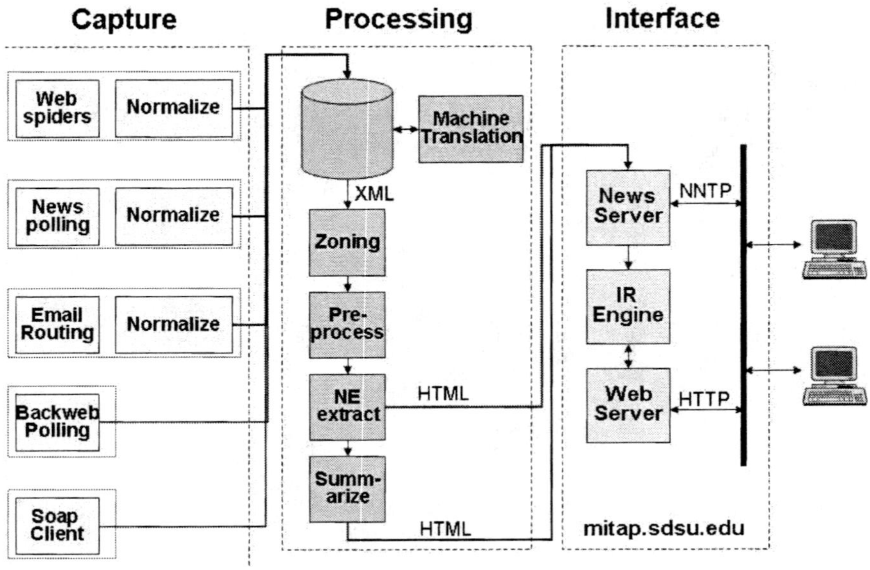

FIGURE 4. Schematic of MiTAP Processing

capturing timely information about disease-related activities, the system can assist in early detection of signs of disease outbreak in open source data, allowing the user to find timely data, do historical searches, look for related materials in a given country, or track trends over time. Figure 3 shows a schematic view of the MiTAP architecture.

The MiTAP system can be divided into three stages: capture, processing, and interface (see Figure 4). The capture phase is responsible for collecting open source, electronic data in multiple languages from local, regional, and national news feeds, newsgroups and electronic mailing lists. Specific sources are scheduled for capture on a daily basis, using source-specific scripts that also record key meta-data (e.g., source, headline, date). The current system is limited to written material (on-line news and e-mail); however, commercial technology is maturing that makes it possible to collect broadcast news (TV and radio) in advanced systems [**18**]. The data from all of these sources are then sent on to the processing phase, where the individual components are responsible for translation, entity extraction (identification of key terms such as disease terms or locations), as well as automated multi-document summarization. The processed documents are then sent to a news server, where they are automatically binned into relevant news groups (by source, by region, or by disease, for example). They are also indexed and archived for later retrieval by an information retrieval or search engine. The user can access the data in a variety of ways: for daily browsing via a news reader and for historical search against the indexed archives via a web client. The data from these sources can be visualized or analyzed via tables, timelines or (eventually) geospatial displays. In addition, we are now creating APIs for programmatic culling of information from the daily capture, for use in a prototype for automated alerting.

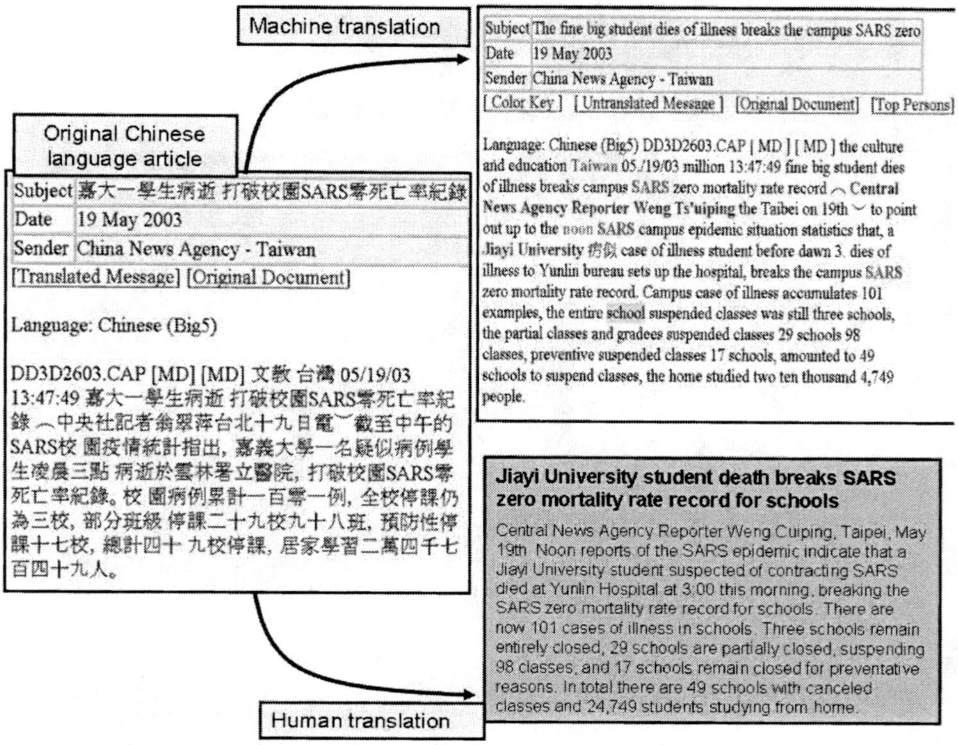

FIGURE 5. Chinese Document with Machine and Human Translations

5. Natural Language Technologies in MiTAP

Natural language processing technologies play a key role in many aspects of the MiTAP system. These include machine translation of foreign language information into English; automated extraction of key terms for improved browsing and visualization; multi-document summarization; automated binning of information into relevant news groups; and support for search against the archived data.

5.1. Translation. Non-English sources are routed to the appropriate machine translation system in MiTAP. This requires identification of the language and the encoding (character set representation) of the document. MiTAP has, to date, used commercial off-the-shelf machine translation systems [**15**]. The quality of translation varies greatly from language to language and its adequacy depends on the intended use of the translated text [**23**]. Translation of European languages, including Russian, is quite good, while the quality of Asian language translation is poorer. The quality can be improved by use of domain-specific lexicons, e.g., for medical terms, although to date, we have not incorporated specialized lexicons into MiTAP. Figure 5 shows a Chinese message (left), with a machine translation (upper right) made with a commercial off-the-shelf translation system, and a human translation (lower right) of the same message. While there are many translation errors, there is still enough information for a user to determine the relevance of the article. The automatic translation, while hard to read, would at least alert

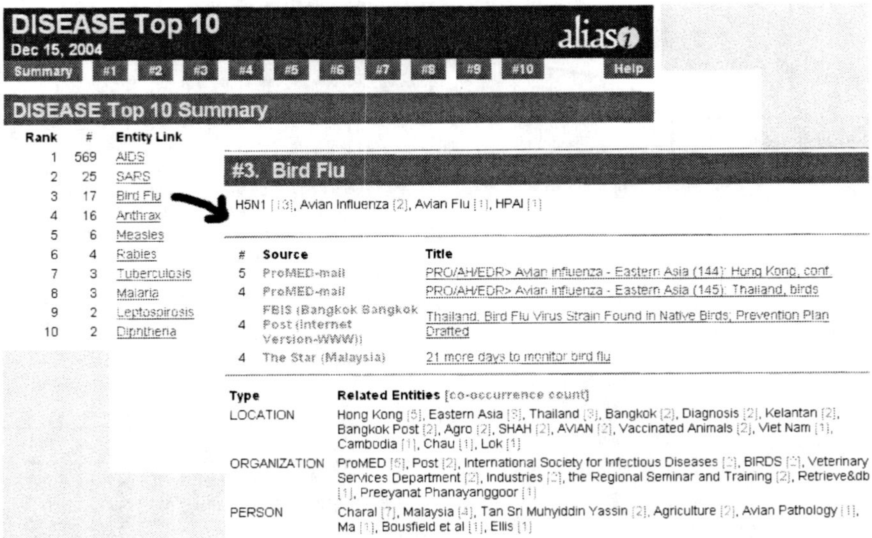

FIGURE 6. Alias-I Daily Top Ten Disease List

the reader that there was relevant information about SARS in the article. This particular article was discovered by a user searching for school closings associated with the SARS outbreak.

5.2. Extraction. After the foreign language articles are translated into English, all English articles (original language and translated documents) are normalized into a common format, tagged for location, organization, disease, date and other entities, summarized, categorized by content, and made available to users via a news server [**12**] and web-based search engine [**13**]. Here "tagging" refers to named entity tagging — the process by which names in running text are identified and "tagged" with appropriate semantic class information. MiTAP currently uses the Alembic natural language processing system for its entity tagging [**1, 21**]. In addition to the standard entities tagged in newswire (person, organization, location, time, date, money, percentages), Alembic has been extended to tag disease names and to terms related to illness.

Once a named entity phrase is identified, the tagger inserts XML annotation into the text. The XML is converted into HTML tags, which are then rendered in different colors or fonts for ease in skimming. There are an increasing number of commercial systems and research systems available for named entity tagging. Evaluation of entity tagging systems shows that they perform tagging on "clean" newswire at about 90-95% balanced precision and recall [**20**][5]. We have estimated tagging accuracy for the MiTAP data to be somewhat lower (in the range of 70-80% accuracy). This range is consistent with recent results reported for biology entity tagging from the biological literature, in the range of 80-85% for the top performing systems[**27**].

[5]Recall is number of entities a system correctly identifies over the total number of entities in the document. Precision is the number of entities a system correctly identifies over the total number of entities identified. Balanced precision and recall (or F-measure) is the harmonic mean of precision and recall: $2 \times P \times R/(P + R)$.

After pre-processing and named entity tagging, marked-up messages are posted to MiTAP and indexed. Within the message, entities are color-coded for easy skimming; for example, disease names are in red, organizations/institutions are in purple, location names in yellow, etc. A list of "Top Persons" and "Top Organizations" is also available as a pull down list at the top of each document for quick browsing. These color coded tags make tagged entities stand out, particularly disease names. Errors also are easy to spot with the color coding. A desirable feature for a future version of the interface would allow users to correct mistagged entities; these corrections could be fed back to the underlying entity tagger, enabling it to improve over time.

Tagging of entity names serves several functions in MiTAP. It supports rapid browsing (e.g., finding disease mentions — tagged in red — in a long text). It also supports the "binning" of information into topic-specific news groups, based on the diseases discussed in an article. Similarly, articles are also binned by region, so that there is newsgroup for, e.g., China, and another one for Korea. However, MiTAP's current entity tagging system does not associate geographic coordinates or information about where a geographic feature is located. This is a major lack: having such "geospatial semantics" would be very useful for processing epidemiological information. It would support both geospatial visualization, and geographic query expansion for better search, so that, e.g., searching for information about events in Guangdong would automatically be expanded to search for mentions of all major cities in Guangdong province. This capability requires disambiguation of a name in its geographic context. For example, there are many cities named "Rome" or "Paris". In order to correctly associate a geospatial location with a geographic name, the name must be associated with the correct region and country. Once this is done, the name can be displayed on a map, using its latitude and longitude. The map in Figure 3 represents an early integrated demonstration built with the MetaCarta system (`http://www.metacarta.com`).[6]

The entity tagging software also supports summarization. For example, Alias I[**2**] uses the entity tagged data and an algorithm that identifies co-reference — repeated reference to the same entity within a document — to produce a ranking of diseases mentioned in the news each day ("Disease Top 10") — see Figure 6. The system counts disease mentions in each article and the number of articles about each disease to produce this list, which is useful to track possible outbreaks or diseases in the news each day. The Alias I summarization system also presents other summary information (location, person, organizations) to provide additional context [**3**].

5.3. Search Interface. Users can access information in MiTAP in two distinct ways: via a search interface or via a browsing interface. The search interface provides access to the tagged articles, as well as the foreign language articles, that have been stored in an archive. For retrospective searching, MiTAP currently uses the Lucene search engine [**13**]. Figure 7 (top) shows the search window; this window allows the user to select the particular sources to search (a pull down menu on the bottom left), to select a date range (menu in middle left), and to specify order of presentation (lower right: by date or by relevance ranking displayed as a

[6]This feature is not part of the current system; however, such a visualization capability, supported by a high quality gazetteer and a capability for disambiguation of geographic place names, would be of great utility to many users of MiTAP.

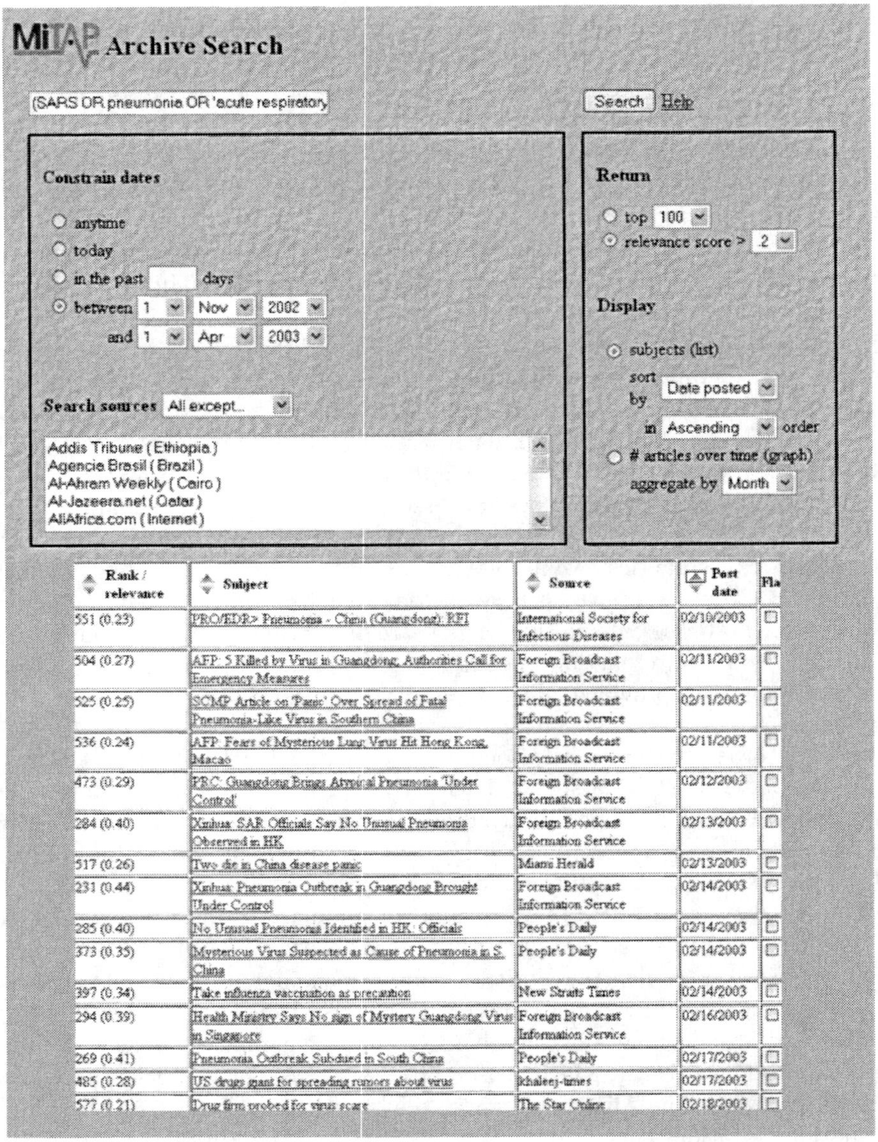

FIGURE 7. Search Interface (Top) and Search Results (Bottom)

list or a graph). The search is created by typing in a Boolean combination of keywords, such as "(China OR Guangdong) AND (SARS OR pneumonia OR 'acute respiratory infection')". For the search shown, the parameters were set to search all sources, from November 2002 to April 2003, shown as a list sorted by date, returning all results with a relevance score greater than 0.2 (set in the right upper panel).

In our current experimental version, we have been working in collaboration with Dr. James Wilson at the Georgetown University Imaging Science and Information Systems Center. This version is designed for automated alerting if results from

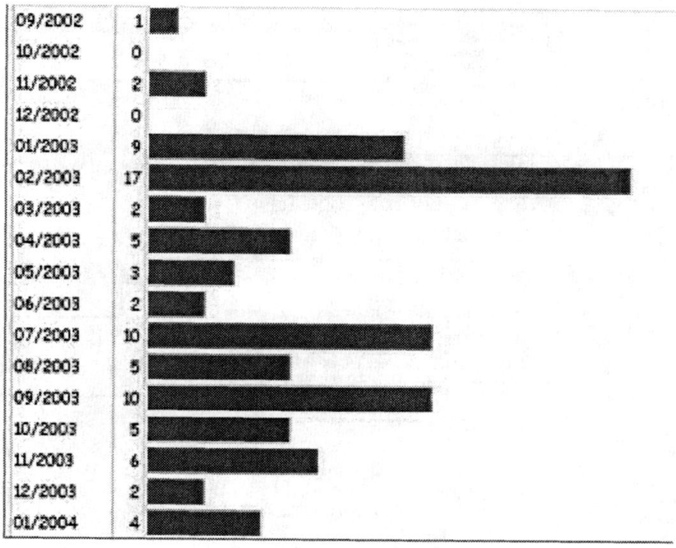

FIGURE 8. Hits per Month for Search "China AND vinegar"

routine searches deviate from an established baseline. In this system, searches can be saved, so that they can be automatically rerun at specified intervals. This version also supports cross-language retrieval, specifically English/Chinese, based on a modified system developed at the University of Maryland (Darwish 2002). This allows a user to specify a query in English. Several bi-lingual English/Chinese lexicons are used to translate the query terms into the "target" language (Chinese), and the archived text is searched to provide a ranked list of Chinese documents. All retrieved Chinese documents are linked to their machine translated, tagged versions. In addition, we are now adding support for direct search against Chinese documents using Chinese keywords.

Results from a search can be retrieved as an ordered list of documents or plotted as a graph against a timeline. Visualizing the data in a graph sometimes reveals patterns, trends, or peaks indicative of interesting activity. The graph of retrieved search results in Figure 8 shows a data spike corresponding to a surge in mentions of disinfectant sales during the SARS outbreak in February 2003 — a month before the WHO announced the epidemic.

5.4. Browsing Interface. The second interface to the system is the browsing interface. For display in this interface, the processed messages are converted to HTML, with color-coded named entities, and routed to newsgroups hosted by a Network News Transport Protocol (NNTP) server, InterNetNews [**12**], as shown in Figure 4. As described above, each message is tagged, and these tags, along with meta-data and pattern-matching techniques, are used to assign each article to one or more specialized news groups.

A major advantage to using the NNTP news server is that users can access the information using a standard mail/news browser such as Netscape Messenger or Outlook Express. There is no need to install custom software, and the instant sense of familiarity with the interface is crucial in gaining user acceptance — little to no training is required. The news server allows access to the data anywhere at

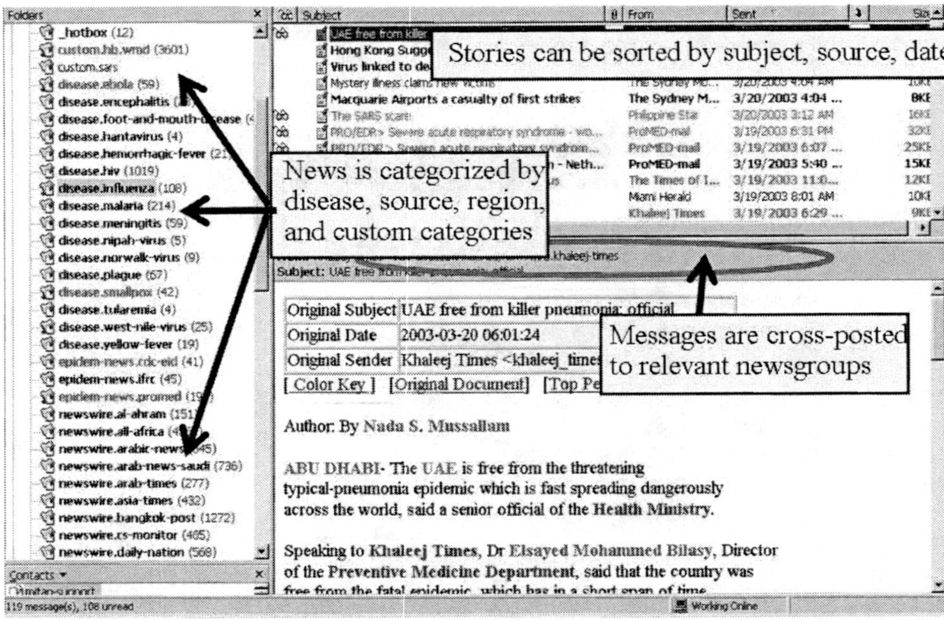

FIGURE 9. MiTAP Browsing Interface Showing Newsgroups (Left), Message Headers (Top) and Message (Bottom)

any time. In addition, where Internet connectivity is unreliable, the news client can be configured to download relevant MiTAP data for later use offline. Mail readers also provide additional functionality such as alerting to new messages on specified topics, flagging messages of significance, and access to local directories that can be used as a private workspace. Other newsgroups can be created as collaborative repositories for users to share collective information.

Figure 9 shows the news browser interface. On the left is a sample of newsgroups that the user has subscribed to, including disease-specific groups, regional groups, and source-specific groups. On the top right is the list of message headlines from a selected newsgroup. Below that is the selected message in which entities are tagged using color-coded fonts.

6. Applications of MiTAP

MiTAP has been collecting data and making it available to authorized users since fall 2001. During this period, we have seen three distinct classes of MiTAP usage emerge: (1) daily browsing; (2) archival search; and most recently, (3) automated alerting.

6.1. Browsing. Access to MiTAP news groups was made available shortly after the Sept. 11, 2001 attack. Since that time, hundreds of users, including medical analysts, government and military officials and members of humanitarian assistance and disaster relief organizations have accessed the system on a regular basis or as needed, to track news around the world. The needs of particular user groups have affected the specific sources being captured. The initial focus was on disease outbreak; after Sept. 11, the focus moved to the situation in the Middle

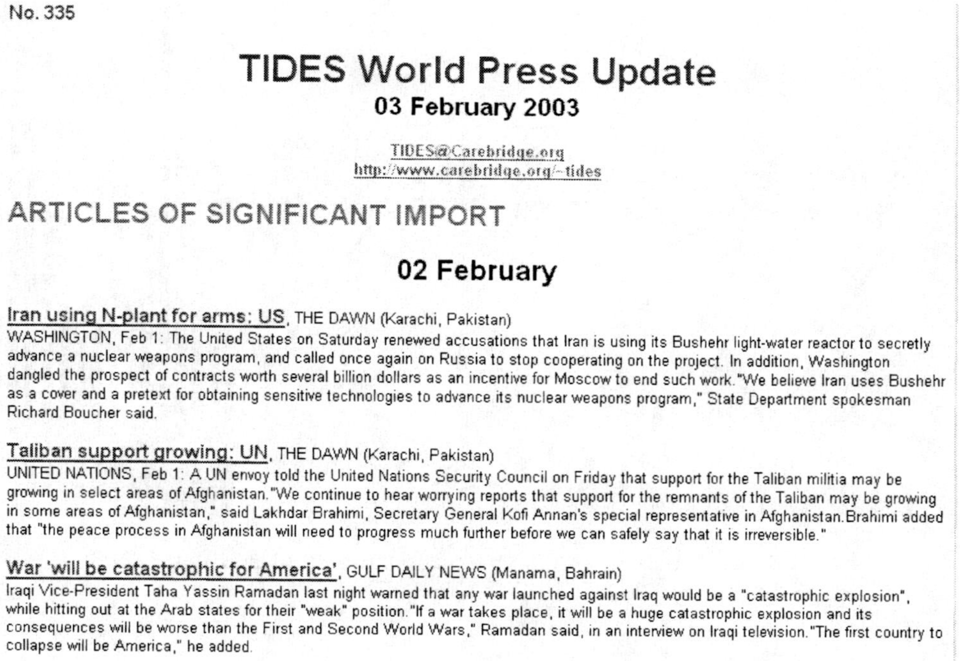

No. 335

TIDES World Press Update

03 February 2003

TIDES@Carebridge.org
http://www.carebridge.org/~tides

ARTICLES OF SIGNIFICANT IMPORT

02 February

Iran using N-plant for arms: US, THE DAWN (Karachi, Pakistan)
WASHINGTON, Feb 1: The United States on Saturday renewed accusations that Iran is using its Bushehr light-water reactor to secretly advance a nuclear weapons program, and called once again on Russia to stop cooperating on the project. In addition, Washington dangled the prospect of contracts worth several billion dollars as an incentive for Moscow to end such work."We believe Iran uses Bushehr as a cover and a pretext for obtaining sensitive technologies to advance its nuclear weapons program," State Department spokesman Richard Boucher said.

Taliban support growing: UN, THE DAWN (Karachi, Pakistan)
UNITED NATIONS, Feb 1: A UN envoy told the United Nations Security Council on Friday that support for the Taliban militia may be growing in select areas of Afghanistan."We continue to hear worrying reports that support for the remnants of the Taliban may be growing in some areas of Afghanistan," said Lakhdar Brahimi, Secretary General Kofi Annan's special representative in Afghanistan.Brahimi added that "the peace process in Afghanistan will need to progress much further before we can safely say that it is irreversible."

War 'will be catastrophic for America', GULF DAILY NEWS (Manama, Bahrain)
Iraqi Vice-President Taha Yassin Ramadan last night warned that any war launched against Iraq would be a "catastrophic explosion", while hitting out at the Arab states for their "weak" position."If a war takes place, it will be a huge catastrophic explosion and its consequences will be worse than the First and Second World Wars," Ramadan said, in an interview on Iraqi television."The first country to collapse will be America," he added.

FIGURE 10. TIDES World Press Update

East, and eventually, to the war in Iraq; our current focus has returned to disease outbreak.

A version of the system was used between November 2001 and February 2003 to prepare the TIDES World Press Update, a daily report distributed worldwide (Figure 10). The MiTAP news interface made it possible for a team of expert consultants working for Carebridge (`http://www.carebridge.org/`) to spend one to two hours a day browsing some 1000 MiTAP articles, preparing the TIDES World Press Update, which was "designed to improve our understanding of the forces shaping public perceptions globally, with particular current attention to South and Central Asia, the Middle East and the Islamic world." [7] The same team of consultants has since produced several other newsletters from MiTAP data. More recently, the system was refocused in support of the war in Iraq, with the consultants preparing a daily TIDES Iraq Reconstruction Report (TIRR) as well as a weekly Global Threat Update.

Neither the TIDES World Press Update nor the TIDES Iraq Reconstruction Report addressed issues of disease outbreak explicitly, although TIRR had a special section on Public Health. However, these publications provide a model for how the capture and presentation of open source news can be used to provide a broad perspective on world events. The text mining and natural language processing capabilities in MiTAP have been a major factor in allowing a user to scan a range of resources and select the most interesting entries for further dissemination. The

[7] The TIDES World Press Update was edited by Mark Prutsalis of the TIDES World Press Reports.

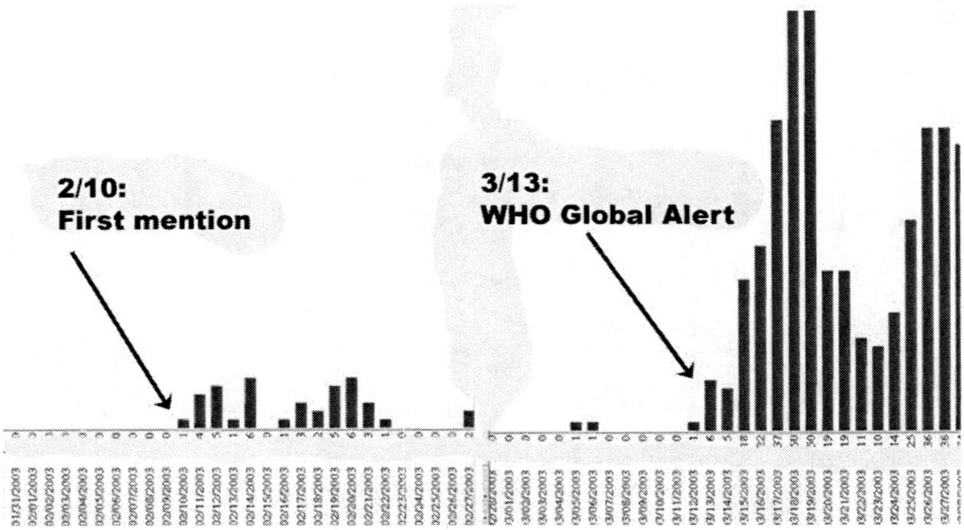

FIGURE 11. Mentions of SARS from Beginning of February, 2003 to End of March, 2003

TIDES World Press Reports team of consultants relied extensively on MiTAP's binning mechanism, a labor-saving device allowing them to select just 1% of collected articles for inclusion in the newsletters. This model applies equally well to monitoring disease outbreak; indeed, GPHIN currently provides this kind of capability to the public health community, with plans to enhance its multilingual capabilities in the future.

6.2. Archival Search. Ad hoc searching against the archives constitutes the second major class of MiTAP applications. For example, we used the archive for a retrospective analysis of the SARS outbreak, to look for early evidence of the outbreak. Search for early mentions was complicated by the fact that the disease had not yet been identified; the term SARS did not become standard usage until late February. To capture the earlier events, the search included the terms " 'acute respiratory infection' OR pneumonia" as well as a geographic constraint: "China OR Guangdong".

The earliest explicit mention of the outbreak found in the archives was reported in ProMED on Feb. 10 (see text of the message in Figure 1); by Feb. 11 there were 3 mentions from Chinese papers (South China Morning Post, Xinhua, China Daily) plus another ProMED posting. From that point on, there was sporadic coverage, followed by a lull, with a sudden huge jump when WHO issued its global alert on March 13. The MiTAP archives contain a (partial) record of how the SARS outbreak was reported in the (English language) press, as shown in Figure 11. In the graph, the number of articles retrieved by the keyword search for each date appears below the bars in the graph; below that are the dates.

6.3. Automated Alerting. We are now involved in a third type of activity, in collaboration with Dr. James Wilson. This activity involves generation of automated alerts to the public health community, based on detecting specific indicators of a severe and uncontrolled outbreak, such as reports of people dying, or hospital closings. The collection is automatically searched each day for occurrences of documents with these indicators. These are fed into a statistical model, which will trigger an alert when a combination of indicators exceeds the expected background occurrence rate. If an alert is raised, the analyst will be able to drill down into the system, to examine the underlying evidence (the news stories, and other sources, as they are added). We are now in the process of evaluating the sensitivity and specificity of the model's ability to detect a potential uncontrolled outbreak using news data from several countries. Once the model is validated, the goal is to monitor the daily message stream (in multiple languages) for advanced warning of disease outbreak.

7. Future Directions: Text Mining for Monitoring Disease Outbreak

The original hypothesis behind the creation of MiTAP was that global tracking of disease outbreak could be improved through the collection of open source information, particularly *local* information — by capturing data in local languages, from a variety of sources, including, eventually, broadcast news data (radio, TV). The goal was for MiTAP to provide users with "one-stop shopping" for this information, organized in an intuitive way, so that a user could quickly locate the information of interest.

In the process of creating this prototype, we have learned some valuable lessons, both about the state of the underlying technology and about ways in which imperfect technology can nonetheless be very useful.

7.1. Lessons Learned About Technology. The three stages of processing — capture, processing and interface — have each presented their unique challenges.

Capture of online news sources turns out to be a non-trivial problem. Each source is formatted somewhat differently, and sources may change their formatting or even their organization of materials over time. A capture script is required for each source to collect important meta-data (e.g., source, date, by-line information), and content, without capturing undesirable text, such as advertisements or banners. Currently, adding a new source requires that a person write a new capture script for that source. This may also require correct handling of character set encodings for foreign language materials. Since capture occurs at the front-end of this process, any failure in the capture of source material can disrupt the entire process. Writing and maintaining capture scripts has turned out to quite labor intensive.

Processing of foreign languages raises language-specific issues that can affect performance or even feasibility for a particular language. These issues include:

- Detection and handling of character set encodings, particularly for languages, like Chinese, that have multiple encodings;
- Indexing strategies for information retrieval. Indexing for retrieval is generally done on words, after removing "stop" words (small frequently occurring words such as prepositions in English), and after "stemming." For English, stemming is easy and highly optimized (for example, removal of the plural "s" on nouns, or "-ed" on verbs). However, different languages present new challenges. For example, not all languages have word boundaries (e.g., Chinese, Japanese, Thai). For Chinese, one successful strategy

has been to index on pairs of characters; for Japanese, the accepted practice is to use a word segmentation program, which may itself introduce errors. Arabic presents a different problem, because vowels are not explicitly written, but can change the meaning of a word. Languages with many inflections (many different endings for nouns and verbs) require more complicated stemming algorithms. These are known problems in information retrieval that affect the quality (and even feasibility) of the information retrieval for the particular language.

- Commercial machine translation quality varies considerably from language to language. Translation quality for Chinese, for example, is generally good enough to determine the topic of the article, but not necessarily the detailed contents. Quality for the Romance languages is generally quite good. User satisfaction will depend on how the translation is used: a user expecting a fluent translation may find the current Chinese translations unsatisfactory; however a user who just wants to get a sense of what an article is about may be quite satisfied.

Interface transparency is critical to users:

- People are familiar with news browsers, so this provided a very lightweight and quite successful interface for browsing.
- The news groups provided an intuitive and flexible method of organizing several thousand new messages a day. However, the binning methods need to be improved, to group only articles that are really about a particular region or a disease. There are many "false positives" that appear in the various news groups. Allowing users to customize their own newsgroups for tracking a specific topic would also be useful.
- Search is less transparent, even to sophisticated users. Boolean search queries (made up of terms connected by "AND" and "OR") are familiar and fairly easy for most users to construct and to debug, even though they do not always produce the best results. Thus, the most sophisticated technology may not always be the most appropriate, if the goal is to achieve maximum transparency, with users in control of the system.

7.2. Good Use of Imperfect Technologies. Perhaps one of the most interesting lessons we learned is that imperfect technologies may still be very useful. We found this was true for the natural language technologies involving retrieval of relevant documents, translation of foreign language material, and extraction or tagging of key kinds of information.

- Retrieval: search technologies are very approximate. A good search might return 6 relevant articles out of the top ten (60% precision). Recall is even more of a problem, since to achieve high recall, the system would have to return many false positives. However, search is generally "good enough" to find things of interest and to detect trends retroactively (see Figure 11). Whether search is good enough to provide any kind of quantitative input that could drive an alerting system remains the topic of ongoing research.
- Translation: a translation may be quite poor, but it is still better than no translation, if it lets a user distinguish whether there is useful information in a story or not.

- Extraction: the extraction used in MiTAP was quite errorful; however, it was still good enough that users preferred to see the articles with the color-coded entries, to draw their eye to interesting parts of the story.

7.3. Challenges During Development. From the initial conception of the MiTAP experimental prototype in 2001 to its current multiple instantiations, we have faced many challenges. In particular, the diversity of our growing user base — from researchers to lay people, from medical analysts to humanitarian organizations — has forced us to accommodate multiple users with multiple needs and multiple use cases. We have considered such issues as system accessibility and usability, human factors, the organization of large amounts of data, and the need to manage user expectations vis a vis imperfect human language technologies.

The adoption of the web and news servers to house the processed data greatly facilitated user access — especially for remote users where training is not possible and/or for users in restricted environments where installing new software is not permitted. The system is available from anywhere at any time, making it easy for users from around the world to access MiTAP data from any computer. The use of email-like formatted articles streamlines integration of MiTAP data into existing work practices/environments and other analytic tools, and allows data to be annotated and otherwise manipulated as easily as email.

Along with new users came new requests for different domains, different data sources, and different geographic regions. Very quickly, the number of data sources increased from a handful of sources to almost one hundred. This required us to shift focus from how to capture the data to how to organize, manipulate, visualize, browse and search overwhelming quantities of data. We created new newsgroups and customized tracking, allowing different users with different interests to create their own "view" into the data by subscribing to only those newsgroups of relevance. We improved our filtering of incoming material and modified the binning algorithm for newsgroups, to allow for more flexible pattern matching. With so much more data available, we began to explore visualization tools, such as timelines and geospatial displays, and we investigated the use of a variety of multidocument summarization tools, including Columbia University's Newsblaster (`http://www1.cs.columbia.edu/nlp/newsblaster/`) as well as Alias I's Top 10 lists. Users provided feedback and guidance in the development of a color scheme for highlighting terms that would continue to draw attention to relevant entities without competing for the attention of the user and without becoming an eyesore.

One of our greatest on-going challenges has been to manage user expectations relative to the use of imperfect human language technologies. Different users have different needs and different expectations; this has been particularly true for machine translation. Some users have examined the output of machine translation and claimed that it was useless since the sentences were poorly constructed and did not make much sense. Another user explained that, prior to MiTAP, he used to receive random hard copies of foreign language data with a few keywords and terms circled and translated by a human. If he deemed a particular article to be relevant to his interests, he would send the hard copy to a busy team of human translators who would later translate the article and return it up to two weeks later. With the MiTAP system, this same user was able to examine the machine translated articles and identify a relevant subset — even with poor translation — that was either useful enough as is or he could send the original foreign language version to the human translators for better translation. Either way, the user claimed he was able to access more foreign language information in a more timely manner and had more control over identifying relevant articles.

This same issue has appeared with respect to searching over foreign language text: should this text be searched in English, against the translated text? Or should it be searched via (human) translation of keywords against the original documents, returning the original documents (and associated translations). The second method is far more likely to produce reliable results, since it does not depend on the correctness of the translation. But the translations must still be good enough to allow the user to confirm that the search has returned the desired information.

7.4. Open Research Questions. Our work to date has focused on creating a proof-of-concept system. We are only now at the stage where medical practitioners can begin systematic experiments to determine whether the system can really support improved monitoring of disease outbreaks.

We envision experiments along several lines:

- To determine whether routine collection of open source media (in local languages) can provide better insight into emerging health problems in specific regions. Clearly this paradigm requires that there be some online information sources, and that these provide information that it is not readily available in the global (English language) press. It will require more robust capture, better binning, more accurate search and improved extraction and visualization of critical data, such as geographic locations.
- To determine whether the quality of language processing is good enough for languages other than English, so that English-only public health practitioners find the system useful, at least to find articles of relevance. Furthermore, if human translation is required, does the system cut down on the amount of translation that is required? Does the system speed up the process of flagging important information?
- To determine whether adding additional local sources (particularly broadcast news sources) could improve timely capture of critical information, without overwhelming any practitioner who might wish to use the system. This would require high quality transcription of speech, translation, and more accurate binning, extraction and summarization of critical information.

MiTAP has taken a significant step down the path towards a proof-of-concept system for the capture and access of global information about disease outbreak, although there remains a great deal more to do. MiTAP has demonstrated that it is possible to capture and make accessible large amounts of online information in multiple languages. Technology is emerging to facilitate capture of broadcast news in English and in other languages. For example, DARPA's Enhanced TIDES Iraq Reconstruction Report (eTIRR) effort uses both expert Arabic-English translation services from the National Virtual Translation Center (NVTC) (`http://www.nvtc.gov`) as well as machine-translation (Language Weaver: `http://www.languageweaver.com`) via BBN Technologies (`http://www.bbn.com`) for many Arabic broadcast and internet news sources. Both machine translation and speech transcription (necessary for transcribing news broadcasts) are required to realize the vision of rapid capture of local information. These technologies are errorful processes; however, our anecdotal experience to date indicates that while the results of a transcription or translation may be hard for a human reader to understand, they may nonetheless contain enough information (in the form of key words or phrases) to carry information for keyword based searching, or to alert the human reader that a particular story needs to be carefully transcribed and translated.

Bringing these sources of information together in an end-to-end system concept creates a rich testbed for quantitative evaluation of text mining capabilities, including transcription, translation, information extraction, search and topic detection, and tracking algorithms (`http://www.nist.gov/speech/tests/tdt/`).

The MiTAP resources also provide a testbed for epidemiological modeling. Given sporadic and highly incomplete data, this raises many questions: Is it possible to use the data in some systematic way for early detection of outbreaks? Does collecting this kind of open source information provide value-added to the existing mechanisms, both formal (WHO, CDC) and informal (GPHIN, ProMED)? And if there is potential value-added, what additional tools must be put in place to make the system useable and useful to public health personnel?

We believe that MiTAP will continue to provide an excellent testbed for multidisciplinary research, involving public health personnel, epidemiologists, researchers in mathematical modeling and text mining, and system engineers. These are the different perspectives and skills that must be combined to provide a much-needed early warning system for global disease outbreak.

Acknowledgements. Many people have contributed to the development of MiTAP. We would like to specifically acknowledge the contributions of MITRE staff, including Conrad Chang, Andy Chisholm, David Day, John Henderson, Janet Hitzeman, Ann Huang, Scott Mardis, Tom McEntee, Keith Miller, William Morgan, Florence Reeder, Lee Tilton, Marc Ubaldino, Steve Wohlever, George Wilson, and Guido Zarrella. We would like to acknowledge the original vision for MiTAP, which came from Gary Strong, who was, at that time, the program manager for the DARPA TIDES program. We would especially like to thank Cmd. Eric Rasmussen, US Navy, for his vision and patient help in shaping MiTAP. We thank Mark Prutsalis, of TIDES World Press Reports, who made many valuable contributions in helping us to understand how such a system could be used in a production environment. We also thank Allen Sears, CNRI, for his continued advice and support, as well as Charles Wayne, DARPA for his support. Finally, we would like to acknowledge our current collaborator, James Wilson at the Georgetown University Imaging Science and Information Systems Center, whose vision is pushing forward towards a new set of capabilities for global disease outbreak monitoring.

References

1. Aberdeen, J., Burger, J., Day, D., Hirschman, L., Robinson, P., and Vilain, M. MITRE: Description of the Alembic System as Used for MUC-6. In *Proceedings of the Sixth Message Understanding Conference (MUC-6)*, pages 141–155, Columbia, MD, 6–8 November 1995.
2. Alias I, Inc. New Technology for Information Access, 2002 `http://www.alias-i.com`
3. Baldwin, B., Moore, M., Ross, A., Shah, D. Trinity Information Access System. In *Proceedings of Human Language Technology Conference (HLT 2002)*, San Diego, CA.
4. Chapman, W.W., Christensen, L.M., Wagner, M.M., Haug, P.J., Ivanov, O., Dowling, J.N., Olszewski, R.T. Classifying Free-text Triage Chief Complaints into Syndromic Categories with Natural Language Processing. *Artificial Intelligence in Medicine*, 2004 (in press).

5. Damianos, L., Ponte, J., Wohlever, S., Reeder, F., Day, D., Wilson, G., Hirschman, L. MiTAP for Bio-Security: A Case Study. AI Magazine, Volume 23, No. 4, pages 13–29, 2002.
6. Damianos, L., Ponte, J., Wohlever, S., Reeder, F., Day, D., Wilson, G., Hirschman, L. MiTAP, Text and Audio Processing for Bio-Security: A Case Study. In *Proceedings of IAAI-2002: The Fourteenth Innovative Applications of Artificial Intelligence Conference*, Edmonton, Alberta, Canada, July 28 – August 1, 2002.
7. Damianos, L., Wohlever, S., Kozierok, R., Ponte, J. MiTAP for Real Users, Real Data, Real Problems In *Proceedings of the Conference on Human Factors of Computing Systems (CHI 2003)*, Fort Lauderdale, Florida, April 5–10.
8. Darwish, K. PSE: A Small Search Engine written in Perl 2002 `http://tides.umiacs.umd.edu/software.html`
9. Friedman, C., Alderson, P.O., Austin, J.H, Cimino J.J. and Johnson S.B. A General Natural-Language Text Processor for Clinical Radiology. JAMIA 1(2) 161–174. 1994
10. Friedman, C., Knirsch, C.A, Shagina, L., Hripcsak, G. Automating a Severity Score Guideline for Community-Acquired Pneumonia Employing Medical Language Processing of Discharge Summaries. AMIA 256–260. 1999.
11. Hitt, E. Early inklings about SARS: An informal infectious disease reporting system shows the value of broad access. *The Scientist*, March 24, 2003. `ttp://www.`te-scientist.com.
12. INN: InterNetNews, Internet Software Consortium 2001, `http://www.isc.org/products/INN`.
13. The Jakarta Project, 2001 `http://jakarta.apache.org/lucene/docs/index.html`.
14. Leahy S. SARS: Pandemic fears in an interlinked world. *Asia Times* April 25, 2003.
15. Miller, K., Reeder, F., Hirschman, L., Palmer, D. Multilingual Processing for Operational Users, *NATO Workshop on Multilingual Processing at EUROSPEECH*, 2001.
16. Morens D.M., Folkers G.K., Fauci A.S. The challenge of emerging and re-emerging infectious diseases. *Nature* 2004 Jul 8;430(6996):242–9.
17. Olszewski, R. Bayesian Classification of Triage Diagnoses for the Early Detection of Epidemics. Recent Advances in Artificial Intelligence. *Proc of the 16th Internl FLAIRS Conf.* 412–416, AAAI Press, 2003.
18. Palmer, D., Bray, P., Reichman, M., Rhodes, K., White, N., Merlino, A., Kubala, F. Multilingual Video and Audio News Alerting In *Companion Volume to Proceedings of HLT-NAACL*, Boston, MA, May 2–7, 2004, pages 245-246.
19. ProMED-mail. Pneumonia - China (Guangdong): RFI. ProMED-mail 2003; 10 Feb: 20030210.0357 `http://www.promedmail.org`. Accessed 21 December 2004.
20. Sundheim B. Overview of the Results of the MUC-6 Evaluation. In *Proc. of the Sixth Message Understanding Conference.* pages 13–31, Morgan Kaufman, 1995
21. Vilain, M. and Day, D. 1996. Finite-state phrase parsing by rule sequences. In *Proceedings of the 1996 International Conference on Computational Linguistics (COLING-96)*, Copenhagen, Denmark, 5–9 August 1996.
22. Wayne, C. Multilingual Topic Detection and Tracking: Successful Research Enabled by Corpora and Evaluation, In *Proceedings of Language Resources and Evaluation Conference (LREC)* 2000, pages 1487–1494.
23. White J.S. and Taylor K.B. A Task-Oriented Evaluation Metric for Machine Translation. In *Proc. of the First Language Resources and Evaluation Conference*, Granada, 1998
24. World Health Organization. Severe Acute Respiratory Syndrome: Status of the Outbreak and Lessons for the Immediate Future. Geneva, May 2003. `http://www.who.int/csr/media/sars_wha.pdf`
25. Woodall, J., Aldis R. Gaps in Global Surveillance. Occasional Papers No. 1 BioWeapons Prevention Project. December, 2003. `http://www.bwpp.org/publications/occasional/op001-global-surveillance.pdf`
26. Woodall J, Calisher C.H. ProMED-mail: background and purpose. *Emerg Infect Dis.* 2001;7(3 Suppl):563
27. Yeh, A., Morgan, A, Colosimo. M., and Hirschman, L. BioCreAtIvE task 1A: gene mention finding evaluation, to appear in *BioMed Central BioInformatics*, 2005.

THE MITRE CORPORATION, 202 BURLINGTON ROAD, BEDFORD, MA 01730, USA
E-mail address: `lynette@mitre.org`

DIMACS Series in Discrete Mathematics
and Theoretical Computer Science
Volume **70**, 2006

Generalized Contingency Tables and Concept Lattices

David Ozonoff, Alex Pogel, and Tim Hannan

ABSTRACT. We present two new concepts in epidemiology, the generalized and closed set contingency tables, and discuss some of their mathematical foundations, derived from lattice theory (Ganter and Wille, 1999). As the names suggest, they are a generalization of the conventional contingency table or cross-classification. Development of this idea leads to some new research directions in epidemiology and new methods of data analysis, and this paper represents the first step towards introducing the basic concepts.

1. Conventional contingency tables

Contingency tables, or cross-tabulations ("cross tabs"), are a mainstay of data analysis and one of the elementary constructions in preparing data for exploration and scrutiny. Table construction requires at least three study design-based operations. First, a collection of n subjects is selected, with the sampling method giving rise to different kinds of contingency tables (cross-sectional, cohort, case control). Second, "variables of interest" are selected (e.g., sex, age, case status, exposure status) and a way to express those variables (a classification scheme) specified. Third, the value of the variable for each subject (their age, sex, etc.) is ascertained, i.e. a measurement is made. This may require taking an interval measure and scaling it into categories (e.g., age categories), a scaling operation. These operations are the subject of a large literature, both classical and contemporary [**9**].

To make the underlying machinery as simple and clear as possible, we will ignore the difference between a factor (such as sex) and its levels (male, female), considering each level as a characteristic feature of a subject. We thus convert all interval, ordinal, and continuous variables to indicator variables, referring to them as attributes (or sometimes the equivalent word, features). This corresponds to

---

2000 *Mathematics Subject Classification.* Primary 62P10 Applications to biology and medical sciences; Secondary Galois correspondences, closure operators.

Key words and phrases. contingency table, concept lattice.

This publication was made possible by grant number 5 P42 ES07381 from the National Institute of Environmental Health Sciences, NIH..

All the authors wish to thank the National Science Foundation and its support to DIMACS for making this collaboration possible.

TABLE 1. Subjects classified by sex (M,F), handedness (R,L) and age (< 65, 65+).

	M	F	R	L	<65	65+
Case1	1	0	0	1	0	1
Case2	0	1	1	0	1	0
Case3	1	0	0	1	0	1
Case4	1	0	1	0	1	0
Case5	0	1	1	1	1	0
Case6	0	1	0	1	1	0
Case7	1	0	1	0	0	1

TABLE 2. One-attribute frequency table.

Males	4
Females	3
Right-handed	4
Left-handed	4
<65	4
65+	3

common language: subjects have attributes or features, such as being young, being female, etc., a more natural usage for our purposes than "variable values." Having or not having the attribute can be coded with ones and zeroes. The raw data for a contingency table consists of a listing of each subject and his or her attributes (for an example, see Table 1). A one-dimensional contingency table is merely a frequency table, i.e., a table that gives the number of subjects with each attribute (Table 2).

Most contingency tables are two-dimensional, i.e., they cross-classify two attributes. When we cross-classify two attributes by two other attributes (e.g., we consider male/female by young/old) we arrive at the familiar 2×2 table. If we cross-classify r attributes by c attributes, we have an $(r \times c)$ contingency table. Usually the attributes are disjoint, so each subject is placed into one of the rc cells, and presenting the number of subjects in each of the cells determines the contents of the contingency table. A useful picture here is a scatterplot, which plots the values of one variable against another (say, age versus height). We can divide the age category (the x-axis) into two halves (growing, adult) and the height into two categories (short, tall), as shown in Figure 1. If we count up the number of points in each quadrant, we get a 2×2 contingency table. Similarly, if we divide the age axis into r categories and the height category into c categories and again count subjects, we get an $r \times c$ contingency table.

A population of n subjects classified according to k features could give the number of subjects with various combinations of feature values. Thus a cell of a three-way contingency table of 524 people classified by sex (M, F), 5 age categories, and 5 race categories would have 50 cells ($2 \times 5 \times 5$). For a three-way table, we have a cube, and generalizing up to higher dimensions, we get "hypercubes".

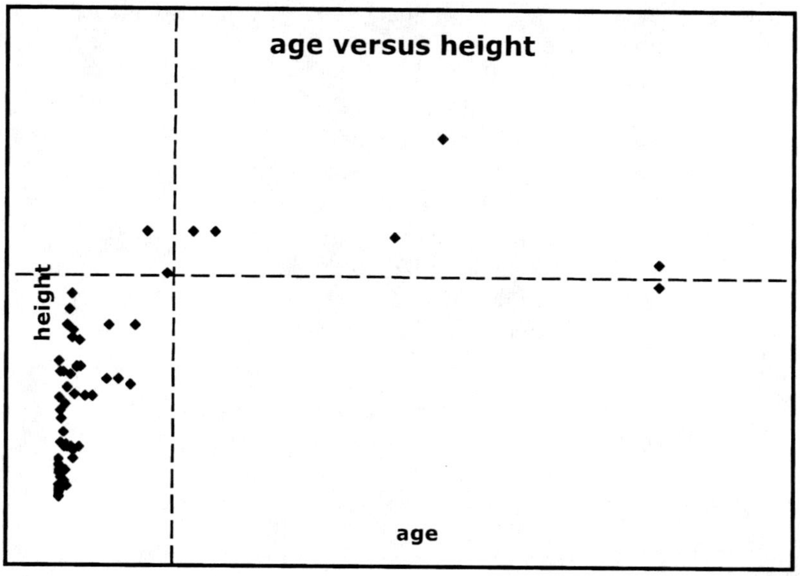

FIGURE 1. Scatterplot divided into quadrants (giving rise to a 2 x 2 table).

Note that it is usually assumed that this process partitions the attribute space, i.e., the features are mutually exclusive and exhaustive of that space. We can relax this to provide a further generalization. While it is usual to cross features that are mutually exclusive (age 0 – 4 years, 5 – 19 years, etc.) one could have feature values that are nested or related in some other way (e.g., age $\leq$ 5, age $\leq$ 19, etc., or overlapped) or not exhaustive (e.g., right-handed, omitting categories of left-handed and ambidextrous). Moreover, one could also cross features with themselves. Admittedly it is not very informative to cross all subjects who are male with all subjects who are male, but it is useful for the sake of generality. We can also cross mutually exclusive features (e.g., cross all subjects who are male with all subjects who are female). This is not only theoretically useful for generalization, but may also be of practical interest if one were unsure if "hybrid" cases (e.g., hermaphrodites) exist, or for detecting miscodes.

As an example, consider the set of seven people classified by sex (M/F), age (< 65/65+), and handedness (R/L) of Table 1. "Yes" is coded as 1 and "no" coded as 0 for each. Note that subject 5 is both right-handed and left-handed, i.e., is ambidextrous.

The simplest contingency table is the one-way table giving the counts of subjects with each attribute (Table 2), but this can be extended to include paired attributes taken in combination:

A more usual (but equivalent) way to exhibit the same data is via a two-way contingency table:

While this shows us some paired combinations at once, we do not have all of them, since age paired with handedness is not represented.

TABLE 3. A two-attribute frequency table. The ambidextrous subject is counted twice.

Right-handed males	2
Left-handed males	2
Right-handed females	2
Left-handed females	2
Males <65 y.o.	1
Females <65 y.o.	3
Males 65 and older	3
Females 65 and older	0

TABLE 4. Handedness and age by sex.

	R	L	<65	65+
M	2	2	1	3
F	2	2	3	0

TABLE 5. An unusual (but possible) two-way contingency table.

	M	F	L	R	<65	65+
M	4	0	2	2	1	3
F	0	3	2	2	3	0
L	2	2	4	1	2	2
R	2	2	1	4	2	1
<65	1	3	2	2	4	0
65+	3	0	2	1	0	3

2. Generalizing the contingency table

To remedy the lack of some paired combinations, we could make two-way contingency tables with arbitrary, or even all, attributes on each axis (thereby getting *all* paired combinations):

Extending this, we could make a generalized (global) contingency "table" (here a six-dimensional hypercube) with all feature values on all axes. This would give us all feature values "crossed" with all other feature values, even with themselves. This produces a great many cells, in this case $6^6 = 46,656$. But M crossed with itself (the set of all males who are also males) just gives back the same set of males, so wherever we have "self-crossed" cells we can reduce it to just one cell determined by the repeated attribute. For example, if we were doing a three-way contingency table with the data in Table 1 (think of a cube with six attributes per side), the cell $\{M, M, R\}$ would be the same as $\{M, R\}$ in terms of the subjects it contained, while $\{M, M, M\}$ would have the same number of subjects as $\{M\}$. In this way the number of meaningfully different cells in this case is reduced to $2^6 = 64$, the number of all possible combinations of the attributes when order doesn't matter and there are no repeats.

$\{\{\}, \{<65\}, \{65+\}, \{F\}, \{L\}, \{M\}, \{R\}, \{<65, 65+\}, \{F, <65\}, \{F, 65+\}, \{F, L\},$
$\{F, R\}, \{L, <65\}, \{L, 65+\}, \{M, <65\}, \{M, 65+\}, \{M, F\}, \{M, L\}, \{M, R\},$
$\{R, <65\}, \{R, 65+\}, \{R, L\}, \{F, <65, 65+\}, \{F, L, <65\}, \{F, L, 65+\}, \{F, R, <65\},$
$\{F, R, 65+\}, \{F, R, L\}, \{L, <65, 65+\}, \{M, <65, 65+\}, \{M, F, <65\}, \{M, F, 65+\},$
$\{M, F, L\}, \{M, F, R\}, \{M, L, <65\}, \{M, L, 65+\}, \{M, R, <65\}, \{M, R, 65+\},$
$\{M, R, L\}, \{R, <65, 65+\}, \{R, L, <65\}, \{R, L, 65+\}, \{F, L, <65, 65+\},$
$\{F, R, <65, 65+\}, \{F, R, L, <65\}, \{F, R, L, 65+\}, \{M, F, <65, 65+\}, \{M, F, L, <65\},$
$\{M, F, L, 65+\}, \{M, F, R, <65\}, \{M, F, R, 65+\}, \{M, F, R, L\}, \{M, L, <65, 65+\},$
$\{M, R, <65, 65+\}, \{M, R, L, <65\}, \{M, R, L, 65+\}, \{R, L, <65, 65+\},$
$\{F, R, L, <65, 65+\}, \{M, F, L, <65, 65+\}, \{M, F, R, <65, 65+\}, \{M, F, R, L, <65\},$
$\{M, F, R, L, 65+\}, \{M, R, L, <65, 65+\}, \{M, F, R, L, <65, 65+\}\}$

FIGURE 2. Names of the cells in the Generalized Contingency Table (the powerset, $\mathcal{P}(S)$ = the set of all subsets of S). The first entry, $\{\}$, is the empty set, i.e., the set with no members, also denoted $\emptyset$.

This suggests that a way to think about all "cell contents" of a contingency table (which together determine any table) is to consider the set of all unique subsets of the attribute set A, which is called the powerset of A, denoted $\mathcal{P}(A)$ (see Figure 2). The powerset is a mathematical object that plays a part in the theory we are building here. From the epidemiological perspective, it represents all the unique commonalities (conjunctions) of attributes that might be present in the dataset, i.e., the complete set of possible conjunctive commonalities among members of the population that are the basis for epidemiological analysis.

Table 2 describes the number of subjects (the cell "contents") associated with the one-element subsets (the entries $\{<65\}$, $\{65+\}$, $\{F\}$, $\{L\}$, $\{M\}$, $\{R\}$ in $\mathcal{P}(S)$ in Figure 2); Tables 3 and 4 each show some of the two-element subsets ($\{M, R\}$, $\{M, L\}$, $\{F, R\}$, $\{F, L\}$, $\{M, <65\}$,$\{F, <65\}$, $\{M, 65+\}$, $\{F, 65+\}$); and Table 5 shows all of the two-element subsets (and also includes redundant cells, such as $\{M, M\} = \{M\}$, and thus includes Tables 2, 3 and 4).

Figure 2 lists all the unique (conjunctive) combinations of attributes (paying no attention to order and without repeats).[1] If we were to attach to each the number of subjects with that combination of attributes, we would arrive at the *generalized contingency table*. For example, the contents of $\{M, L\}$ give the number of all subjects who have the attributes of being male and left-handed in common (here two subjects), while $\{M, <65, 65+\}$ is the size of the set of all males who are both less than 65 years old and 65 years old or greater, which in this case is obviously zero, but note that for any given dataset it could be non-zero (if there were a miscode).

The three operations used to construct a conventional table are all visible in the generalized contingency table, giving the n subjects (sampling), the number of possible cells (variable selection or classifying), and the distribution of the sampled subjects into the appropriate cells (measurement). The number of subjects does not depend on the number of cells (e.g., the number of cells, 4, in a 2×2 table

[1] All further references to combinations of attributes are assumed to be conjunctive combinations.

does not depend on the number of sampled subjects), nor is the manner in which subjects are distributed into each cell (measurement) fixed by either the sampling or the classification. The three operations jointly determine the contingency table, a fact we will formalize shortly.

The generalized contingency table includes a conventional contingency table (e.g., a $2 \times 2 \times 2$ table), but it also includes *all* the possible cells that might be in *any* contingency table of the dataset (hence the name). The table cells designate attributes and combinations of attributes (variable selection) that might be held or shared in common by sampled subjects in a dataset. The contents of the table cells are a record of the number of subjects that actually do share the attributes in a specific dataset (measurement). In the more general case we do not require or even expect the attributes to be mutually exclusive, so that the marginal totals will almost never equal the total number of subjects with a particular attribute. The generalized contingency table contains all the cells in a conventional table and is itself a mathematical object, the powerset, of more interest, versatility and consequence.

3. Lattice structure in a data set

In epidemiological analyses we usually begin with a table similar to Table 1, the raw data generated in the field when we assign to each subject the characteristics or attributes of interest (age, sex, case status, exposure history, etc.). We then ask simple and natural questions about what attributes people who share certain other attributes have in common, for example, what did everyone who got sick have in common compared to those who didn't get sick, etc. This suggests a natural role for mathematical concepts and formalisms that study commonalities and comparisons. The branch of mathematics called lattice theory is well suited to formalizing just such commonalities and comparisons.

We have already noted that the cells of the generalized contingency table can be identified with elements of a well-known mathematical object called the powerset of the set of the attributes, i.e., the set of all subsets of the attribute set. There are many such subsets (which we will call generalized contingency table cells), in general $2^{|A|}$, the number of subsets of A, where $|A|$ is the size of A. Thus for the raw data in Table 1 with six attributes ($A = \{M, F, R, L, <65, 65+\}$), there are $2^6 = 64$ cells in the generalized contingency table, including those with no features, one feature, and two, three, four, five, and six features; all of these cells are listed in Figure 2.

The number of subjects *specified by* a particular subset (sometimes called the *support* of the particular subset and referred to as *prevalence* in epidemiology[2]) plays no part in the number of subsets, *which is always* $2^{|A|}$. We may not be interested in most of these cells, since, for example, the prevalence of any combination with mutually exclusive attributes is zero. However, the mutual exclusiveness of these attributes is a feature of the data, since it might include a subject that is of both

[2]Epidemiologists often use the term prevalence both to refer to the raw number of subjects associated with a particular attribute set and the proportion of the population with that attribute set. This lack of precision rarely causes confusion in practice.

TABLE 6. Dataset of Table 1 with fewer attributes.

	M	R	L	65+
Case1	1	0	1	1
Case2	0	1	0	0
Case3	1	0	1	1
Case4	1	1	0	0
Case5	0	1	1	0
Case6	0	0	1	1
Case7	1	1	0	1

sexes because we are studying hermaphrodites, or more commonly because the data have been miscoded. The fact that particular cells *are* empty of subjects is a reflection of the data, not pre-ordained or logically necessary.[3]

We can simplify things further in the case of mutually exclusive categories (for example, a conventional study where the data are clean and one knows that a person is either male or female, or younger than 65 or is 65 or older). Thus, in an instance where only Male or Female genders are of interest, a subject coded zero for Male is a Female (not a male). Note that the fact that this smaller Table 6 can be interpreted to contain exactly the same information as the larger Table 1 is itself a reflection of the structure in the data. We will return to this idea shortly.

We see that the set of all males consists of cases 1, 3, 4, and 7. The attribute they all have in common is that they are all male. The set of females consists of subjects 2, 5, and 6. This comes from knowledge of the context that informs the analyst that a subject is either male or female (not male). Examining the set of righthanders, $\{2, 4, 5, 7\}$ and the set of lefthanders, $\{1, 3, 5, 6\}$, we see that L and R are are not mutually exclusive attributes because case 5 satisfies both. In order to make a more compact notation, we introduce here the $o(-)$ operator on $\mathcal{P}(A)$: for $X \subseteq A$,

$$o(X) = \{s : s \text{ is a subject satisfying } X\}.$$

Now we can write $o(R) = \{2, 4, 5, 7\}$ and $o(L) = \{1, 3, 5, 6\}$.

In each instance the subjects do not have anything *more* in common than being male, righthanded or lefthanded: adding any other attribute will not describe a common feature of the subjects. The same cannot be said, however, of the individuals 65 years old and older. The subjects s satisfying 65+ ($o(65+) = \{1, 3, 7\}$) do have at least one other attribute in common: they are all male. Using the $o(-)$ operator, we see that

$$o(65+) = \{1, 3, 7\} = o(\mathrm{M}, 65+) \subset o(\mathrm{M}) = \{1, 3, 4, 7\}).$$

Thus *in this dataset*, if we know that someone is 65+, we also know they are male (but not conversely). So in some sense the contingency table cell {M,65+} is richer or more informative than the single cell 65+: it reveals more of the attributes of the subjects it represents, which are the same subjects as in the less specified cell, 65+.

[3]That a cell *should be* empty can be considered pre-ordained, a consequence of our semantic interpretation of the attribute combination it represents, but this is not intrinsic to the mathematical representation we consider here.

This is not the only example in this very simple dataset: if one knows a subject is in $o(M, L)$, one also knows they are in $o(M, L, 65+)$. And similarly,

$$o(R, 65+) = o(M, R, 65+), \quad o(L, 65+) = o(M, L, 65+), \quad \text{and}$$

$$o(M, R, L) = o(M, R, L, 65+) \ ,$$

e.g., if a case is in $o(R, 65+)$, then that case is also in $o(M, R, 65+)$ (note that the reverse inclusion comes free – if a subject satisfies M and R and 65+, then they certainly satisfy R and 65+ – so only one direction of the equality is noteworthy). Out of $2^4 = 16$ possible cells (combinations of M, R, L and 65+), only 10 of them,

$$\{\} \quad \{M\} \quad \{R\} \quad \{L\} \quad \{M, 65+\} \quad \{M, R\}$$

$$\{M, L, 65+\} \quad \{R, L\} \quad \{M, R, 65+\} \quad \{M, R, L, 65+\}$$

maximally represent different sets of subjects, with any other combination (not listed) representing the same subjects as a more specified set already on the list (e.g., $o(R, 65+) = \{7\}$ as does $o(M, R, 65+) = \{7\}$). Note that the last of these cells' contents, $o(M, R, L, 65+)$, is empty, i.e., the dataset has no subjects with all four of these attributes. This is a characteristic of this particular dataset.

Thus some of the sets (the ten sets in the example) are distinguished from others in that they represent unique groupings of subjects not represented by any more specified combinations of attributes. Thus $o(R) = \{2, 4, 5, 7\}$ is not represented by any more specified combination of attributes, but $o(65+) = \{1, 3, 7\}$ is also represented by the more specific set $o(M, 65+) = \{1, 3, 7\}$. Mathematical lattice theory starts with a structural description of the set of all of these maximally specified sets of subjects and then provides various properties of this set. For example, one key property that has been established is that this special subset of the generalized contingency table cells contains all the information needed to construct the original data [**4**].

Mathematically these distinguished sets are called closed sets. The other (non-closed) sets, like $\{M, L\}$, can be viewed as incomplete in that they represent subjects that have more in common than they are given credit for. Thus $\{M, L\}$ is in the powerset of A, but it is not a *closed* set in the powerset of A *with respect to the given dataset.* Said a different way, for a particular dataset, not all of the unique combinations of attributes are always needed to describe the dataset. This means that while the number of possible combinations of attributes might be large (2^n), the number of relevant ones is usually much smaller and the closed sets are exactly those which maximize information in this sense. We discuss an example in the next section.

The list of cells of the generalized contingency table results from variable specification alone. Measurement of the sampled subjects fills the cells with content (defines the $o(-)$ operator) and induces the closed set structure. The combination of variable specification, measurement, and sampling can be formalized as a binary relation I (described below) that is used to partition the powerset $\mathcal{P}(A)$ into equivalence classes. Members of the same equivalence class are different combinations of attributes that, in the dataset under study, represent exactly the same subjects.

In linear statistical models this can produce an extreme form of collinearity where the two variables or combinations of variables are not just linearly related but

TABLE 7. Closed sets (bold), the non-closed sets that represent the same subjects, and the subjects represented.

Closed set	Equivalence Class	Subjects
{}	$\emptyset = \{\ \}$	{1,2,3,4,5,6,7}
{M}	**{ M }**	{1,3,4,7}
{R}	**{ R }**	{2,4,5,7}
{L}	**{ L }**	{1,3,5,6}
{M,R}	**{M,R}**	{4,7}
{R,L}	**{R,L}**	{5}
{M,65+}	{65+}, **{M,65+}**	{1,3,7}
{M,L,65+}	{M,L},{L,65+},**{M,L,65+}**	{1,3}
{M,R,65+}	{R,65+},**{M,R,65+}**	{7}
{M,R,L,65+}	{M,R,L},{R,L,65+}, **{M,R,L,65+}**	$\emptyset$ ={}

identical. However here the underlying effect does not depend on any parametric form, and the analog to collinearity exists in any statistical procedure involving categorical variables. Thus it is a generalization of collinearity since it holds for any conceivable model form. Consider the equivalence classes of our small example shown in Table 7. Including the variables M, R and L and their interactions would not entail any collinearity because M, R, L, {M, R}, {M,L}, { R,L} and {M, R, L } all represent different sets of subjects (each come from a different equivalence class). But M, L and 65+ and their interactions would create a severe problem because 65+ and {M,65+} come from the same class, and {M,L}, {L,65+} and {M,L,65+} come from the same class. Thus there are only five *different* sets of subjects to represent the eight parameters (including the intercept) of each variable and its interactions.

The mathematical formulation leads naturally to a set of useful techniques which have not yet been applied in epidemiology. Mathematically, the raw data listings from which contingency tables are derived consist of a set S of objects (the result of sampling), a set A of attributes (indicator variables, the result of classifying), and a binary relation I (a subset of the Cartesian product $S \times A$, the result of measurement) that indicates which objects s have which attributes a, by the membership of the particular ordered pairs (s, a) that are members of I. The mathematical formulation that I is a subset of the Cartesian product of S and A (written $I \subseteq S \times A$) expresses a natural epidemiological idea of "a subject possessing an attribute."[4] Thus the binary relation I consists of all the individual categorical determinations we make on each subject as to their age, sex, handedness, etc. In other words, I is equivalent to a raw data table such as Table 1 or 6.

Beginning in the 1970s mathematical lattice theorists developed Formal Concept Analysis (FCA) using a mathematical notion of "concept" [**4**]. It is based on a

[4]In our example a typical member of the relation I, e.g. (case 1, M)$\in I$, states that an object belonging to the set S (here case 1) satisfies an attribute belonging to the set A (here male), and similarly the information (case 2, M) $\notin I$ states that an object belonging to the set S (here case 2) does *not* have an attribute belonging to the set A (here male). Other examples of elements of I include (case 2, R) and (case 7, 65+), while neither (case 2, L) nor (case 5, 65+) are elements of I.

TABLE 8. Raw data table rearranged to show closed set $\{M, L, 65+\}$.

	R	M	L	65+
Case2	1	0	0	0
Case1	0	**1**	**1**	**1**
Case3	0	**1**	**1**	**1**
Case4	1	1	0	0
Case5	1	0	1	0
Case6	0	0	1	0
Case7	1	1	0	1

general observation (1930s) that a natural set of mappings arises when sets S and A are connected by a binary relation I [**2**]. Here is a more formal mathematical description, followed by an illustration of its epidemiological content.

To each subset X of S, we associate the set $a(X)$ of all attributes the subjects in X have in common, and to each subset Y of A, we associate the set $o(Y)$ of all subjects that have every attribute in Y. Remembering that each cell of the generalized contingency table is a combination of attributes, we fill the cell with a number by counting the subjects with the indicated combination of attributes. More formally, the table cells are filled with subject counts via the composition of the map $o : \mathcal{P}(A) \to \mathcal{P}(S)$ with the cardinality ("size") function $|(-)| : \mathcal{P}(S) \to \mathbb{Z}$, where $\mathbb{Z}$ is the set of non-negative integers. The closed sets discussed above are those subsets Y of A such that $a(o(Y)) = Y$ and these sets are called intents of formal concepts in FCA or closed sets in lattice theory. By taking all closed sets together, we obtain a closure system, which is always a complete lattice, that is, an algebraic structure determined by a partial order in which an arbitrary subset has both a supremum (least upper bound) and infimum (greatest lower bound). The elements of this closure system (also called a topped intersection structure [**3**]), are the cells of the closed set contingency table, and observing its order structure allows us to view the hierarchical structure of contingency table cells. Once we associate a set of objects with each cell of the closed set contingency table, using the $o(-)$ operator, we have the *concept lattice* that is found in FCA.

One view of this definition (Table 8) is realized within a data table by shuffling rows and columns so that object-attribute relations are maintained but the 1s are placed together in a block. Here we see the closed set $\{M, L, 65+\}$ in the data of Table 6 with a block of ones marked:

We cannot add any attribute column (here there is only one, R) or any rows (there are four more) that will make this block bigger. With other rearrangements we can get other blocks. Here is the closed set $\{M, R\}$.

These blocks represent collections of cases and all the things that these cases, and only these cases, have in common. This exposes the underlying motivation for using the word "concept" for this situation in Formal Concept Analysis.[5] It is in analogy with the idea that the "concept" of a bird, for example, is represented

[5]When the underlying binary relation is converted into a symmetric relational structure, the result is a bipartite graph, and in this case these object set-attribute set pairs are also called *bicliques* in graph theory.

TABLE 9. Raw data table rearranged to show closed set $\{M, R\}$.

	R	M	L	65+
Case2	1	0	0	0
Case1	0	1	1	1
Case3	0	1	1	1
Case4	**1**	**1**	0	0
Case7	**1**	**1**	0	1
Case5	1	0	1	0
Case6	0	0	1	0

by the set of those creatures we call birds, along with all the things birds, and only birds, have in common: lays eggs, air breather, warm-blooded, etc. (see the expanded example in [**6**]). In the less encompassing case of a single dataset, the concepts represent the set of such unique commonalities present in that dataset, given the descriptions of cases in terms of their attributes.

We summarize with the following formal definitions.

DEFINITION 3.1. The *generalized contingency table* for n subjects, each of whom can have k possible attributes, is a function from the powerset of the k attributes to the set of non-negative integers whose value is the number of subjects (prevalence) in each of the subsets of the powerset of the attributes (this function value is $|o(X)|$ for attribute set X).

Remark: The definition generalizes the idea of contingency tables in two respects. It makes no assumptions that the attributes are mutually exclusive or exhaustive, and it considers all combinations of attributes. Thus the cells of the generalized contingency table are a superset of the cells of all other conventional contingency tables. The powerset is a mathematical object that itself forms a complete lattice, called the lattice of sets.

As noted above, the data may also be sufficiently structured that we can look at a much smaller complete lattice within the lattice of sets that contains all information of the dataset:

DEFINITION 3.2. The closed set contingency table for a specific dataset of n subjects, each with k possible attributes, consists of a function from the set of closed (attribute) sets determined by the data table (via the condition $a(o(X)) = X$) to the set of non-negative integers whose value at each closed attribute set X is again $|o(X)|$, the number of subjects determined by the set X.

Remark: While the generalized contingency table will always have exactly 2^k different domain elements, the number of closed set contingency table cells depends on the data. Usually this will be very much smaller than 2^k. The difference between the two is not because there are insufficient subjects to fill the cells with unique values, since if there are $|S|$ subjects with $|A|$ attributes, all cells of the generalized contingency table can theoretically be distinctly filled whenever $|S| \geq |A|$, i.e., whenever the number of subjects exceeds the number of attributes. Rather, the difference is due to the fact that the closed set contingency table restricts the

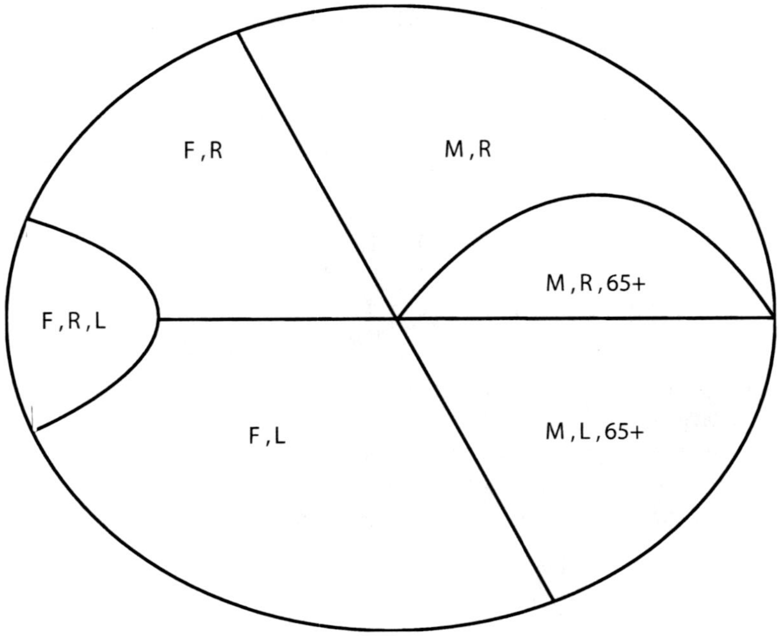

FIGURE 3. Venn diagram of data structure in Table 6. Right-handed and left-handed partition the males but overlap in the females (not males). The 65+ subjects are all contained in the Male group and all left-handed males are 65+ and some right-handed males are 65+.

domain of the map $|o(-)|$ to those sets of attributes that are maximally specified with respect to the given dataset.

4. Depicting the Closed Sets with Venn and Hasse Diagrams

The closed set contingency table that is contained in the generalized contingency table gives an important view of the data not produced by more conventional data analysis schemes. In particular, it reveals structure and relationships between complex combinations of attributes, something that requires preconceived or trial and error inquiries with usual methods. Even in a tiny dataset like that in Table 6, the search for these blocks in a data table is cumbersome and unintuitive for the analyst to perform, but algorithms have been devised over the past twenty years that yield all the blocks quickly. In this section we consider the views of the data given by Venn diagrams and Hasse diagrams, and argue that the Hasse diagram gives a very compact view of the hierarchical relationships between concepts generated from a dataset.

First consider a Venn diagram of the dataset we have considered so far (Figure 3). Here the latent structure of the small dataset in Table 6 is visually presented although it is not particularly easy to grasp, even in this very simple and small dataset. The eye tends to see many sub-collections in this diagram, some that are not present in the original dataset. For example, the top rectangle labeled "F (=

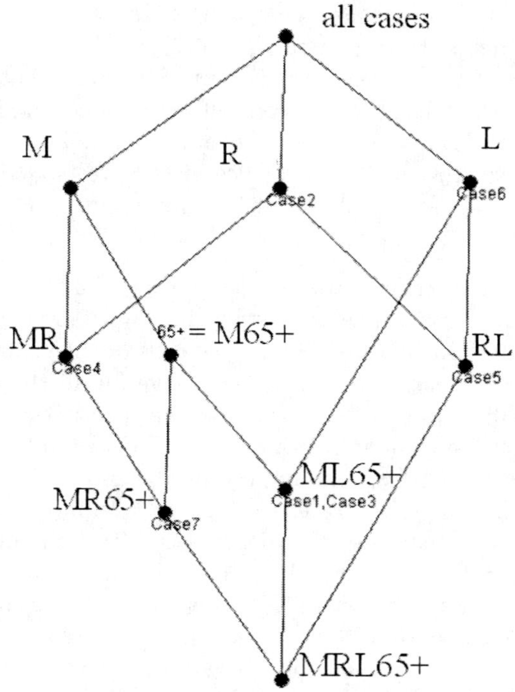

FIGURE 4. Lattice of Table 6 and its 10 closed sets (Table 7); each of these combinations of attributes represents different sets of subjects; any particular subject will usually be in several such sets.

not M)" represents the zero entries under the M column of Table 6. The Venn diagram forces on us not only the variables in the dataset (M, R, L, 65+) but also their negations (not M, not R, not L, not 65+) and all their conjunctions (M and not R, not R and not L, etc.), with each a separate "piece" of the diagram. There are a great many such pieces and combinations of regions. The Venn diagram, while more visually informative than the raw data table, rapidly becomes too complicated for even fairly small datasets. On the other hand there are only eight proper closed sets (plus the whole set and the empty set to equal ten), each corresponding to a maximally specified generalized contingency table cell. We can improve on the Venn diagram by depicting only the closed sets (which have all the information) in a diagram that shows how they are related to each other. The picture is obtained by connecting with a line closed sets that include (on the level of cases) other closed sets as subsets, the larger set of cases being above. Where two of these lines meet below there is a set intersection of the set of cases associated with the closed sets above. The diagram can be generated by a computer, using algorithms developed in the last fifteen years for the computation and effective visualization of the closure system generated from a data table [**1**], offering a view of both local and global structures in the data. Figure 4 shows what the diagram looks like for our small dataset of Table 6. In the diagram the concepts labeled "caseX" represent the first subset of cases in which caseX first appears, while the attribute names above the concept indicate the attribute set that determines that set of cases.

Using Table 7, for example, we see that the closed "empty set" is at the top (representing all subjects; third column, Table 7), while the closed sets M, R and L represent subjects that are each contained in the top set but not in each other. Hence they are just below the top and connected by a line. Similarly for the closed sets {M,R} and {R,L}. Here 65+ is not shown as a node because it is not a closed set, and the closed set in whose equivalence class it rests, {M,65+}, is below M because the subjects represented by {M,65+} are completely contained in the set of subjects represented by M, etc.

Note that in Table 6 there were originally $4 \times 4 \times 4 \times 4 = 256$ combinations of variables (including repeated values) of which $2^4 = 16$ are combinations without repeats (the powerset, which we are calling the cells of the generalized contingency table). But only ten of these (the closed sets) contain all the information in this dataset. In this small example, the savings are not so striking, but if we consider a larger dataset the results may be dramatic. For example we recently looked at a dataset consisting of 89 water samples and 66 properties of the samples. In comparison to the 2^{66} ($> 10^{19}$) combinations of attributes (and an even larger number of possible combinations of subjects), only 3175 distinct combinations of subjects were present in the data. They are the closed sets. Among these 66 attributes some are related, for example, the attribute that stipulates which of the ten towns the sample came from. Thus these ten attributes have only ten legitimate combinations instead of $2^{10} \approx 1000$, since a sample can come from only one of the ten towns. However this reduction from 1000 to 10 is itself a reflection of structure in the data, in this case the fact that the ten town attributes are mutually exclusive. Even if we make these *a priori* estimates, the number of possible combinations is still greater than 3×10^7 so that the number of closed sets is still four orders of magnitude smaller, again a reflection of a great deal of additional structure in the data.

For large datasets we can simplify the picture further in various ways by including only those closed cells that have a sufficient prevalence to warrant our attention (for example, that have five or more subjects in them). It is known mathematically that this kind of truncation does not alter the picture above the cutoff point. The resulting pictures are called "iceberg lattices" because of the way they represent the part that "sticks up" above the cutoff level [**10**]. In the water sample set, if we focus only on cells that refer to groups of cases that comprise 5% (respectively, 20%) or more of the whole set, then there are only 2427 (resp., 818) such maximally specified combinations.

The generalization of a contingency table gives us a view of all combinations of subject attributes relevant for our dataset, not just those taken pairwise or some other fairly low dimensional combination forced upon us by the fact that paper is a two-dimensional object. We get a visual version from the lattice diagram of the closed sets induced by the binary relation I, i.e., induced by the operation of measuring the sampled population.

The basic idea behind the lattice diagram of closed sets (called a Hasse diagram in mathematics) is that it spatially displays the order relations in a set of objects. Order relations (here we are talking partial orders [**3**], for example, $\subseteq$, the set theory symbol for "is included in") can be visualized by drawing a line between a larger

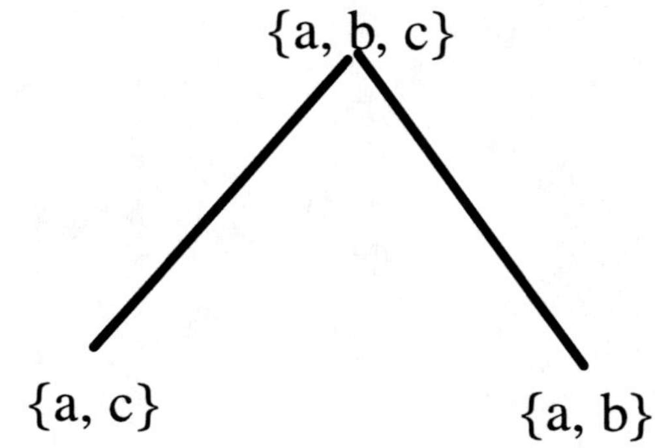

FIGURE 5. Example of a Hasse diagram involving three sets.

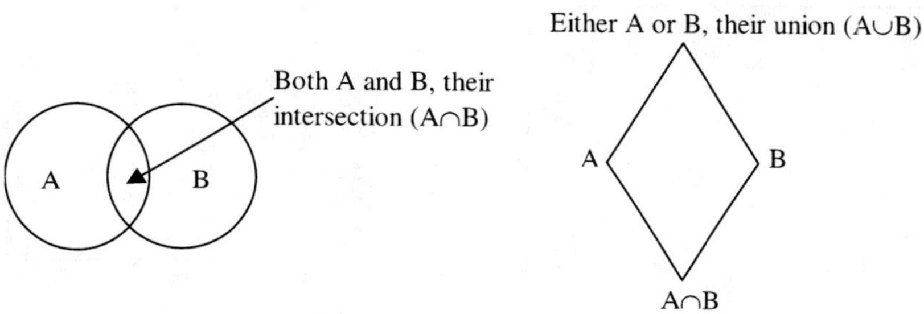

FIGURE 6. Venn diagram (left) and its Hasse diagram.

object, above, and a related (smaller) object below. Thus we would portray the relation between the sets, $\{a, b, c\}$, $\{a, b\}$ and $\{a, c\}$, where the second and third are contained in the first, in this way:

In Figure 5 notice that both $\{a, c\}$ and $\{a, b\}$ are contained in the set above ($\{a, b, c\}$) and are hence connected to it with a line, but that neither is contained in the other ($\{a, c\}$ is not completely contained in $\{a, b\}$ nor is $\{a, b\}$ contained in $\{a, c\}$). We can use Venn diagrams to help us develop a visual vocabulary:

While a Venn diagram can give some indication of the number of objects in sets A and B and their common elements (intersection), e.g. by using the relative sizes of the circles or other shapes, the Hasse diagram is only a depiction of the order structure, i.e., what is contained or not contained in sets, with no indication of the sizes of the sets involved. In Figure 6 we don't know if there are two cases in the overlap or two hundred cases, only that there is some overlap.

One way to add this prevalence information to the diagram is to add a zero-to-one scale to the left of the diagram, where the height corresponds to the proportion of total cases contained in the set. We call this depiction "support push" because prevalence is also called support in the FCA literature. We will generally use the epidemiologic term prevalence, meaning here prevalence proportion (sometimes called prevalence rate although it is not truly a rate). Here is an example:

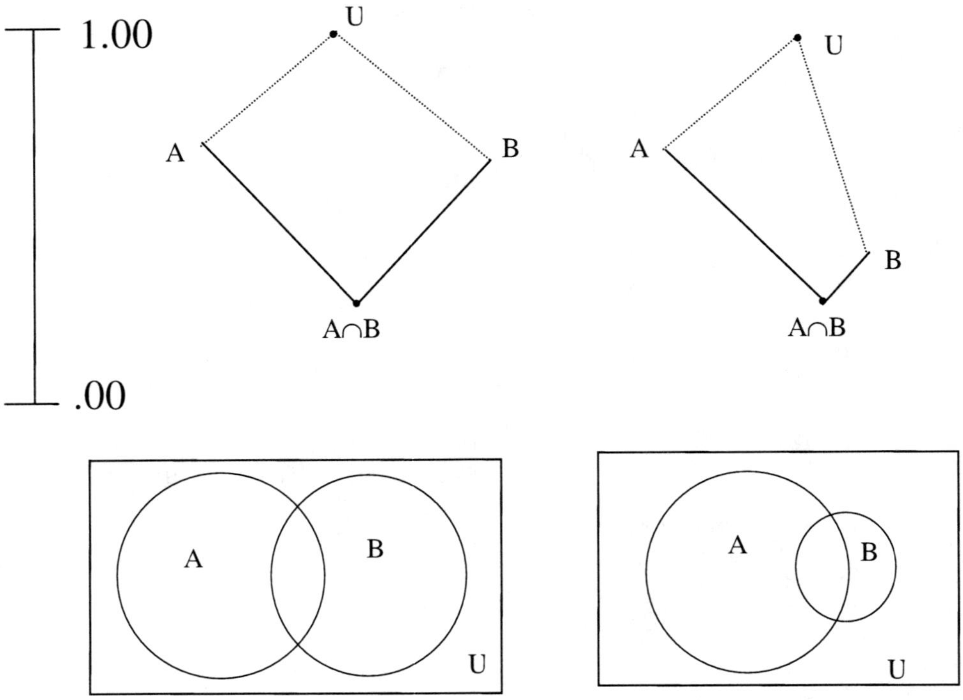

FIGURE 7. We call the Hasse diagrams at top the symmetric vee and the "checkmark". Here they are shown with the corresponding Venn diagrams.

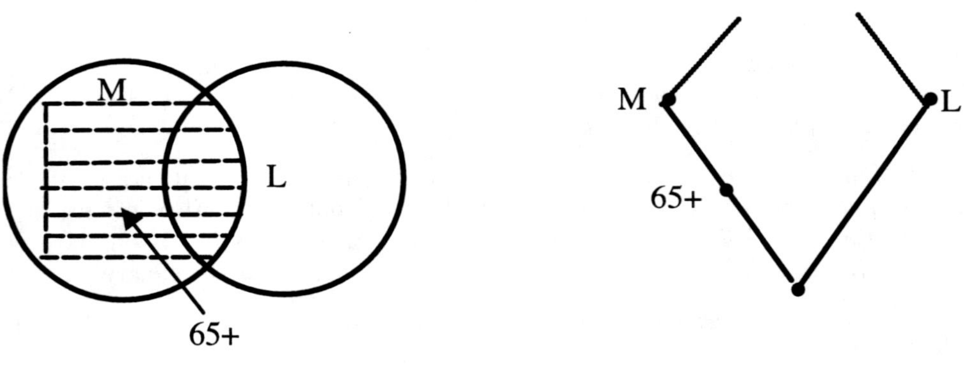

FIGURE 8. A Venn diagram and its associated Hasse diagram; only bottom half shown.

Two overlapping sets (for example, right-handed males) where the proportion of subjects in each category is roughly equal will meet below in a symmetric vee, whereas if the sets are unequal in size they will produce a checkmark-like configuration (here a backwards checkmark). These configurations are depicted in Figure 7. If we add a third set, a number of configurations are possible. Consider the diagrams in Figure 8, for example, which depict the Male, Left-handed, 65+ situation of Table 6:

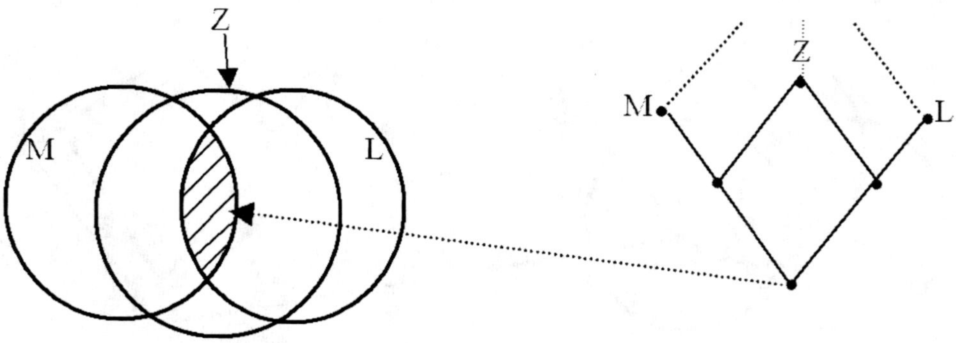

FIGURE 9. A Venn diagram depicting three sets, with its associated Hasse diagram (bottom half).

It is easy to see in either of these diagrams that if you are 65+, then you are Male, and if you are Male and Left-handed (M, L), then you are also 65+. The right diagram shows that 65+ is "less than" M (meaning the set of subjects represented by 65+ is contained in the set of subjects represented by M) while the subjects who have maleness and left-handedness in common (the M,L meeting point at the bottom of the vee) are contained in 65+ (and of course also contained in each of M and L). We can read these statements like implications: being ML implies 65+ (and of course also M), i.e., *if* you are a left-handed male, *then* you are also 65+. Said another way, "implication reads upwards" in the diagram.

Another example, shown in Figure 9, involves an attribute Z. The diagram shows (reading upwards) that all subjects who are M and L (bottom of the vee) are also Z (reading upwards). Note that being M and Z does not imply L, nor does being Z and L imply M. The relative sizes are given by the heights. All of these are facts visible on the Venn diagram at left, but even with as few as three attributes the Venn diagram is becoming harder to read while the lattice diagram shows them immediately. Moreover, the lattice diagram at right can be produced automatically by computer from the raw data table, an important advantage for complex datasets. Of course, such 100% implications are not so common in real-world datasets, so we are also interested in "near implications," also known as association rules. [6] Consider Figure 10.

Notice that now the implication is not 100%. If you are M, L, you are very likely to be Z (the two lower points are close in height), but there are some subjects who are M, L but not Z (Z is not on an upward path from their meeting point). However where M, L, and Z all meet is not much below the M, L meet, which indicates the "almost" overlap. As can be seen at right, the M, L intersection is now larger than the overlap of M, L, and Z (the tip of the lower vee) which is contained in it. The closer together in height these bottom nodes are, the more overlap there is and hence the "nearer" to a full implication (i.e. the nearer to stating that 100% of M, L are also Z).

[6] It has been observed by various authors ([**13**], [**7**]) that the computation of association rules includes, and can be organized by, the computation of the concept lattice. The equivalence relation on the power set of the attribute set that is given by the concept lattice computation induces induce a partition, and related reduction, of the full set of association rules.

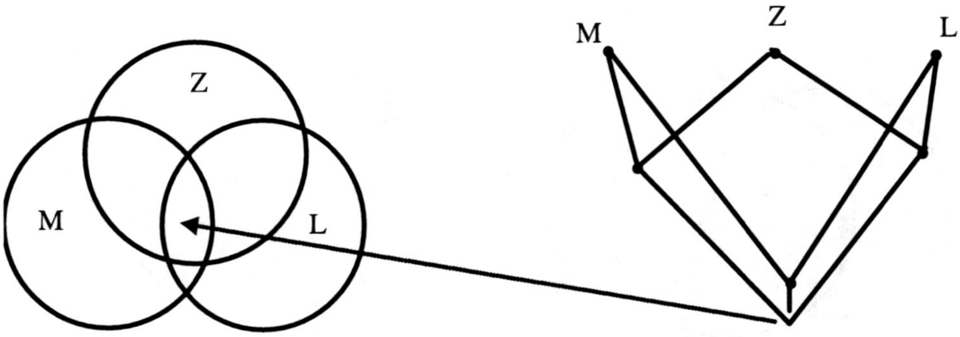

FIGURE 10. A Venn diagram and its associated Hasse diagram, with support push.

TABLE 10. Data tables for Figures 9 and 10.

	M	L	Z
c1	0	0	1
c2	0	1	1
c3	1	0	0
c4	1	1	1
c5	1	1	1
c6	1	0	1
c7	0	1	0
c8	0	0	1

	M	L	Z
c1	0	0	1
c2	0	1	1
c3	1	0	0
c4	1	1	0
c5	1	1	1
c6	1	0	1
c7	0	1	0
c8	0	0	1

These examples also illustrate another reason to add prevalence (support) information to the pure order information of the conventional Hasse diagram. The data tables in Table 10 will produce the examples in Figures 9 and 10, respectively:

The tables are identical except for the change from a one to a zero in attribute Z in case 4. This small change clearly makes a qualitative difference in the topology of the Hasse diagrams, but by incorporating the degree of overlap or mismatch using height, we add information on the magnitude of the visually qualitative change not present in the order-only Hasse diagram, where height has no quantitative meaning. This is one of the innovations presented in this paper (also see [**8**]).

Clearly prevalence has epidemiologic significance. Prevalence is the proportion of subjects that have that attribute or combination of attributes in the dataset. It is proportional to the number of such subjects, which is also called prevalence (or relative support in the FCA literature). We can take two nodes whose attributes overlap, for example as shown in Figure 11, and use them to construct a 2×2 table in the following way.

Figure 12 shows a 2×2 table constructed from this configuration, with the prevalence data in boxes:

One can see that the four corners of the diamond are sufficient to fill in all the cells of the table. Further, we need not include negations of features of interest to capture all the relevant information regarding the 2×2 table. This means a further

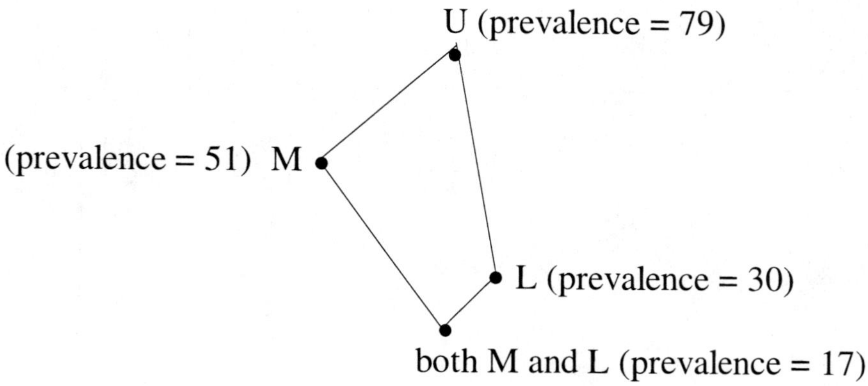

FIGURE 11. Some hypothetical nodes in the lattice diagram of a raw data table.

	L	not L	
M	17	34	51
not M	13	15	28
	30	49	79

FIGURE 12. 2×2 table constructed from the diamond configuration of two nodes in Figure 11.

simplification beyond that already offered by the reduction from the generalized contingency table to the closed set lattice of that table.

Looking at certain configurations in terms of the more familiar tables also allows us to see their meaning more clearly. The general case involves two attributes that overlap to some extent. As an example, in a sample of all subjects (U), a subset is male (M) and a subset consists of substance abusers (S):

If we write $|U|$, $|M|$ and $|L|$ for the number of subjects U, the number of males, M, and the number of substance abusers, S, we can construct corresponding tables for each of these diagrams:

It is easy to see from the tables that relationship III shows a perfect correlation between being male and being a substance abuser, and relationship IV shows that all substance abusers are males. Diagram II, where M and S meet at the empty set, shows they are mutually exclusive, while diagram I shows they overlap, with the degree of overlap indicated by the relative height of their meet (the element directly below M and S in the diagram).

In these generic cases every pair of closed sets determines a 2×2 table, with the entries indicated in Figure 13 and Table 11 completely determining the table. Thus the diagram also implicitly depicts conventional epidemiological effect measures for each pair of closed set attribute combinations (in this case combination M and combination S). It is a simple matter to have the computer calculate measures (e.g.,

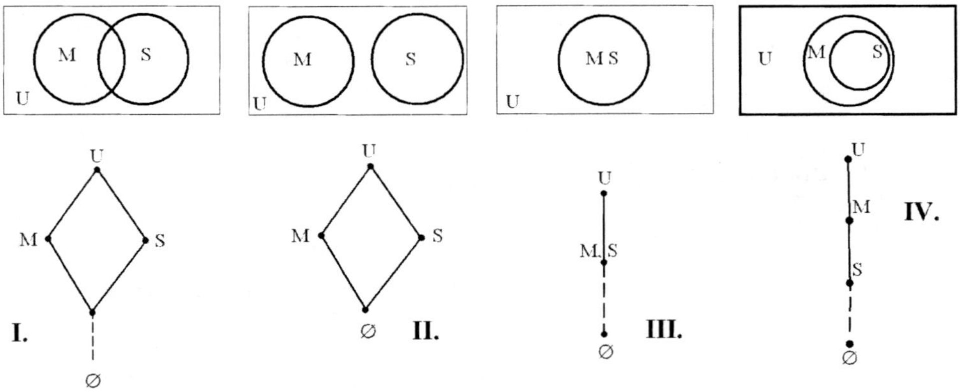

FIGURE 13. Venn and lattice diagrams for some hypothetical attribute relationships; the symbol $\emptyset$ stands for the "empty set," i.e., there are no subjects in the set. Relative heights are not shown on this diagram but are easily obtained in the computer realization. U stands at height 1.00, while $\emptyset$ stands at height 0.00.

odds ratio, relative risk, or prevalence ratio, as appropriate) with a mouseclick for any pair of nodes on the diagram.[7]

5. Next Steps

We have presented here the basis for some new mathematical objects, the generalized and closed set contingency tables, that may be of use in data analysis. Computer-aided visualization of the lattice structure of a dataset needs to be interpreted in epidemiologic terms. To that end we are in the process of developing a "visual vocabulary" that links diagrammatic represenations of data structures to epidemiologic measures, and we are using it on real-world epidemiologic datasets to see the utility of these methods in practice.

[7]Lattice viewing and rule capture are two basic components of the Seqer software package being developed at the Physical Science Laboratory of New Mexico State University.

TABLE 11. 2×2 tables for the diagrams of Figure 11.

	S	not S	
M	|MS|	|M|-|MS|	|M|
not M	|S|-|MS|	|U|-|M|-|S|+|MS|	|U|-|M|
	|S|	|U|-|S|	|U|

I.

	S	not S	
M	0	|M|	|M|
not M	|S|	|U|-|M|-|S|	|U|-|M|
	|S|	|U|-|S|	|U|

II.

	S	not S	
M	|S|	0	|S|
not M	0	|U|-|M|-|S|+|MS|	|U|-|S|
	|S|	|U|-|S|	|U|

III.

	S	not S	
M	|S|	|M|-|S|	|M|
not M	0	|U|-|M|	|U|-|M|
	|S|	|U|-|S|	|U|

IV.

References

1. For an extensive reference list of FCA application papers see: http://www.mathematik.tu-darmstadt.de/ags/ag1/Literatur/literatur_en.html
2. Birkhoff, G.: "Lattice Theory", American Mathematical Society, Providence, R.I., 1st edition, 1940.
3. Davey, B. and Priestley, H., "Introduction to Ordered Sets and Lattices, 2nd Edition", Cambridge University Press, Cambridge, 2002.
4. Ganter, B. and Wille, R.: "Formal Concept Analysis: Mathematical Foundations", Springer, NY, 1999. ISBN 3-540-62771-5
5. Freese, R.: "LatDrawWin, a lattice drawing applet", Available at the URL: www.math.hawaii.edu/~ralph/LatDraw.
6. Hannan, T., Miller, L., and Pogel, A.: "The Visualization of Weighted Lattices", at the Workshop on Applications of Lattice Theory to Computer Science, July 2003, at DIMACS, Piscataway, NJ. Available at the URL: http://dimacs.rutgers.edu/Workshops/Lattices/slides/pogel.ppt
7. Pasquier, N., Bastide, J., Taouil, R., and Lakhal, L.: Discovering Frequent Closed Itemsets for Association Rules. In Lecture Notes in Computer Science (LNCS) **1540**, Springer-Verlag (1999) 398-416.
8. Pogel, A., Hannan, T. and Miller, L. Visualization of Concept Lattices Using Weight Functions, Supplementary Proceedings of the International Conference on Conceptual Structures (Huntsville, AL), Shaker, 2004.
9. Rothman K.J., Greenland S., "Modern Epidemiology", Lipponcott-Raven, 1998.
10. Stumme, G., Taouil, R., Bastide, Y., Pasquier, N. and Lakhal, L.: "Computing iceberg concept lattices with Titanic", Data and Knowledge Engineering (Elsevier), 42 (2002), 189-222.
11. Wille, R.: "Why Can Concept Lattices Support Knowledge Discovery in Databases?", Technische Universitat Darmstadt, Fachbereich Mathematik, Preprint Nr. 2158, June 2001. Available at http://wwwbib.mathematik.tu-darmstadt.de/Math-Net/Preprints/Listen/pp01.html
12. Yevtushenko, S., et al: "Concept Explorer", Open source java software available at the URL: http://sourceforge.net/projects/conexp, Release 1.2, 2003.
13. Zaki, M., and M. Ogihara, M.: "Theoretical Foundations of Associations Rules", in Proceedings of 3rd SIGMOD'98 Workshop on Research Issues in Data Mining and Knowledge Discovery (DMKD'98), Seattle, Washington, USA, June 1998.

Department of Environmental Health, Boston University School of Public Health, Boston, MA 02118, USA

E-mail address: dozonoff@bu.edu

Physical Science Laboratory, New Mexico State University, Las Cruces, NM 88003, USA

E-mail address: Alex.Pogel@psl.nmsu.edu

Physical Science Laboratory, New Mexico State University, Las Cruces, NM 88003, USA

E-mail address: thannan@nmsu.edu

DIMACS Series in Discrete Mathematics
and Theoretical Computer Science
Volume **70**, 2006

Graph Partitions and Concept Lattices

James Abello and Alex Pogel

ABSTRACT. The contingency table plays an important role in epidemiology and naturally generalizes to the concept lattice (see [**13**] in this Volume). This is a mathematical object that reveals hierarchical structure in data and has been used in a variety of knowledge discovery applications. The simple purpose of employing the concept lattice as a replacement for a traditional (low-dimensional) contingency table is to increase the number of features that an epidemiologist may consider when cross-classifying a population. In general, the concept lattice grows quite rapidly. However, graph-theoretic methods exist that can focus attention on subsets of the data that are particularly rich in interconnections. Therefore, in response to this growth, we propose a natural solution: use graph-theoretic decomposition methods to focus attention on particularly relevant portions of the concept lattice for a given dataset. This paper presents connections between two decomposition methods, *rooted level aware breadth first search* and *peeling*, and the concept lattice. In many instances, these results allow the concept lattice to be analyzed by sections. While the work presented here is primarily theoretical, we are currently using our results to drive the development of a collection of software tools that will be used to analyze real data sets.

1. Introduction

A fundamental epidemiological tool is the two-dimensional contingency table. It has recently been established that a natural generalization of the two-dimensional contingency table is the generalized contingency table and its minimal representation, the concept lattice. Besides presenting all the cell counts in a generalized contingency table, the concept lattice also provides a hierarchical structure of the data. This hierarchical representation is the foundation on which most of the knowledge discovery applications have been built [**16, 8**], especially since it has been shown that this is a natural structure in which to discover implications in the data [**10**].

2000 *Mathematics Subject Classification.* Primary 06A15 Galois correspondences, closure operators ; Secondary 05C90 Applications.

The authors thank Lance Miller and David Millman for their implementation of software related to this research. We also thank the National Science Foundation and DIMACS for their support making this collaboration possible.

For a detailed discussion of the connection between epidemiology and concept lattices, we refer the reader to [**13**] (in this Volume). We stress that our intention in employing the concept lattice in place of the traditional (low-dimensional) contingency table is to increase the number of features that an epidemiologist may consider when cross-classifying a population, and to allow investigations of data to be more data-driven, and less query driven. We feel these are important advances to work toward, especially given the great monetary and energy expenses associated with the collection of epidemiological data. For these advances to be converted into real, usable tools for epidemiologists, there are a few important steps to be taken, in sequence: theoretical development, software implementation, distribution, evaluation and improvement. The goal of this paper is to begin to establish some of the necessary theoretical development.

In testing the concept lattice construction with real datasets, rather than small, artificial datasets, we have seen that the lattice can grow quite rapidly. In some cases it approaches the theoretical upper bound which is exponential in the number of attributes. An important step of lattice-centered data analysis involves viewing a lattice on a computer monitor, as hand-calculations are only reasonable in the smallest of examples – see [**11, 17**] for some automated lattice drawing tools. Even with automated drawing tools, the quick growth of the lattices presents two challenges. The first issue is whether the automated drawing tools can provide a diagram at all, since the underlying algorithms are often at least quadratic in the number of concepts. Assuming that a diagram can be created in a reasonable amount of time, the second issue arises from the observation that hundreds, or thousands, of concepts in a diagram immediately tax the human viewer's ability to absorb information from the presented layout. More generally, the concept lattice computation simply generates too large a number of concepts to easily manage, regardless of whether the concepts are viewed or not. These complexity concerns create a need for some control to be exercised with regard to how many concepts are computed at a time, a problem discussed in [**14**] and [**7**].

In response to these issues, we propose a natural solution: use graph-theoretic decomposition methods to focus attention on special portions of a given dataset. Thus we examine various decomposition methods, along the lines of [**5**], to apply to the given input binary relation that is the usual initial datum for the concept lattice construction. In this paper we first discuss the rooted level-aware breadth first search through the binary relation, and then turn to the decomposition of the binary relation into subrelations determined by iterative stages of a process called graph peeling. We have considered some of the lattice theoretical aspects related to the application of these graph-theoretic decomposition methods. This paper presents advances in the connection between decompositions of the data and decompositions of the corresponding lattice specifically to induce partitions of the corresponding concept lattice. In the sense that we apply graph-theoretic methods to concept analysis, this work is similar to [**6**]. While the work presented here has some theoretical flavor, it is motivated by the software development work reported in [**3**]. We report on some of the steps we have taken towards a software package that can be used to examine real data.

First we introduce some notions from graph theory and Formal Concept Analysis, establishing that the concept lattice is, in graph-theoretic terms, equivalent to the lattice of maximal bicliques of the bipartite graph obtained by symmetrizing the object-attribute pairs of the input binary relation. Next, we find that a rooted breadth-first search decomposition of a graph-connected binary relation leads to a closely related partition of the concept lattice. This result is used to describe how the concept lattice can be unfolded in stages, according to the information gathered during the breadth first search. Finally, we turn our attention to a process called graph peeling, and present the first steps of a similar investigation of the relationship between peeling and the concept lattice. We also discuss some first conclusions regarding the practical use of peeling in conjunction with the concept lattice.

In summary, our investigation is based on the principle that we can determine inexpensively computed decompositions of the input data (the binary relation), which we foresee will at times help to organize the computation and search of the concept lattice.[1] On the application side, we see the rooted level-aware breadth first search and peeling as two possible methods of offering glimpses of the full concept lattice, by allowing portions of the lattice to be viewed independently. This paper presents initial structural results and application strategies as a starting point of a larger programme.

2. Definitions

Although some of the definitions appearing throughout this section do not require that the sets involved be finite, we make a standing assumption that all sets under consideration are finite.

2.1. Graph Theoretical Notions. In this subsection we introduce the necessary graph theoretical terminology.

DEFINITION 1. *A (loopless) graph* $\mathfrak{G}$ *is a pair* (V, E) *such that* V *is a nonempty set and* E *is a subset of* $\mathcal{P}_2(V)$*, the set of all two-element subsets of* V*; elements of* V *are called vertices, while elements of* E *are called edges, and the two vertices associated with a particular edge are called the endpoints of the edge.*

DEFINITION 2. *If* x *is a vertex in a graph* $\mathfrak{G} = (V, E)$*, its neigborhood is*

$$N(x) = \{y \in V : \{x, y\} \in E\}.$$

In epidemiological terms, the neighborhood of a vertex is the set of all data elements that are related to the vertex (by acquaintance, by recent contact, by genetic history, etc). The *subgraph induced* by a subset S of V is the graph $\mathfrak{G}_S$ whose edge set E_S consists of those edges with both endpoints in S.

DEFINITION 3. *A bipartite graph (bigraph) is a graph* $\mathfrak{G} = (V, E)$ *for which there exists a non-trivial partition* $\{V_L, V_R\}$ *of* V *such that for each* $e \in E$,

$$e \cap V_L \neq \emptyset \quad \textit{and} \quad e \cap V_R \neq \emptyset.$$

[1]This strategy should be understood in contrast with approaches that use general properties of the structure of the input data. For example, [**14**] incorporates the usual support thresholding used in association rule mining into an algorithm for computing generators (key sets) for frequent closed itemsets, using a pruning method [**1**]; the general property used there is that the set of all key sets is an order ideal of the power set of the attribute set.

In words, V is partitioned into two independent nonempty sets: each edge connects an element in one block of the partition to an element in the other block. We call V_L the set of *left vertices*, and we call V_R the set of *right vertices.* If E contains all possible edges between V_L and V_R, $\mathfrak{G}$ is called a complete bipartite graph. A complete bipartite graph $\mathfrak{G}_S$ that is an induced subgraph of $\mathfrak{G}$ is called a *biclique* of $\mathfrak{G}$. A biclique is *maximal* if it is not contained in a larger biclique.

2.2. Formal Concept Analysis Notions. We follow the definitions introduced in [**10**], and repeat a few here, especially when there are graph-theoretical interpretations of interest.

DEFINITION 4. *A formal context is a triple $\mathbb{K} = (O, A, E)$ of nonempty sets, where $E \subseteq O \times A$. If a formal context $\mathbb{K}$ satisfies $O \cap A = \emptyset$, then we say it is bigraph inducing. The bipartite graph $\mathfrak{G}_K$ of a bigraph inducing formal context $\mathbb{K} = (O, A, E)$ is*

$$\mathfrak{G}_K = (O \cup A, \{\ \{o, a\} : oEa\ \})\ .$$

The edge set of the bigraph $\mathfrak{G}_K$ is called the symmetrization of the binary relation E.

DEFINITION 5. *Given a formal context (O, A, E), for each subset P of O and for each $H \subseteq O \times A$, we define the operator $(\ \ )^H$ on $\mathcal{P}(O)$ and $\mathcal{P}(A)$, as follows: for $P \subseteq O$, let*

$$P^H = \{a \in A : \forall p \in P, pHa\ \}$$

and dually, for $B \subseteq A$, let

$$B^H = \{o \in O : \forall b \in B, oHb\ \}.$$

When a formal context $\mathbb{K} = (O, A, E)$ is fixed in a discussion, we write P' in place of P^E, and B' in place of B^E. Also, P'' is shorthand for $(P')'$. Suppose that O is a set of patients, while A is a set of features of the population. In this case, the epidemiological interpretation of P^H is that it is the set of all features that the patients in set P have in common. Dually, B^H is the set of patients that share every feature of the set B. We have used the relation H (a subset of E, and possibly equal to E) in this definition, instead of the full relation E, in order to speak of subrelations, once we begin to decompose the data. The following statement is an immediate consequence of the definitions, and is recorded for later reference:

LEMMA 6. *Let $\mathbb{K} = (O, A, E)$ be a formal context and suppose $H \subseteq E$. If $B \subseteq A$, then $B^H \subseteq B^E$. If $P \subseteq O$, then $P^H \subseteq P^E$.*

DEFINITION 7. *A formal context $\mathbb{K} = (O, A, E)$ is graph-connected provided it is bigraph inducing and the binary relation $E \cup E^{-1}$ on $O \cup A$ is connected in the usual sense, i.e. for all $x, y \in O \cup A$, there exists a path from x to y using ordered pairs from $E \cup E^{-1}$.*

We observe that if a bigraph inducing formal context $\mathbb{K} = (O, A, E)$ is graph-connected, then the induced bipartite graph $\mathfrak{G}_{\mathbb{K}}$ is connected. If a bipartite graph is connected, then the partition of its vertex set is unique, so in the case of a graph-connected formal context $\mathbb{K} = (O, A, E)$ such that $|O| \neq |A|$, we can recover $\mathbb{K}$ from $\mathfrak{G}_{\mathbb{K}}$. The important point is that if we induce a bigraph from a formal context, then various standard graph decomposition methods immediately come to mind and can be considered as a way to ameliorate the inherent complexity present in the formation of concepts.

Suppose $\mathbb{K}$ is bigraph inducing. Then, using graph terminology regarding the graph $\mathfrak{G}_K$, we see that $P' = \bigcap_{p \in P} N(p)$, i.e. P' is the intersection of the $\mathfrak{G}_K$-neigbourhoods of all the elements in P. Further, if both P and P' are nonempty, then $P \cup P'$ is the vertex set of a nonempty biclique in the bipartite graph $\mathfrak{G}_K$. If both P'' and P' are nonempty, then the union $P'' \cup P'$ is the vertex set of a maximal biclique of $\mathfrak{G}_K$ and every maximal biclique of $\mathfrak{G}_K$ arises this way, for some subset P of O. Dually, $B' = \bigcap_{a \in B} N(a)$ is the intersection of the $\mathfrak{G}_K$-neigbourhoods of all the elements in B. Similar comments regarding cliques and bicliques of the bipartite graph $\mathfrak{G}_K$ apply here as well.

The elements of the concept lattice associated with $\mathbb{K} = (O, A, E)$ are the pairs $(P, B) \in \mathcal{P}(O) \times \mathcal{P}(A)$ such that $P' = B$ and $B' = P$; such pairs are called *concepts* of the formal context $\mathbb{K}$, and P is called the *extent* and B the *intent* of the concept. In graph terminology, a formal concept of a bigraph inducing $\mathbb{K}$ with nonempty intent B and nonempty extent P will generate a maximal biclique with vertex set $P \cup B$ in the bigraph $\mathfrak{G}_K$. Let $\mathfrak{B}(\mathbb{K})$ be the set of all concepts of the formal context $\mathbb{K}$, ordered by inclusion in the first coordinate, i.e. $(P, B) \leq (Q, C)$ if and only if $P \subseteq Q$. This ordering makes $(\mathfrak{B}(\mathbb{K}), \leq)$ a complete lattice, i.e. a partially ordered set $(L, \leq)$ in which every subset of L has a least upper bound and a greatest lower bound in L. Thus we call the ordered set $(\mathfrak{B}(\mathbb{K}), \leq)$ *the concept lattice* of $\mathbb{K} = (O, A, E)$ (we usually omit the ordering $\leq$ and denote the lattice simply by $\mathfrak{B}(\mathbb{K})$). See **[13]** for an epidemiological view of this construction. There it is explained that the concept lattice represents a maximal reduction of the generalized contingency table.

Given a formal context $\mathbb{K} = (O, A, E)$, if $P \subseteq O$ and $B \subseteq A$, then the formal context $\mathbb{K}_{P,B} = (P, B, E \cap (P \times B))$ is called a *subcontext* of $\mathbb{K}$. Each restriction of either the domain or codomain to a proper subset induces maps between concept lattices. In particular, Propositions 31 and 32 of **[10]** state that subsets $P \subseteq O$ and $B \subseteq A$ induce order embeddings

$$\mathfrak{B}(\mathbb{K}_{P,A}) \to \mathfrak{B}(\mathbb{K}), \quad \mathfrak{B}(\mathbb{K}_{O,B}) \to \mathfrak{B}(\mathbb{K}) \quad \textit{and} \quad \mathfrak{B}(\mathbb{K}_{P,B}) \to \mathfrak{B}(\mathbb{K})$$

such that the first map is $\bigvee$-preserving, the second is $\bigwedge$-preserving, and the third could be given by either mapping,

$$(X, Y) \mapsto (X'', X') \quad \textit{or} \quad (X, Y) \mapsto (Y', Y'')$$

but these need be neither $\bigvee$- nor $\bigwedge$-preserving. Since our key purpose is to decompose lattices in practice, a technical goal of this paper is to provide conditions on concepts of subcontexts (determined by the Level-Aware Breadth First Search and Peeling) which imply that these operators are simply the identity map on such concepts. Stated in more intuitive terms, we seek conditions that are sufficient to ensure that concepts of the subcontext are "real", i.e. that they are concepts of the full context $\mathbb{K}$.

2.3. Association Rules: Confidence and Support. We conclude this section with two important functions used in data mining activity involving association rules **[1]**. As in Formal Concept Analysis, the input data involves binary attribute values assigned to a set of objects, i.e. a formal context. Given a set A of attributes, an association rule is a pair (X, Y) (often written $X \to Y$) with X, Y subsets of A, interpreted to say "in (some) cases where X holds, Y also holds" (near implication), or "in the event of X, event Y also occurs" (conditional event).

Two functions used to formulate evaluation criteria for association rules, and to control the size of sets of association rules that are created during data mining activity based on a formal context $\mathbb{K} = (O, A, E)$, are $conf_{\mathbb{K}}(-)$ (confidence) and $supp_{\mathbb{K}}(-)$ (support), given by

$$conf_{\mathbb{K}}(\ (X,Y)\ ) = \frac{|X' \cap Y'|}{|X'|} \qquad and \qquad supp_{\mathbb{K}}(\ (X,Y)\ ) = \frac{|X' \cap Y'|}{|O|}$$

[Recall that X' is the mathematical notation introduced earlier for the set of subjects which satisfy *every* property in the set X.] Support outputs the percent of overall evidence in the formal context for which the rule is positively witnessed, while confidence outputs the percent of those instances in the formal context where the hypothesis holds for which the conclusion also holds (with the appropriate qualifications, this is clearly equivalent to conditional probability).

Suppose we consider a grocery shopping context $\mathbb{G}$, where O is the set of shopping carts observed at checkout and A is the set of items the carts contained (e.g., cart #141 may have contained beer, diapers, pretzels and milk). If we consider the rule "beer $\to$ pretzels" and find that

$$supp_{\mathbb{G}}(beer \to pretzels) = 0.22 \qquad and \qquad conf_{\mathbb{G}}(beer \to pretzels) = 0.84$$

then of all the observed carts, 22% bought both beer and pretzels, and of those carts that contained beer, 84% of them also contained pretzels.

We define a function $Csupp_{\mathbb{K}} : \mathfrak{B}(\mathbb{K}) \to [0,1]$, called the *concept support* function, by assigning to each concept $D = (P, B)$ of $\mathbb{K} = (O, A, E)$ the value $Csupp_{\mathbb{K}}(D) = \frac{|P|}{|O|}$. Then the support of an association rule (X, Y) is the concept support of the concept generated by $X \cup Y$, that is

$$supp_{\mathbb{K}}(\ (X,Y)\ ) = Csupp_{\mathbb{K}}((X', X'') \wedge (Y', Y'')) = Csupp_{\mathbb{K}}(\ (X' \cap Y', (X' \cap Y')')\ )\ .$$

Also note that the support of a valid implication $X \to Y$ (i.e. an association rule (X, Y) with 100% confidence) is the concept support of the concept (X', X'') generated by the premise X.

The connection between the computation of concepts and the derivation of association rules has been observed by many authors, e.g. [**14, 18**], and we will provide some observations regarding the connection of graph decompositions with association rules in a later section.

3. LABFS and Concept Lattices

Formal Concept Analysis includes a variety of decomposition and construction methods. Many of these constructions are lattice-theoretic or universal-algebraic in nature and origin. Here we present a new decomposition of concept lattices, via the translation of a traditional graph-theoretic decomposition method that has been successfully applied to provide an overview of sparse massive data sets [**5**]. After the Breadth First Search decomposition method on bigraphs is presented, it is then extended to a given formal context (O, A, E) by applying it to the symmetrization of the binary relation E. Finally, we present theorems regarding the relationship between the decomposition of the formal context and the decomposition of the concept lattice.

3.1. Level-Aware Breadth First Search. The *rooted level-aware breadth first search* (abbreviation: LABFS) decomposition of a connected bigraph fixes a vertex as a root and partitions the vertex set by graph-theoretic distance from the root. Given a connected bigraph $\mathfrak{G} = (V, F)$, we fix some $r \in V$ and consider the function $d_r : V \to \mathbb{N} \cup \{0\}$, where $d_r(v)$ is the graph-theoretic distance from v to r (the minimum path length from v to r). Now we partition V by setting $L_i(r) = d_r^{-1}(\{i\})$, for each $i \in \mathbb{N} \cup \{0\}$. Clearly $V = \bigsqcup_{i \in N \cup \{0\}} L_i(r)$, where $\sqcup$ denotes disjoint union. The element r is called *the root* of the LABFS decomposition, and in general the induced partition of V will depend on r. While it is always true that $L_0(r) = \{r\}$, beyond that we cannot say much more about the partition. There are bigraphs with choices of r such that $V = L_0(r) \sqcup L_1(r)$ and there are bigraphs with choices of r such that

$$V = \bigsqcup_{i=0,1,2,\ldots,|V|-1} L_i(r) ,$$

where each $L_i(r)$ is nonempty. Note that all the partition blocks (and later, subrelations) that we consider in the sequel are dependent on the choice of r, so we will write expressions such as $L_1(r)$ as L_1.

The following statement is easy to prove:

LEMMA 8. *Let $\mathfrak{G} = (V, F)$ be a connected bigraph, and let a root $r \in V$ be given. For $i \in \mathbb{N} \cup \{0\}$, let $L_i = d_r^{-1}(\{i\})$ and let $F_i = \{\{u, v\} : u \in L_i, v \in L_{i+1}\} \cap F$. Then*

(1)
$$V = \bigsqcup_{i \in \mathbb{N} \cup \{0\}} L_i \quad \textit{and} \quad F = \bigsqcup_{i \in \mathbb{N} \cup \{0\}} F_i,$$

(2) *If $\mathfrak{G} = (V, F)$ is a connected bigraph, say, with root r in the right vertex set V_R, then $\{L_{2j}\}_{j \in \mathbb{N} \cup \{0\}}$ is a partition of V_R and $\{L_{2j+1}\}_{j \in \mathbb{N} \cup \{0\}}$ is a partition of V_L.*

From the LABFS partition of the induced connected bigraph $\mathfrak{G}_{\mathbb{K}}$ of a graph-connected formal context $\mathbb{K} = (O, A, E)$, we construct partitions of O and A and a covering of the binary relation E which will be used to understand large lattices by suitable smaller lattices. For the rest of this section, we define *r-rooted formal context* $\mathbb{K}$ to mean that $\mathbb{K} = (O, A, E)$ is a bigraph inducing, graph-connected formal context with distinguished element $r \in A$, and we let $\mathfrak{G}_{\mathbb{K}}$ be the induced (connected) bipartite graph. Given an r-rooted formal context $\mathbb{K}$, the partitions in Lemma 8 induce corresponding partitions of O and A, (via intersection with O and A respectively), all depending on the fixed choice of root r in A,

$$O = L_1 \sqcup L_3 \sqcup L_5 \sqcup \ldots \quad \textit{and} \quad A = L_0 \sqcup L_2 \sqcup L_4 \sqcup \ldots ,$$

	a-1	a-2	a-3	a-4	a-5	a-6	a-7	a-8	a-9	a-10
o-1	X			X			X			X
o-2				X						
o-3		X				X			X	
o-4	X									
o-5							X	X		
o-6			X				X			
o-7					X					
o-8				X					X	
o-9		X					X			
o-10		X	X	X	X			X		X
o-11	X									
o-12			X						X	
o-13						X				
o-14		X			X					
o-15				X					X	
o-16		X						X		
o-17				X						
o-18		X			X	X	X			X
o-19	X							X		X
o-20		X								
o-21			X			X				
o-22				X						
o-23		X					X			X
o-24	X									
o-25								X		
o-26		X			X					
o-27						X			X	
o-28			X	X					X	
o-29						X				X
o-30			X					X		

	a-1	a-7	a-4	a-10	a-8	a-3	a-2	a-5	a-6	a-9
o-1	X	X	X	X						
o-4	X									
o-11	X									
o-19	X			X	X					
o-24	X									
o-5		X			X					
o-6		X				X				
o-9		X					X			
o-18		X		X			X	X	X	
o-23		X		X			X			
o-2			X							
o-8			X							X
o-10			X	X	X	X	X	X		
o-15			X							X
o-17			X							
o-22			X							
o-28			X			X				X
o-29				X					X	
o-16					X		X			
o-25					X					
o-30					X	X				
o-12						X				X
o-21						X			X	
o-3							X		X	X
o-14							X	X		
o-20							X			
o-7								X		
o-13									X	
o-26							X	X		
o-27									X	X

FIGURE 1. The formal context $\mathbb{C}$, in LABFS-specific tabular form at right.

and Lemma 1 also implies that the relation E can be expressed via subrelations of E that are between blocks of the partitions of O and A.

Now, in place of the disjoint edge sets F_i in Lemma 8, we clearly have disjoint sets E_i of ordered pairs, where $E_i = \{\ (o,a) : o \in O, a \in A, \{o,a\} \in F_i\ \}$ but because of our interest in the concept lattice, we want to further define subrelations S_i of E, for $i \in \mathbb{N} \cup \{0\}$, by setting

$$S_i = (L_{i+1} \times (L_i \cup L_{i+2})) \cap E \qquad \textit{and} \qquad S_i = ((L_i \cup L_{i+2}) \times L_{i+1}) \cap E$$

for i even and i odd, respectively. Note that these subrelations will not be disjoint. We call S_i the ith *LABFS subrelation* of $\mathbb{K} = (O, A, E)$.

Consider the following graph-connected formal context $\mathbb{C}$ with 30 objects and 10 attributes, presented in tabular form at left in Figure 1. The object names have the form "o-i", for object i, and the attribute names have the form "a-j", for attribute j. If we choose root "a-1", and determine the sets corresponding to the various levels, and also shuffle the objects and attributes in the tabular presentation to reflect the levels, then the resulting tabular representation of $\mathbb{C}$ is shown at right in Figure 1.

At right, in the tabular representation corresponding to the LABFS decomposition we can read that there are levels L_0, L_2 and L_4 consisting of attributes and seen grouped in order at the column headings, and levels L_1, L_3 and L_5 consisting of objects, identified by the groupings at the row headings.

For example, L_1 is the attribute set {a-7,a-4,a-10,a-8}. Further, the subrelations E_i and S_i are easy to read off from the diagram: the subrelations S_i appear as consecutive rectangles, placed successively from the top left of the diagram down toward the bottom right, each with a line splitting its interior, indicating that the local object set (alternatively, local attribute set, depending on parity) is a union of two levels, namely L_i and L_{i+2} for the appropriate value of i.

In the following Lemma, we summarize the partitions we have established for a given graph-connected formal context.

LEMMA 9. *Let $\mathbb{K} = (O, A, E)$ be an r-rooted formal context. If, for $i \in \mathbb{N} \cup \{0\}$, we define L_i and S_i as above, then*

$$A = \bigsqcup_{i\in\mathbb{N}\cup\{0\}} L_{2i}, \quad O = \bigsqcup_{i\in\mathbb{N}\cup\{0\}} L_{2i+1}, \quad E = \bigsqcup_{i\in\mathbb{N}\cup\{0\}} E_i, \quad \textit{and} \quad E = \bigcup_{i\in\mathbb{N}\cup\{0\}} S_i.$$

3.2. LABFS-Induced Decomposition of the Concept Lattice. Figure 1 indicates (by example) that we can find concepts of the full context by looking within three consecutive levels. We make this rigorous by establishing a connection between the concept lattices of subrelations determined by the LABFS decomposition and the full concept lattice of the original relation.[2] While the intuitive content of this sequence of statements through Theorem 14 is very simple, the rigorous statement of the results allows the more difficult Corollary 16 to be expressed correctly.

DEFINITION 10. *Let $\mathbb{K} = (O, A, E)$ be an r-rooted formal context. We say concept $(P, B) \in \mathfrak{B}(\mathbb{K})$ is in r-concept level i provided*

$$\forall j < i, \quad (P \cup B) \cap L_j = \emptyset \quad \textit{and} \quad (P \cup B) \cap L_i \neq \emptyset\,.$$

Thus (P, B) is in concept level i provided that L_i is the first partition block, from the r-rooted LABFS decomposition of $\mathbb{K} = (O, A, E)$, that $P \cup B$ meets. To match traditional FCA notation, we let $\mathfrak{B}_i(\mathbb{K})$ denote the set of all concepts in concept level i.

The next sequence of statements establishes that the entire extent and intent of every concept of $\mathbb{K} = (O, A, E)$ must be included in three consecutive levels of the partition $\{L_0, L_1, ..., L_n\}$ of $O \cup A$.

LEMMA 11. *Let $\mathbb{K} = (O, A, E)$ be an r-rooted formal context and let X be a nonempty subset of $O \cup A$. For $X \subseteq L_i$ and $i \geq 0$, it follows $X' \subseteq L_{i-1} \cup L_{i+1}$.*

PROPOSITION 12. *Given an r-rooted formal context $\mathbb{K} = (O, A, E)$,*

$$\mathfrak{B}(\mathbb{K}) = \bigsqcup_{i\in\mathbb{N}\cup\{0\}} \mathfrak{B}_i(\mathbb{K}).$$

Also, if $(P, B) \in \mathfrak{B}_i(\mathbb{K})$, then

$$\begin{array}{ll} P \subseteq L_{i+1}, \quad B \subseteq L_i \cup L_{i+2} & \textit{if } i \textit{ is even,} \\ B \subseteq L_{i+1}, \quad P \subseteq L_i \cup L_{i+2} & \textit{if } i \textit{ is odd.} \end{array}$$

PROPOSITION 13. *Let $\mathbb{K} = (O, A, E)$ be a graph-connected formal context, and let a root $r \in A$ be given. Then $\mathfrak{B}_i(\mathbb{K}) \subseteq \mathfrak{B}(S_i)$.*

---

[2]The proofs of these statements can be found in [**3**].

Thus, the ith r-concept level of an r-rooted formal context is included in the set of formal concepts of S_i, its ith LABFS subrelation. Unfortunately, the reverse inclusion does not hold, but the following theorem shows that the set of non-trivial concepts in $\mathfrak{B}(S_i)$ that intersect L_i consists of formal concepts of $\mathbb{K}$ that are in the r-concept level i along with those ordered pairs (P, B) that generate (in $\mathbb{K}$) formal concepts in the r-concept level $i-1$.

THEOREM 14. *Let* $\mathbb{K} = (O, A, E)$ *be an r-rooted formal context. If* $(P, B) \in \mathfrak{B}(S_i)$, *with* $P \neq \emptyset$, $B \neq \emptyset$ *and* $L_i \cap (P \cup B) \neq \emptyset$, *then*

(1) *If* $(P \cup B) \cap L_{i+2} \neq \emptyset$, *then* $(P, B) \in \mathfrak{B}_i(\mathbb{K})$.
(2) *If* $(P \cup B) \cap L_{i+2} = \emptyset$, *then*
There exists $(Q, C) \in \mathfrak{B}_{i-1}(\mathbb{K})$ *such that* $P \subseteq Q$ *and* $B \subseteq C$, *or* $(P, B) \in \mathfrak{B}_i(\mathbb{K})$.

If the concept lattice is stripped of its least and greatest element, and we consider the symmetrization of the resulting order relation of the stripped lattice, then the concept levels determined (by definition) from a rooted LABFS of the associated formal context are equivalent to the levels determined by a rooted LABFS of the symmetrized order structure from the root equal to the concept generated by the root element used in the context. We now give a more rigorous description of this relationship between LABFS of a context and LABFS of its concept lattice.

Recall the standard attribute set embedding $\mu : A \to \mathfrak{B}(\mathbb{K})$ given by

$$\mu(a) = (\{a\}', \{a\}'') ,$$

and the corresponding object embedding γ. To ease the description of the concept lattice of the subrelation generated from the root r and the elements in all the levels up to some level L_i, we extend the usual notation, by defining $\mu[B] = (B', B'')$, for $B \subseteq A$, and similarly, $\gamma[P] = (P'', P')$, for $P \subseteq O$.

DEFINITION 15. *Fix* $\mathbb{K} = (O, A, E)$. *For any subset* $B \subseteq A$, *define*

$$\downarrow_{\mathfrak{B}(\mathbb{K})} \mu[B] = \bigcup_{b \in B} \{C \in \mathfrak{B}(\mathbb{K}) \mid b \in intent(C)\}$$

and for $P \subseteq O$

$$\uparrow_{\mathfrak{B}(\mathbb{K})} \gamma[P] = \bigcup_{p \in P} \{C \in \mathfrak{B}(\mathbb{K}) \mid p \in extent(C)\}.$$

These subsets of $\mathfrak{B}(\mathbb{K})$ are also known as the order ideal of $\mathfrak{B}(\mathbb{K})$ determined by $\mu[B]$ and the order filter of $\mathfrak{B}(\mathbb{K})$ determined by $\gamma[P]$, where γ and μ are the object- and attribute-embedding maps presented in [**10**]. Our purpose in introducing these subsets of $\mathfrak{B}(\mathbb{K})$ is to describe the connection between the unions

$$\bigcup_{j=0,1,\dots,i} \mathfrak{B}_j(\mathbb{K}) ,$$

which are clearly nested as i ranges from 0 to its maximum value, and the concepts of unions of the subrelations S_j. Note that if L_0, L_1, ..., L_{k-1}, L_k is the full list of levels of an r-rooted formal context $\mathbb{K}$, then

$$\mathfrak{B}(\mathbb{K}) = \bigcup_{j=1,\dots,k-1} \mathfrak{B}_j(\mathbb{K}) .$$

COROLLARY 16. *Let $\mathbb{K} = (O, A, E)$ be an r-rooted formal context, such that the intent of $1_{\mathfrak{B}(\mathbb{K})}$ is empty and the extent of $0_{\mathfrak{B}(\mathbb{K})}$ is empty. Let $i \in \mathbb{Z}$ satisfy $i \geq 2$. Define the formal context $\mathbb{K}_i = (O_i, A_i, U_i)$ by setting*

$$U_i = \bigcup_{j=0,1,\ldots,i-2} S_j,$$

and letting O_i and A_i be the domain and codomain of U_i, respectively. Let $\mathcal{C}_i$ be the set of concepts (P, B) of $\mathbb{K}_i$ such that $P \neq \emptyset$ and $B \neq \emptyset$ and $P \cup B \not\subseteq L_{i-1} \cup L_i$. Then $\mathcal{C}_i$ is equal to

$$[(\bigcup_{j<i-2,\ j\ odd} \uparrow_{\mathfrak{B}(\mathbb{K})} \gamma[L_j]) \setminus 1_{\mathfrak{B}(\mathbb{K})}] \cup [\bigcup_{j\leq i-2,\ j\ even} \downarrow_{\mathfrak{B}(\mathbb{K})} \mu[L_j]) \setminus 0_{\mathfrak{B}(\mathbb{K})}] .$$

The most important step in the proof involves the fact that the concepts in $\mathcal{C}_i$ are all in $\mathfrak{B}(\mathbb{K})$ by Theorem 14, because of the condition $P \cup B \not\subseteq L_{i-1} \cup L_i$ and the definition of U_i.

Of course, a corresponding statement can be made for odd values of i. The key point to take from Corollary 16 is that for increasing values of i, the unions that express the concepts in $\mathcal{C}_i$ are nested, so that, as i grows – that is, as the LABFS decomposition of $\mathbb{K}$ unfolds the full relation – the union expresses which are the corresponding concepts in the full concept lattice. The appearance of the levels L_j in the unions expressing $\mathcal{C}_i$ indicates the tight connection between LABFS levels and the concepts they generate.

3.3. Unfolding a Concept Lattice Using LABFS. In practice, the effect of Corollary 16 is that we can choose a root, say, some attribute $r \in A$, and unfold the lattice diagram from the corresponding attribute concept $\mu(r)$. Suppose the rooted LABFS decomposition has been determined, and we have limited our attention to the subcontext generated by the union of the subrelations S_j, as in Corollary 16. The concepts of $\mathfrak{B}(\mathbb{K})$ that can be computed from this subrelation are, first, those non-trivial concepts below $\mu(r)$, the concept determined by the root r. Next we compute those concepts which include objects in L_1 in their extent but exclude r in their intent; this includes the attribute concepts $(\{\alpha\}', \{\alpha\}'')$ with $\alpha \in L_2$, except for those such that $\alpha \rightarrow r$. Next come the concepts which include attributes in L_2 (except for the attribute concepts which have already appeared), and so on, up to L_i, save for those two-part concepts (described in Theorem 14) including only elements from L_{i-1} and L_i which must be verified in the full context $\mathbb{K} = (O, A, E)$. In this section, we first present an example illustrating the unfolding of the concept lattice from a root concept, and follow that with a discussion of the utility of unfolding in the context of viewing association rules via a concept lattice.

Now consider the formal context $\mathbb{F}$ in Figure 2, with 14 objects and 13 attributes, already arranged to display the attr-1–rooted LABFS decomposition. This synthetic data is both sparse and connected. The context is followed by the lattice $\mathfrak{B}(\mathbb{F})$, with 34 concepts and 69 edges.

The concept lattice in Figure 3 is drawn using Concept Explorer [**17**]. After minimal manipulation of the diagram, we see that its structure is that of a 4-fence

	attr-1	attr-2	attr-3	attr-4	attr-5	attr-6	attr-7	attr-8	attr-9	attr-10	attr-11	attr-12	attr-13
obj-1	X	X											
obj-2		X	X										
obj-3			X	X									
obj-4				X	X								
obj-5					X	X							
obj-6					X		X						
obj-7						X	X						
obj-8							X	X					
obj-9								X	X				
obj-10									X	X			
obj-11										X	X	X	
obj-12										X	X		X
obj-13										X		X	X
obj-14											X	X	X

FIGURE 2. A graph-connected formal context $\mathbb{F}$, in LABFS-specific tabular form.

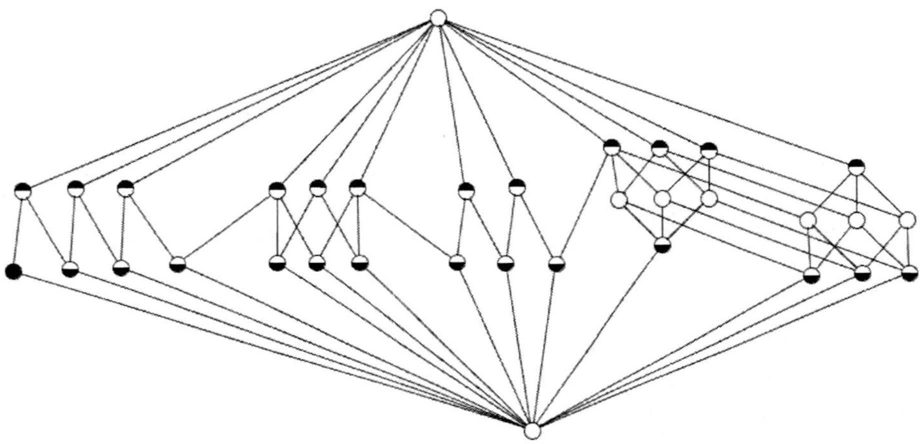

FIGURE 3. The lattice $\mathfrak{B}(\mathbb{F})$ corresponding to the formal context depicted in Figure 2 as drawn by Concept Explorer.

lattice[3] glued at a coatom to a Boolean algebra with 3 atoms, glued at a coatom to a 3-fence lattice with one additional leg, glued at a coatom to a Boolean algebra with 4 atoms (a j-fence lattice is a j-fence with a top and bottom added).

The software supporting our theoretical work is the program DCOMP that implements both the rooted LABFS decompositions we are discussing in this section and also the peeling decomposition to appear in the next section. This software is very primitive and was used only to test theoretical constructions, and is not intended for actual use by epidemiologists. The feature of DCOMP that we use now is its conversion of an input of a formal context and a root to an output of the LABFS decomposition of the relation. After the initial information of data and root is specified, the program also allows the user to output the subcontext generated by

[3]A *fence* is a "zig-zag" ordered set which simply alternates up and down relations, from a minimal element, up to a maximal element, down to a different minimal element, up to a different maximal element, and so on. A 4-fence has four minimal elements and four maximal elements.

```
FenceBA-3FenceBA-4.txt
| 27 | 13 | 14 | 32 | 0.175824
Root | # of Vert | # of Edges | # of Levels
attr-1 27 32 20
L0 1 1 1.0 (0,0)          L10 2 3 0.75 (11,12)
L1 1 1 1.0 (1,1)          L11 2 1 0.5 (13,14)
L2 1 1 1.0 (2,2)          L12 1 1 1.0 (15,15)
L3 1 1 1.0 (3,3)          L13 1 1 1.0 (16,16)
L4 1 1 1.0 (4,4)          L14 1 1 1.0 (17,17)
L5 1 1 1.0 (5,5)          L15 1 1 1.0 (18,18)
L6 1 1 1.0 (6,6)          L16 1 3 1.0 (19,19)
L7 1 1 1.0 (7,7)          L17 3 6 0.66 (20,22)
L8 1 2 1.0 (8,8)          L18 3 3 1.0 (23,25)
L9 2 2 0.5 (9,10)         L19 1 0 0 (26 26)
```

FIGURE 4. The LABFS overview of $\mathbb{F}$, produced by DCOMP.

	attr-1	attr-2	attr-3	attr-4	attr-5	attr-6	attr-7
obj-1	X	X					
obj-2		X	X				
obj-3			X	X			
obj-4				X	X		
obj-5					X	X	
obj-6					X		X
obj-7						X	X
obj-8							X

FIGURE 5. The subcontext $\mathbb{F}_{0-11}$ of $\mathbb{F}$, viewed in ConExp.

levels L_i through L_j, for $i < j$. The concept lattice of the output subcontext can then be viewed in Concept Explorer [**17**]. Figure 4 shows the output of DCOMP on the input of the context in Figure 2, and its functions also include the determination of the context generated by subrelation $S_0 \cup S_1 \cup \ldots \cup S_9$, and finally the conversion of that subcontext to the input format of Concept Explorer.

In its command line window, DCOMP displays the statistics associated with each new level, and between new levels and the previous level. The display shows the number of new vertices in level L_i, the number of edges from level L_i to level L_{i+1}, and the density of edges relative to the maximum possible $|L_i \times L_{i+1}|$. This feature provides an overview of the LABFS results, relative to root r (in the example shown, $r =$attr-1), so that sparser sections of the data can be distinguished from less sparse sections. In Figure 4, DCOMP indicates the portions of the binary relation that form a fence: the consecutive levels reading "$Li \quad 1 \quad 1 \quad 1.0 \quad (j, j)$" indicate levels of the LABFS that have one new vertex, one edge to level L_{i+1}, density 1.0, and where the new vertices range from j to j in the index list.

After the LABFS overview, DCOMP allows the user to output the subcontext generated by levels L_i to L_j. For example below, by requesting levels L_0 through L_{11}, the subrelation $S_0 \cup S_1 \cup \ldots \cup S_9$ is saved to a file, and similarly by requesting levels L_{11} through L_{19}, the subrelation $S_{11} \cup S_{12} \cup \ldots \cup S_{19}$ is saved to a file. If requested, DCOMP also converts a given context to the input format of Concept Explorer (briefly, ConExp), so its lattice can be viewed.

	attr-8	attr-9	attr-10	attr-11	attr-12	attr-13
obj-8	X					
obj-9	X	X				
obj-10		X	X			
obj-11			X	X	X	
obj-12			X	X		X
obj-13			X		X	X
obj-14				X	X	X

FIGURE 6. The subcontext $\mathbb{F}_{11-19}$ of $\mathbb{F}$, viewed in ConExp.

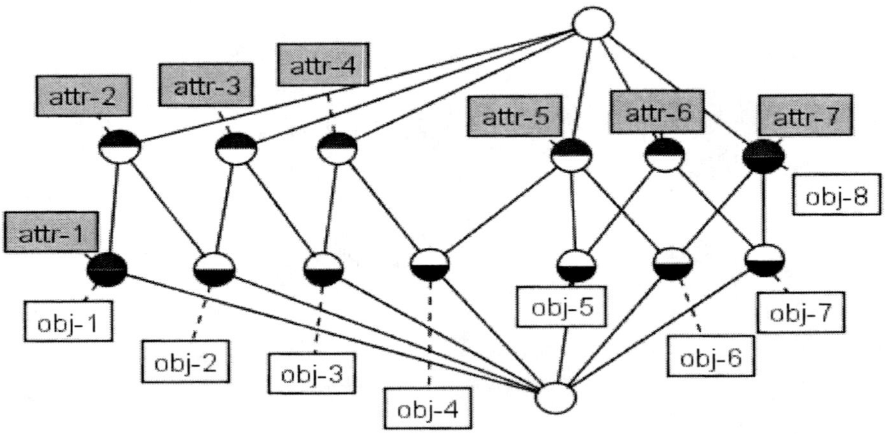

FIGURE 7. The lattice of the subcontext $\mathbb{F}_{0-11}$ in Figure 5, viewed in ConExp.

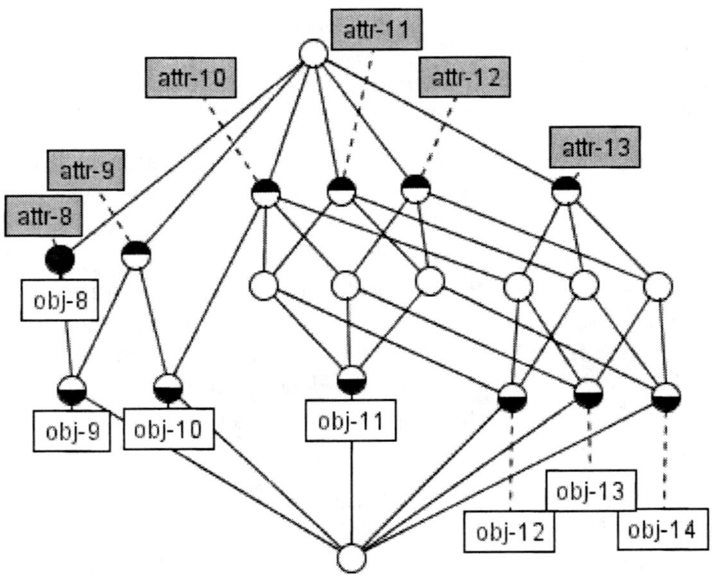

FIGURE 8. The lattice of the subcontext $\mathbb{F}_{11-19}$ in Figure 6, viewed in ConExp.

In Figure 7, note that the concept generated by obj-8 in the subcontext is not the same concept generated in the full context of Figure 2 (it does not include attr-8 as it should), but all other concepts are concepts of the full context. As stated above, only concepts determined exclusively from elements of the last two levels need to be checked for their standing in the full context – all others are "real". A similar comment applies to Figure 8, so that the only concept from the full concept lattice $\mathfrak{B}(\mathbb{F})$ that does not appear in the lattice $\mathfrak{B}(\mathbb{F}_{0-11})$, nor in $\mathfrak{B}(\mathbb{F}_{11-19})$, is the object concept $(\{\text{obj-8}\}'', \{\text{obj-8}\}')$.

Through this example we have shown how DCOMP can be used to view various portions of a lattice, as defined by reference to a chosen root. It should be clear by this point that had we successively viewed the lattices of the subcontexts $\mathbb{F}_{0-3}$, $\mathbb{F}_{0-4}$, $\mathbb{F}_{0-5}$, $\mathbb{F}_{0-6}$ and so on, concluding with the subcontext $\mathbb{F}_{0-19}$, that we would see the full concept lattice unfold before us from the chosen root.

We have not yet implemented a lattice viewer that visually contrasts actual concepts (of the full context) with those that may only be two-part concepts (again, as in Theorem 14). Thus in viewing the lattices of subcontexts we are left to determine which concepts are concepts of the full subrelation. However, flagging the actual concepts should not pose any great challenge, since the results we have presented provide sufficient information to compute only those concepts of induced subcontexts that are in the full concept lattice.

3.4. Rooted LABFS and Association Rules. From the artificial example just considered and Theorem 14, it is apparent that these results regarding the LABFS decomposition may allow (depending on the depth of the relation) an efficient localized computation of the concept lattice. A judicious choice of a root will impact the level of lattice unfolding, and since the complexity of LABFS is linear on the number of edges of the corresponding graph, we foresee that inexpensive searches will help make this choice. The sparser the data, the more useful we expect the LABFS decomposition to be in providing such localization. If in addition the diameter of the associated graph is large then by choosing antipodal roots one expects more lattice unfolding.

On the other hand, the worst-case context $(\{1, 2, 3, ..., n\}, \{1, 2, 3, ..., n\}, \neq)$ is not decomposed at all by LABFS, as any element chosen as root will yield only levels L_0, L_1 and L_2, so the only subrelation is S_0, and it is not a proper subrelation.

The translation of LABFS into the concept lattice allows the lattice to be unfolded from a root attribute. If we determine a subrelation from levels L_0, L_1, L_2, and L_3, then all concepts with the root in their intent will be present, and all these concepts are concepts of the full lattice. Further, any concepts with attributes from L_2 in their intent will have their full extents represented, since we extended as far as L_3, though they may be missing attributes in their intent. An association rule, say $\{\alpha, \beta, \delta\} \to \rho$, has its confidence value $conf_{\mathbb{K}}(\ \{\alpha, \beta, \delta\} \to \rho\ )$ determined by dividing the cardinality of the concept extent $\{\alpha, \beta, \delta\}'$ by the cardinality of the concept extent $\{\alpha, \beta, \delta, \rho\}'$. Suppose we compute $\mathbb{K}_3(\rho)$ from a given context $\mathbb{K}$. If we are focused on what (nearly) implies ρ, there are two advantages offered by working in $\mathbb{K}_3(\rho)$ instead of $\mathbb{K}$: first, only attributes related to ρ through some objects will appear in $\mathfrak{B}(\mathbb{K}_3(\rho))$, e.g. $\alpha, \beta, \delta \in A$ with $\{\alpha, \beta, \delta, \rho\}' \neq \emptyset$; second, the presence of the full ($\mathbb{K}$-)extents for the related concepts $\mu[\{\alpha, \beta, \delta, \rho\}]$ and $\mu[\{\alpha, \beta, \delta\}]$ in $\mathbb{K}_3(\rho)$ ensures that

$$conf_{\mathbb{K}}(\ \{\alpha, \beta, \delta\} \to \rho\ ) = conf_{\mathbb{K}_3(\rho)}(\ \{\alpha, \beta, \delta\} \to \rho\ )\ .$$

A similar observation regarding support can be made as long as we divide by the cardinality $|O|$ of the full object set instead of the cardinality of $O_j(\rho)$, the object set of $\mathbb{K}_j(\rho)$.

Thus, limiting our attention to only levels L_0, L_1, L_2 and L_3 corresponds to a query mode for considering association rules that have the root in their conclusion. Beyond these first three levels, DCOMP can indicate how many objects and attributes will be picked up, and the user can decide how deeply to go before truncating to a subcontext. If this is not possible, another root can be chosen for separate examination.

3.5. Discussion. The determination of the LABFS decomposition(s) associated with a formal context provides an overview of the data – crucial when the data is large, since the lattice will be too large to view (or even possibly to store) – and the results we have presented provide sufficient information to compute only those concepts of LABFS-induced subcontexts that are in the full concept lattice.

We make one final note regarding the dependence of the depth of the LABFS output on the nature of the input. Even in the presence of very sparse connected data, a complementary attribute will disallow a LABFS decomposition from having any significant depth. Specifically, if a formal context includes complementary attributes α and ζ, and a root $\beta \in A$ is chosen which does not imply α and does not imply ζ (this will be the case for most epidemiological data, since, e.g., it is often recorded whether a member of a population is Male or Female), then the LABFS decomposition will present at most levels L_0, L_1, ..., L_4. This is because $L_1 = \{\beta\}'$ will include at least one object that satisfies α and at least one object that satisfies ζ, so L_2 must include the attributes α and ζ, which in turn forces L_3 to include all the remaining objects, and then L_4 must include any remaining attributes that did not appear in L_0 or L_2.

Generalizing these comments, note that if there are k attributes such that their neighborhoods correspond to a partition of the set of objects this means that they are mutually independent in the sense that there are no implications among them, and we could present a similar characterization of the depth of LABFS under assumptions that mirror those mentioned for a complementary pair. This suggests their identification and removal as a preprocessing step before applying LABFS. In any event, LABFS will be more effective if the root is chosen to maximize the number of levels in the decomposition. In graph theoretical terms this corresponds to choosing the root so that the number of levels is as close as possible to the diameter of the data bigraph. The results presented in this section constitute a first step in the larger program of decomposing the data bigraph in an efficient manner that translates into decompositions of the corresponding concept lattice. These techniques become imperative when the concept lattice becomes so large that it does not fit in random access memory, so that external memory algorithms are required [**4**]. Moreover, even if it fits in random access memory a fine graded decomposition allows its visual exploration on a monitor screen, the screen certainly being smaller than memory by several orders of magnitude [**2**].

4. Graph Peeling and Concept Lattices

In this section we recall the notion of graph peeling, apply it to graph-connected bigraphs, and discuss some relationships with the corresponding concept lattices. We conclude by applying peeling to an epidemiology dataset, in order to provide an indication of the potential applications we see for this research.

4.1. Peeling and Cardinality Conditions. Let $\mathbb{K} = (O, A, E)$ be a formal context. For each i, we define $\mathbb{K}_i = (O_i, A_i, E_i)$ to be the subcontext of $\mathbb{K}$ generated by *iteratively deleting* all elements that are related to i or less elements. Thus $\mathbb{K}_0 = (O_0, A_0, E_0)$ consists of the set O_0 of objects related to one or more attributes, the set A_0 of attributes related to one or more objects and E_0 is the induced subrelation $E \cap O_0 \times A_0$. For this first case no iteration is necessary, and if $\mathbb{K} = (O, A, E)$ is graph-connected then clearly no deletions occur. For the $i = 1$ case, the iterative deletion is necessary since some elements of degree 2 (or higher) may be related only to elements of degree 1, and only one step of deletion will not delete these elements. To be very clear on this point, we make a formal definition:

DEFINITION 17. *Given $\mathbb{K} = (O, A, E)$ and $i \geq 1$, consider the following sets:*

$$O_{i,1} = \{g \in O : |g'| > i\} \qquad A_{i,1} = \{a \in A : |a'| > i\}$$

$$O_{i,2} = \{g \in O_{i,1} : |g' \cap A_{i,1}| > i\} \qquad A_{i,2} = \{a \in A_{i,1} : |a' \cap O_{i,1}| > i\}$$

$$O_{i,3} = \{g \in O_{i,2} : |g' \cap A_{i,2}| > i\} \qquad A_{i,3} = \{a \in A_{i,2} : |a' \cap O_{i,2}| > i\}$$

and in general

$$O_{i,n} = \{g \in O_{i,n-1} : |g' \cap A_{i,n-1}| > i\} \qquad A_{i,n} = \{a \in A_{i,n-1} : |a' \cap O_{i,n-1}| > i\}.$$

for all $n \geq 2$.[4] *We set*

$$O_i = \cap_{n\geq 1} O_{i,n} \qquad A_i = \cap_{n\geq 1} A_{i,n} \qquad \text{and} \qquad E_i = E \cap (O_i \times A_i)\ ,$$

and finally, $\mathbb{K}_i = (O_i, A_i, E_i)$, which we call the ith peeled subcontext of $\mathbb{K}$.

DEFINITION 18. *The core of formal context $\mathbb{K} = (O, A, E)$ is that peeled subcontext $\mathbb{K}_N = (O_N, A_N, E_N)$ such that N is the greatest integer for which $O_N \cup A_N$ is non-empty.*

---

[4]Since we are only considering finite bigraphs, there exists some M such that $O_{i,M} = O_{i,M+1}$ and $A_{i,M} = A_{i,M+1}$.

With the definitions given above, we can also consider the subcontext $\mathbb{K}_{i,j} = (O_i, A_j, E_{i,j})$, where $E_{i,j} = E \cap (O_i \times A_j)$. It has been shown that $\mathbb{K}_i$ is the largest subcontext of $\mathbb{K} = (O, A, E)$ such that every element has degree $i+1$ or greater. In graph theoretical terms, it is the largest induced subgraph such that each vertex is of degree greater than or equal to $i+1$.

PROPOSITION 19. *If $X \subseteq A_i$ and $|X| > i$, then $X^E = X^{E_i}$. Dually, for $Y \subseteq O_i$, if $|Y| > i$, then $Y^E = Y^{E_i}$.*

PROOF. Suppose $X \subseteq A_i$ and $|X| > i$. Since $E_i \subseteq E$, Lemma 6 directly states that $X^{E_i} = X^E$. For the converse, suppose $g \in X^E$. Then $|g^E| > i$ and in particular g is related to $i+1$ or more elements of X, all of which are in A_i, so $g \in O_i$, since $\mathbb{K}_i$ is the largest subcontext of $\mathbb{K}$ in which every element has degree $i+1$ or greater. Thus $g \in X^{E_i}$ and thus $X^E \subseteq X^{E_i}$. □

COROLLARY 20. *For any $A, B \subseteq A_i$ with $|A| > i$, we have*

$$conf_{\mathbb{K}}(A,B) = conf_{\mathbb{K}_i}(A,B) \ .$$

PROOF. Suppose $A, B \subseteq A_i$ with $|A| > i$. By definition,

$$conf_{\mathbb{K}}(A,B) = \frac{|A^E \cap B^E|}{|A^E|} = \frac{|(A \cup B)^E|}{|A^E|} \ .$$

Since $|A| > i$, it follows that $|A \cup B| > i$, so by Proposition 19,

$$\frac{|(A \cup B)^E|}{|A^E|} = \frac{|(A \cup B)^{E_i}|}{|A^{E_i}|} = conf_{\mathbb{K}_i}(A,B) \ .$$

□

COROLLARY 21. *For $X \subseteq A_i$, if $|X| > i$, then for any $j \leq i$, $X^E = X^{E_{j,i}}$.*

PROOF. Suppose $X \subseteq A_i$ with $|X| > i$. For $j \leq i$, $E_i = E_{i,i} \subseteq E_{j,i} \subseteq E$, so repeated application of Lemma 6 yields

$$X^{E_i} = X^{E_{i,i}} \subseteq X^{E_{j,i}} \subseteq X^E \ .$$

As $|X| > i$, we conclude from Proposition 19 that $X^{E_i} = X^E$, whence $X^{E_{j,i}} = X^E$. □

In order to discuss the strength of the Proposition, we will employ the complete bipartite graph from k vertices to k vertices. For the purposes of constructing examples, we create concrete versions of the complete binary relation by setting $\mathcal{K}_k = (U(k), V(k), \nabla_{k,k})$, where $U(k) = \{o_1, o_2, ..., o_k\}$, $V(k) = \{a_1, a_2, ..., a_k\}$, and $\nabla_{k,k} = U(k) \times V(k)$, ($\nabla_{k,k}$ is the all-relation from $U(k)$ to $V(k)$).

Example 1. Consider the binary relation $\mathcal{L} = (U(k+1) \cup \{g\}, V(k+1), F)$ where

$$F = \nabla_{k+1,k+1} \cup (\{g\} \times \{a_1, a_2, ..., a_k\}) \ .$$

If we set $X = \{a_1, a_2, ..., a_k\}$, then $X \subseteq V(k+1)_k$ and $g \notin (U(k+1) \cup \{g\})_k$ (since $g' = \{a_1, a_2, ..., a_k\}$), so $g \notin X^{F_k}$, but $g \in X^F$. Thus $X \subseteq V(k+1)_k$ and $|X| = k$, but $X^F \neq X^{F_k}$, which shows the cardinality condition in Proposition 19 cannot be weakened.

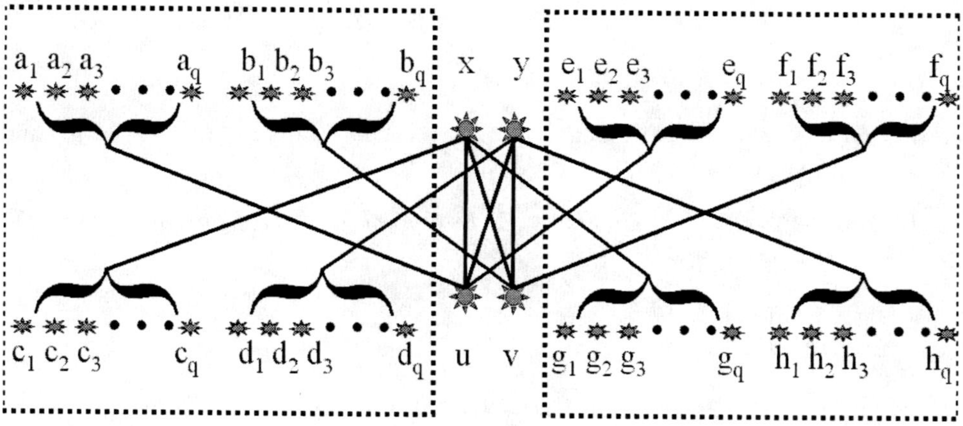

FIGURE 9. A binary relation built from two copies of $\mathcal{K}_{k+1}$.

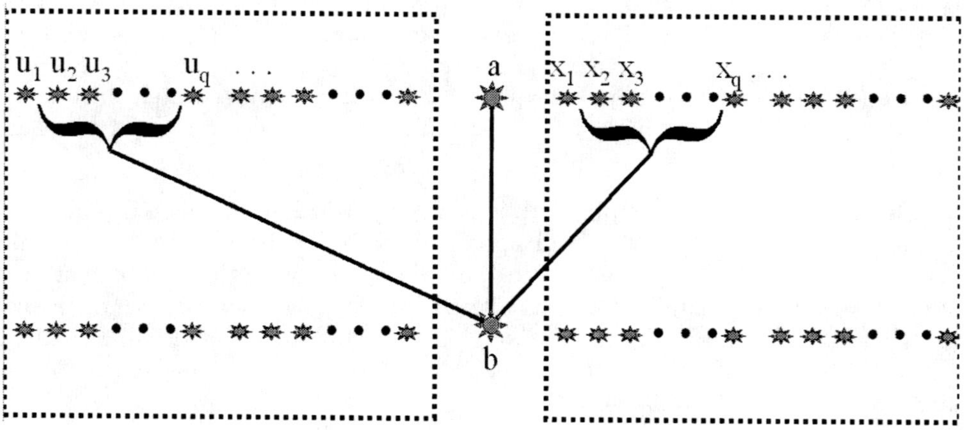

FIGURE 10. Another binary relation built from two copies of $\mathcal{K}_{k+1}$

Example 2. Now we consider two copies of $\mathcal{K}_{k+1} = (U(k+1), V(k+1), \nabla_{k+1,k+1})$, depicted in Figure 9 in dotted boxes at left and right (without the all-relation shown), where $q = \lceil \frac{k+1}{2} \rceil$, with four additional elements x, y, u and z appended. Suppose E is the binary relation depicted in the Figure 9.

If we set $X = \{x, y\}$, then the fact that $E_k = E$ (the kth peeled subcontext is the same as the original since all elements have degree $k+1$ or greater) implies that $X^E = X^{E_k}$, but $|X| = 2$, so this shows the converse does not hold for $k = 2, 3, 4, \ldots$.

Example 3. The last two examples show that Proposition 19, involving only a cardinality condition, cannot be strengthened. Even under the assumptions of Proposition 19, it does *not* follow that $(X^E)^E = (X^E)^{E_k}$. Consider the combination of two copies of $\mathcal{K}_{k+1}$ in Figure 10, this time with only two additional elements a and b appended (again $q = \lceil \frac{k+1}{2} \rceil$).

Suppose the binary relation depicted here is (O, A, E). Setting

$$X = \{u_1, u_2, u_3, ..., u_q, x_1, x_2, x_3, ..., x_q\} ,$$

we have $b \in X^E = X^{E_k}$ (in fact $\{b\} = X^E = X^{E_k}$), but $a \in (X^E)^E) = b^E$ and $a \notin (X^E)^{E_k}$, since $a \notin A_k$.

PROPOSITION 22. *Let $\mathbb{K} = (O, A, E)$ be a graph-connected formal context. For $B \subseteq A$, if $|B^E| > k$ and $|B^{EE}| > k$, then*

(1) $B^E \subseteq O_k$ *and* $B^{EE} \subseteq A_k$
(2) $(B^E, B^{EE}) = (B^{E_k}, B^{E_k E_k}) \in \mathfrak{B}(\mathbb{K}_k)$

Thus, for $(H, N) \in \mathfrak{B}(\mathbb{K})$, if $\min\{|H|, |N|\} \geq k + 1$, *then* $(H, N) \in \mathfrak{B}(\mathbb{K}_k)$.

PROOF. Under the given assumptions, the concept $(B^E, B^{EE}) \in \mathfrak{B}(\mathbb{K})$ yields the subrelation $B^E \times B^{EE}$ of E, and each vertex of this subrelation has degree $k + 1$ or more. Thus $B^E \times B^{EE}$ is also a subset of $E_k = (O_k \times A_k) \cap E$, s $B^E \subseteq O_k$ and $B^{EE} \subseteq A_k$. This proves 1. above. Since $B^E \subseteq O_k$, it follows that $B^E = B^{E_k}$. Thus $(B^E)^{E_k} = (B^{E_k})^{E_k}$, but $(B^E)^E \subseteq A_k$, so $(B^E)^{E_k} = (B^E)^E$, whence $(B^{E_k})^{E_k} = (B^E)^E$, and this proves 2. Finally, the last statement follows by setting $B = N$ and applying 2. □

This Proposition gives simple conditions through which we can identify concepts of the full formal context that will appear in their "real" form in the concept lattice of one of the peeled subcontexts, i.e. will appear with their full extent and intent. Note that Example 2 above, with $B = \{x, y\}$, so that $B^E = \{u, v\}$ and $(B^E)^E = \{x, y\}$, satisfies both $B^E \subseteq O_k$ and $(B^E)^E \subseteq A_k$ but does not satisfy either $|B^E| > k$ nor $|B^{EE}| > k$ for any $k > 1, 2, 3, ...$ Again this shows that a direct converse is not available.

Note that Proposition 22 indicates that we can naturally partition the concept lattice of $\mathbb{K} = (O, A, E)$ using the subcontexts determined via the peeling decomposition, by assigning concept $(H, N) \in \mathfrak{B}(\mathbb{K})$ to concept peeling level j provided that j is the greatest value such that $(H, N) \in \mathfrak{B}(\mathbb{K}_j)$. More theoretical work is needed to determine the connection between $\mathfrak{B}(\mathbb{K})$ and $\mathfrak{B}(\mathbb{K}_j)$, and this is a topic we will address in later reports.

4.2. Experimentation With Peeling Applied to Epidemiological Data. Having laid out some initial theoretical statements relating peeling and the concept lattice, we now turn our attention to our *first experiments* regarding the practical utility of the peeling decomposition. The software implementing the peeling algorithm is PEEL, a part of the program DCOMP mentioned in the previous section. The user first loads data (recorded as an edge list or in tabular form using 0 and 1 values to present relations) – in this figure we have loaded a binary relation 18858 × 80, representing colon-rectum cancer cases and their properties, that is a fragment of the SEER cancer registry – and then can choose from the options shown in Figure 11.

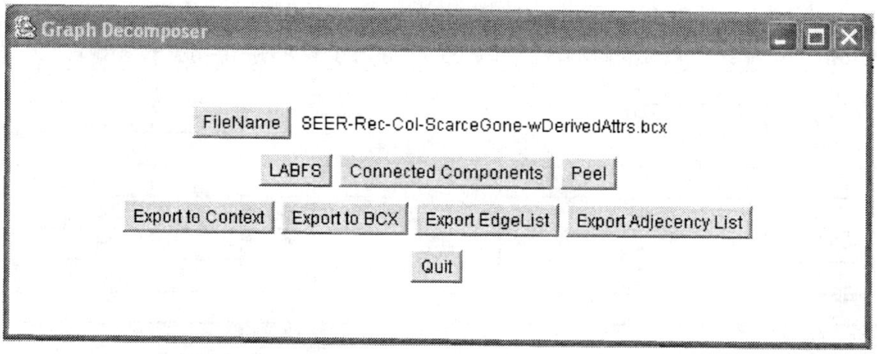

FIGURE 11. The functions available in DCOMP.

The user can apply rooted LABFS to the data, can peel the data, and can export the data to a ConExp readable formal context, or to a Seqer readable formal context (a .bcx file).[5]

In the program, the user requests the PEEL interface, and then enters a pair of values $< i\ j >$, with $i \leq j$. The program will then output the subcontext with domain $(O_{i-1} \setminus O_i) \cup (O_{j-1} \setminus O_j)$, codomain $(A_{i-1} \setminus A_i) \cup (A_{j-1} \setminus A_j)$, and binary relation

$$[(O_{i-1} \setminus O_i) \times (A_{j-1} \setminus A_j)) \cap E] \cup [(O_{j-1} \setminus O_j) \times (A_{i-1} \setminus A_i) \cap E].$$

More intuitively, the "level i" vertices are those vertices that survived the level 1 peeling, the level 2 peeling, the level 3 peeling, etc, up to the level $i-1$ peeling, but will be deleted exactly when the condition "iteratively delete vertices of degree i or less" is invoked, and similarly for "level j", while the only edges that peeling will produce from the $< i\ j >$ command are those from level i to level j (not including edges within level i, nor within level j.

Along with the SEER data, we also considered the well-known Mushroom Database from the UCI KDD Repository [**12**]. This dataset, consisting of 8124 mushrooms and 119 properties of mushrooms, has density 0.193, and yields 32086 concepts. The iceberg lattices[6] of this dataset were considered in [**14**], where it was found that, e.g., there are only 7, 12, and 30 concepts with 85%, 70%, and 55% or greater support, respectively. We applied the peeling decomposition to this dataset and found that the core yielded a reduction to 8031 mushrooms and 110 of their properties. In other words, only 93 mushrooms were deleted, while 9 properties were deleted. Another dataset we considered consisted of properties of all cases of violent death in the state of Massachusetts in year 2000, with 992 cases and 24 of their attributes (provided by D. Ozonoff and available from the authors); we call this the Violent Deaths dataset. This dataset has density .290. Once peeled to its core, we have 951 cases and 22 attributes remaining, with 0.318 density, so again this is an unremarkable reduction.

---

[5]Both ConExp and Seqer are concept lattice viewers, with the latter software developed at the Physical Science Laboratory of New Mexico State University.

[6]An iceberg lattice is a concept lattice with all concepts not meeting a support threshold deleted, where the threshold is user defined. Trimming a concept lattice in this way is equivalent to pruning a table of rules to the set of rules that meet or exceed a user-defined support threshold.

Support Cutoff	Size of Corresponding Iceberg Lattice
0%	32086
10%	4885
20%	1197
30%	427
40%	140
50%	45
55%	30
70%	12
85%	7

Support Cutoff	Size of Corresponding Iceberg Lattice
0%	42695
10%	2382
20%	528
30%	179
40%	74
50%	29
55%	20
70%	80
85%	3

FIGURE 12. Tables showing sizes of iceberg lattices of the mushroom database (left) and the core of the SEER colon-rectum fragment (right).

The fragment of the SEER dataset that we consider (properties of all cases of colon-rectum cancer in the SEER registry database) has 18858 cases and 80 of their attributes. This dataset has density .278. Once peeled to its core, we have only 406 cases remaining and 50 attributes, with 0.5 density. Here we see a drastic reduction of both the object and attribute sets. Further, we note the original total of 42000+ edges has been reduced to a little over 10000 edges. The SEER example indicates that the global density value alone will not tell the story, since peeling does drastically reduce the SEER dataset, even with its 0.27 density. Further research on the degree distribution of the elements of the binary relation should indicate how we can compute whether peeling will provide drastic reduction.

One important aspect of these initial peeling results is that these datasets included a large number or complementary attributes. If we limit the datasets to a subset of attributes with no disjoint attributes, the results are quite different. For example, the mushroom database, restricted to 22 non-disjoint (overlapping) attributes is peeled from 8124 objects to only 43 objects, and 22 attributes to 21 attributes. A similarly limited subset of the Violent Deaths dataset, of size 992×7, is reduced to 51×7 on peeling to the core. Finally, limiting the SEER fragment to 18858×12 yields a core of size 15×11. Thus, we see drastic differences in the effects of peeling between datasets involving complementary attributes and those involving only overlapping attributes. Future work will address optimal handling of $k-$complementary attributes, in both LABFS and peeling decompositions. We believe that relationships discovered within these special subsets of the original dataset will need to be validated against the full dataset, since we have so drastically limited the data. However, we also note that this final step of validation is a far cry from simply querying the full dataset, since we were drawn to special subsets through features of the data itself.

In conclusion, in Figure 12 we report some sizes of the iceberg lattices of the Mushroom database and also of the core of the SEER data already mentioned, to give an idea of what we see might be the next steps of analysis. Note that in the Mushroom database, only 15% of the concepts (4885 of the 32086 total) have 10%

or greater support, and in the core of the SEER data the 10% filter is even more effective, leaving only 5.4% of the full set of concepts.

We make one final note that indicates some of the future challenges we see on the road ahead. Once peeling has reduced our attention to the lattice, or iceberg lattice, of the core, any relationships that are derived within this context must be evaluated within the original, full dataset. The lattice viewer Seqer includes a rule capture component, from within which other datasets can be chosen to evaluate rules against. Thus, if we generate a rule from the core of a dataset, we can validate the rule by computing its value in the full dataset.

References

1. Agrawal, R., Imielinski, T. and A. Swami, A.: "Mining association rules between sets of items in large databases", in ACM SIGMOD Intl. Conf. Management of Data, May 1993.
2. J. Abello, J. Korn: "MGV: A System for Visualizing Massive Multidigraphs", IEEE Transactions on Visualization and Computer Graphics **8** No. 1, January-March 2002.
3. J. Abello, A. Pogel and L. Miller: "Breadth First Search Partitions and Concept Lattices", Journal of Universal Computer Science, Vol. 10, No. 8, 2004.
4. J. Abello, J. Vitter (eds): "External Memory Algorithms", Vol 50 of the AMS-DIMACS Series in Discrete Mathematics and Theorethical Computer Science, 1999.
5. J. Abello, M. Resende, and S. Sudarsky: "Massive Quasi-Clique Detection", In Proceedings of Latin American Informatics, Springer Verlag LNCS, May 2002.
6. A. Berry and A. Sigayret: "Representing a concept lattice by a graph", Proceedings of Discrete Maths and Data Mining Workshop, 2nd SIAM Conference on Data Mining (SDM'02), Arlington (VA), April 2002.
7. A. Berry and A. Sigayret: "Obtaining and maintaining polynomial-sized concept lattices", Proceedings of Workshop FCAKDD (Formal Concept Analysis for Knowledge Discovery in Data bases), ECCAI 02.
8. For an extensive reference list of FCA application papers see: `http://www.mathematik.tu-darmstadt.de/ags/ag1/Literatur/literatur_en.html`
9. Birkhoff, G.: "Lattice Theory", American Mathematical Society, Providence, R.I., 1st edition, 1940.
10. Ganter, B. and Wille, R.: "Formal Concept Analysis: Mathematical Foundations", Springer, NY, 1999. ISBN 3-540-62771-5
11. Freese, R.: "LatDrawWin, a lattice drawing applet", `www.math.hawaii.edu/~ralph/LatDraw`.
12. Hettich, S. and Bay, S. D., The UCI KDD Archive [`http://kdd.ics.uci.edu`]. Irvine, CA: University of California, Department of Information and Computer Science, 1999.
13. Ozonoff, D., Pogel, A., and Hannan, T., "Generalized Contingency Tables and Concept Lattices", this Volume.
14. Stumme, G., Taouil, R., Bastide, Y., Pasquier, N. and Lakhal, L.: "Computing iceberg concept lattices with Titanic", Data and Knowledge Engineering (Elsevier), 42 (2002), 189-222.
15. Stumme, G. and Wille, R.: "A Geometrical Heuristic for Drawing Concept Lattices", Graph Drawing (Springer-Verlag) (1995) 452-460.
16. Wille, R.: "Why Can Concept Lattices Support Knowledge Discovery in Databases?", Technische Universitat Darmstadt, Fachbereich Mathematik, Preprint Nr. 2158, June 2001. Available at `http://wwwbib.mathematik.tu-darmstadt.de/Math-Net/Preprints/Listen/pp01.html`
17. Yevtushenko, S., et al: "Concept Explorer", Open source java software available at `http://sourceforge.net/projects/conexp`, Release 1.2, 2003.
18. Zaki, M., and M. Ogihara, M.: "Theoretical Foundations of Associations Rules", in Proceedings of 3rd SIGMOD'98 Workshop on Research Issues in Data Mining and Knowledge Discovery (DMKD'98), Seattle, Washington, USA, June 1998.

DIMACS Research Institute, Rutgers University, Piscataway, NJ 08854, USA

E-mail address: abello@dimacs.rutgers.edu

Information Sciences, Physical Science Laboratory, New Mexico State University, Las Cruces, NM 88003, USA

E-mail address: Alex.Pogel@psl.nmsu.edu

DIMACS Series in Discrete Mathematics
and Theoretical Computer Science
Volume **70**, 2006

Using Transmission Dynamics Models to Validate Vaccine Efficacy Measures Prior to Conducting HIV Vaccine Efficacy Trials

Kamal Desai, Marie-Claude Boily, Benoît Mâsse, and Roy M. Anderson

ABSTRACT. Mathematical models of disease transmission have proven useful in gaining epidemiological insights into dynamics of infection and informing public health decisions for their control. Such models are now finding applications in the design of expensive clinical trials against HIV to inform statistical parameters, such as sample size, trial duration and efficacy analyses. We illustrate the use of clinical trial simulation to address a methodological problem in estimating efficacy in trials of vaccines against HIV. Because of unknown or poorly understood models of vaccine action, uncertain time-lags in immunity, and the many heterogeneities that influence exposure to HIV, traditional efficacy measures, based on the estimation of hazard rates or on cumulative incidence, produce estimates that exhibit time-dependent biases, even if the true efficacy is constant over time. This motivates the development of a new measure of vaccine efficacy based on hazard regression (HARE), a logspline approach to obtain valid estimates across a range of possible vaccine types, using only information on infection times and baseline properties of the trial patient population. Simulation shows that HARE provides robust vaccine efficacy estimates under a wide range of true efficacies (25% to 75%) and under various models of vaccine action (leaky, all-or-none, Mixed, Distributional) under high or low incidence cohorts (commercial sex workers and male clients of sexually transmitted disease clinics). HARE estimates were generally as valid or better than those obtained with traditional measures, but it does exhibit reduced precision. Given the seriousness of the global HIV pandemic, it is vital that existing statistical frameworks become fully capable of accurately estimating the true efficacy to determine the full potential of candidate vaccines. The analyses presented in this paper offer an avenue for unbiased estimation of vaccine efficacy in large-scale HIV prevention trials, and illustrate the growing need for mathematical models of clinical trial simulation.

2000 *Mathematics Subject Classification.* Primary 92C60 Medical epidemiology ; Secondary 92B15 General biostatistics.

Key words and phrases. logspline, phase 3 clinical trials, AIDS.

KD thanks the Wellcome Trust and Fonds pour la Formation de Chercheurs et l'Aide à la Recherche (FCAR), Quebec for financial support. RMA thanks the Wellcome Trust for research grant support.

1. Introduction

Mathematical models in epidemiology are most often used to gain a better understanding of the transmission dynamics of infections, to interpret epidemiological patterns of diseases, to plan and evaluate health intervention strategies and to guide public health decisions regarding vaccination [**2, 39, 15**]. However, in the case of HIV/AIDS, researchers have turned to mathematical models in recent years to help interpret ambiguous and even contradictory results obtained from trials of HIV interventions given the complex dynamics of HIV [**42, 26, 19**]. Unfortunately, most of these efforts have been done a posteriori, once inconclusive results have already been obtained [**31, 5, 3, 1, 25**].

A better approach would be to employ mathematical models to validate and improve study designs and statistical analysis before they are initiated in order to minimise the chance of obtaining ambiguous or inconclusive results [**15, 1**]. Given the scale of the pandemic and its politically sensitive landscape, this is particularly important in the context of efficacy trials for HIV vaccines and microbicides, which will need to produce informative and unequivocal results so as not to retard product development and licensing [**25, 4, 43, 38, 22, 12**]. Mathematical simulations that mimic the conduct of HIV efficacy trials under different sets of vaccine or microbicidal characteristics and population heterogeneities [**31, 5, 3, 1, 4, 43**] would permit us to test the robustness of trial designs and statistical analysis in situations where the baseline assumptions used to plan trials are violated. For example, time-dependent vaccine efficacy can undermine proportionality of hazards; frailty selection can compromise equality in patients' exposure to HIV between trial arms even after randomisation; co-circulating infections which are cofactors of HIV transmission (e.g. bacterial sexually transmitted infections) confound estimation of protective efficacy against HIV. Under these circumstances, mathematical simulation of clinical trials can help validate trial design parameters such as sample size, follow-up duration, patient visit frequency, choice of statistical endpoints and primary and secondary analyses. Such validation will help ensure adequate statistical power for unbiased and precise statistical efficacy estimation to obtain a clear answer at the end of the trial [**12**].

In this paper, we illustrate, with an example, the use of HIV transmission dynamics models to study methodological questions when planning clinical trials. The study objective is to improve the statistical estimation of HIV vaccine efficacy (VE), which is known to be systematically biased when using standard statistical methods under unknown vaccine properties and population heterogeneities. In particular, we test and validate a new vaccine efficacy measure based on hazard regression (HARE) [**12, 29, 28, 41**], a logspline method for estimation of hazard functions and detection of time-dependent variables. We compare HARE to traditional measures based on comparison of proportions infected per trial arm (cumulative incidence ratio, CIR) or comparison of infection rates using a Cox proportional hazard model (hazard rate ratio, HRR) [**27, 8**].

The paper is divided as follows: First we describe the stochastic mathematical model of HIV transmission used to simulate trials of prophylactic HIV vaccines and the range of scenarios explored. Then, we describe the efficacy measures tested and the statistical analysis. Finally, results on efficacy estimates based on CIR, HRR and HARE obtained under the different scenarios are presented and discussed.

2. Methods

The mathematical model employed encompasses the epidemiological features relevant to HIV transmission and disease progression in a heterosexually mixing population as well as the range of vaccine properties that may be encountered in a HIV efficacy trial. The model has previously been validated for use to explore the potential bias and statistical variability of the traditional efficacy measures based on CIR and HRR in the context of HIV vaccine trials [**12**]. By validation we mean two things. First, the model was able to reproduce the HIV incidence and prevalence observed in field settings based on appropriate epidemiological estimates of the model parameters. Second, when used with the appropriate model of vaccine action, the statistical measures (CIR under Model 2 and HRR under Model 1) produced the valid estimates of vaccine efficacy predicted by theory [**4, 6, 24, 20, 40**] for different ranges of efficacy (including 0% efficacy) in both homogeneous and heterogenous populations. Thus, any biases detected in efficacy estimates can be attributed to the estimation procedure caused by the choice of estimator, frailty or misspecified model of vaccine action, rather than bias in the mathematical model framework itself.

2.1. Transmission Dynamics Model.

2.1.1. *Background Population.* A compartmental stochastic model serves as the template to mirror different features of phase III trial design and HIV transmission (Figure 1). The model consists of five disease states ($h = 1, \dots, 5$) with progression from susceptible ($h = 1$), to three successive infection stages of different duration and degrees of infectiousness ($h = 2, 3$ and 4), to full blown AIDS ($h = 5$). The sexually active population is stratified by sex ($k = 1$ for women, and $k = 2$ for men) and by sexual activity levels ($i = 1, \dots, 6$) representing low ($i = 1, 2$) to high ($i = 3, \dots, 6$) sexually active individuals such as female commercial sex workers (CSW) and male clients of sexually transmitted disease clinics (MCSC). The number of individuals in disease state h, activity class i and of sex k, is noted $X^h_{k,i}(t)$.

2.1.2. *Trial Population and Vaccine Properties.* Upon commencement of the simulated clinical trial, a sample of individuals fulfilling predefined eligibility criteria are drawn from the background population and randomised into controls and vaccinees. The number of controls and vaccinees of disease state h, sex k in activity class i at time t is denoted by $Y^h_{k,i}(t)$ ($h = 1, \dots, 5$) and $Z^h_{k,i}(t)$ ($h = 0, \dots, 10$) respectively. The model is able to represent the different properties of a potential prophylactic vaccine. These are take, degree, time lag and waning [**4, 12, 6, 24, 20**]. Thus, a vaccine may protect against infection only a fraction α of vaccinees (take), leaving the remainder, $1 - \alpha$, completely unprotected. Among those in whom the vaccine "takes", it may reduce susceptibility to infection upon exposure, by a constant fraction, δ (degree). Furthermore, vaccine protection may only last for an average duration (1/waning) or develop after some time delay (time-lag). In the model, vaccinees who take start in state $h = 0$ and remain fully susceptible until they progress to state $h = 1$ at a rate (ℓ=1/time-lag) once protective immunity develops. The number of vaccinees in whom immunization does not take is denoted by $Z^h_{k,i}(t)$ ($h = 6, \dots, 10$). Individuals can also lose their immune protection totally at a "waning" rate (ω) and move directly to $Z^6_{k,i}(t)$.

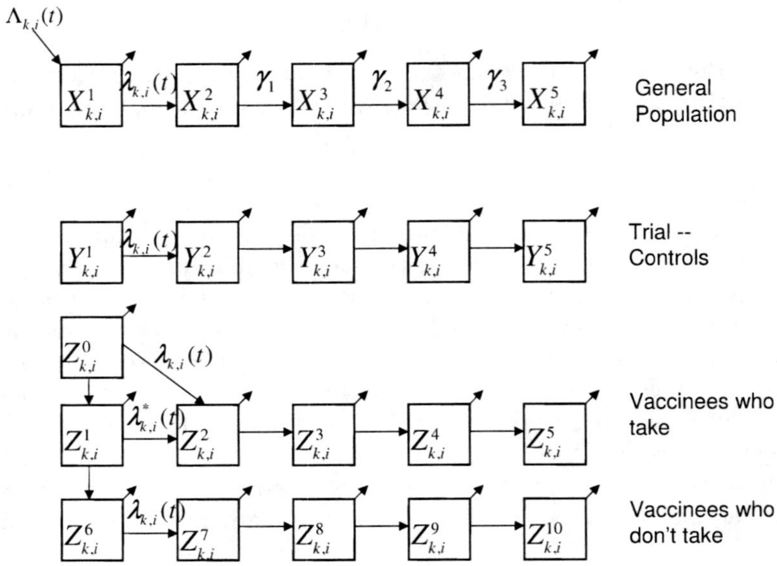

FIGURE 1. Stochastic Mathematical Model representing birth, death, HIV infection and passage between the 3 different stages of HIV infectivity in a sexually active population representing the general population, controls, vaccinees in whom the vaccine provides protection (i.e. takes) and vaccinees who are not protected (i.e. does not take) in an HIV clinical trial. Variables are defined as follows: $\lambda(t)$ is the force of HIV infection in the general population, controls and vaccinees without developed immunity. $\lambda^\star(t)$ is the force of infection in vaccinees with developed immunity. $X^1_{k,i}$, $Y^1_{k,i}$, $Z^1_{k,i}$, $Z^0_{k,i}$ and $Z^6_{k,i}$ are HIV susceptibles respectively in the general population, controls, vaccinees with developed immunity, vaccinees with undeveloped immunity, and vaccinees who don't take (vaccine failures). Similarly, $X^j_{k,i}$, $Y^j_{k,i}$, $Z^j_{k,i}$, $Z^{j+5}_{k,i}$ for $j = 2, 3, 4$ are HIV infecteds. $X^5_{k,i}$, $Y^5_{k,i}$, $Z^5_{k,i}$, $Z^{10}_{k,i}$ are individuals afflicted with full blown AIDS. Description of other parameters and their values are given in Table 2. Forces of infection $\lambda(t)$ and $\lambda^\star(t)$ are detailed in Appendix A.

2.1.3. *Monte Carlo Simulation.* The rate at which any event or transition between states occurs, $R(t)$, in a population of size $N(t) = \sum_{h,k,i} X^h_{k,i}(t)$, is defined by $R(t) = \sum_{r,k,i} R_{r,k,i}(t)$, where r represents the different number of events possible. Given a stratification of two sexes and six sexual activity classes, 492 mutually exclusive events can occur (2 sexes $\times$ 6 classes $\times$ 41 possible events)(Table 1). In the stochastic simulations, a random sequence of individual events is generated. Each of the 492 possible events occurs with probability $P_{r,k,i}(t)$ defined by $P_{r,k,i}(t) = R_{r,k,i}(t)/S(t)$ where $S(t) = \sum_{r,k,i} R_{r,k,i}(t)$. Using RAN2 [**37**], the event chosen at each step of the sequence is determined by a random number generated from a uniform distribution according to the 492 probabilities. The time a person of sex k and class i spends in a specific state r before making a transition is assumed to be exponentially distributed with mean $R^{-1}_{r,k,i}(t)$. Furthermore, the time between any two events is exponentially distributed with mean $S^{-1}(t)$. Therefore, the time of occurrence s of chosen event r can be determined by choosing a random number from a uniform distribution and setting it equal to $F(s)$ in the equation $F(s) = 1 - \exp[-S(t)s]$. Thus by an iterative process, a sequence of events and their time of occurrence is generated. What we obtain at the end of each simulation is a clinical trial data set containing information on time to any of the events for each of the individuals included in the trial [**3, 12**].

2.1.4. *Scenarios and Parameters.* Epidemiological, behavioural and demographic parameters were chosen to represent CSW, MCSC and the general heterosexual population of a sub-Saharan city where the trial is assumed to take place in the early phase of the epidemic (Table 2).

2.1.5. *Trial Design.* All simulated clinical trials represent longitudinal double blind randomised (1:1; placebo: vaccinated) trials with 2000 high risk patients per trial arm and follow-up of two or five years. Most analyses are based on cohorts of CSW with an average initial HIV incidence of 0.06 per annum which rises to 22% per year at year 1, 53% at year 2, 75% at year 3, drops to 67% at year 4, and finishes at 52% at year 5. Trials with cohorts of MCSC with lower incidence rates (incidence rate at years 0 to 5 are on average 6.0%, 8.5%, 5.1%, 2.9%, 2.1% and 1.6% per year) are also explored [**12**].

2.1.6. *Vaccination Scenarios.* We define four scenarios for model of vaccine action. Model 1 defines one extreme where the vaccine reduces the susceptibility to infection of all vaccinees, by a constant fraction (δ=varied, $\alpha = 100\%$). Model 2 defines the other extreme where the vaccine confer total protection to only a fixed proportion of the vaccinees (δ=100%, α=varied). We also define a Mixed Model where a fraction α of takers benefit from a reduction in susceptibility of δ. More generally, we defined a Distributional Model where the reduction in susceptibility varies between "takers". We assume that the "degree" in reduction in susceptibility vary according to a Normal distribution with mean μ_δ and variance σ_δ. In all vaccine scenarios investigated, we assume no time-lag or waning of the immune response over time ($\omega = 0$ and $\ell = 0$). To test the robustness of VE measures, a variety of simulations are performed for the different models of vaccine action and parameter assignments for true vaccine efficacy (25%, 50%, 75%) (see Table 3). For each parameter set or scenario, 50 repetitions were performed in order to be able to assess and compare validity or accuracy (bias) and precision (dispersion around the mean) of estimates.

TABLE 1. Events and Rates in General Population, Controls, and Vaccinees.

(r)	Description of Event	Rate $(R_{r,k,i})$
1	Recruitment into sexually active population	$R_{1,k,i} = \Lambda_{k,i}(t)$
2	Natural death rate (NDR) of susceptibles	$R_{2,k,i} = \mu X^1_{k,i}(t)$
3	NDR of HIV infecteds in first disease state	$R_{3,k,i} = \mu X^2_{k,i}(t)$
4	NDR of HIV infecteds in second disease state	$R_{4,k,i} = \mu X^3_{k,i}(t)$
5	NDR of HIV infecteds in third disease state	$R_{5,k,i} = \mu X^4_{k,i}(t)$
6	Death of AIDS patients	$R_{6,k,i} = (\mu + \nu) X^5_{k,i}(t)$
7	HIV infection of susceptibles	$R_{7,k,i} = \lambda_{k,i}(t) X^1_{k,i}(t)$
8	Progression to second state of HIV infection	$R_{8,k,i} = \gamma_1 X^2_{k,i}(t)$
9	Progression to third state of HIV infection	$R_{9,k,i} = \gamma_2 X^3_{k,i}(t)$
10	Progression to AIDS	$R_{10,k,i} = \gamma_3 X^4_{k,i}(t)$
11	NDR of susceptibles	$R_{11,k,i} = \mu Y^1_{k,i}(t)$
12	NDR of HIV infecteds in first disease state	$R_{12,k,i} = \mu Y^2_{k,i}(t)$
13	NDR of HIV infecteds in second disease state	$R_{13,k,i} = \mu Y^3_{k,i}(t)$
14	NDR of HIV infecteds in third disease state	$R_{14,k,i} = \mu Y^4_{k,i}(t)$
15	Death of AIDS patients	$R_{15,k,i} = (\mu + \nu) Y^5_{k,i}(t)$
16	HIV infection of susceptibles	$R_{16,k,i} = \lambda_{k,i}(t) Y^1_{k,i}(t)$
17	Progression to second state of HIV infection	$R_{17,k,i} = \gamma_1 Y^2_{k,i}(t)$
18	Progression to third state of HIV infection	$R_{18,k,i} = \gamma_2 Y^3_{k,i}(t)$
19	Progression to AIDS	$R_{19,k,i} = \gamma_3 Y^4_{k,i}(t)$
20	NDR of vaccinees before time lag	$R_{20,k,i} = \mu Z^0_{k,i}(t)$
21	NDR of vaccinees after time lag	$R_{21,k,i} = \mu Z^1_{k,i}(t)$
22	NDR of HIV infecteds in first disease state	$R_{22,k,i} = \mu Z^2_{k,i}(t)$
23	NDR of HIV infecteds in second disease state	$R_{23,k,i} = \mu Z^3_{k,i}(t)$
24	NDR of HIV infecteds in third disease state	$R_{24,k,i} = \mu Z^4_{k,i}(t)$
25	Death of AIDS patients	$R_{25,k,i} = (\mu + \nu) Z^5_{k,i}(t)$
26	Development of immunity (time-lag)	$R_{26,k,i} = \ell Z^0_{k,i}(t)$
27	HIV infection before time-lag	$R_{27,k,i} = \lambda_{k,i}(t) Z^0_{k,i}(t)$
28	HIV infection after time-lag	$R_{28,k,i} = \lambda^\star_{k,i}(t) Z^1_{k,i}(t)$
29	Progression to second state of HIV infection	$R_{29,k,i} = \gamma_1 Z^2_{k,i}(t)$
30	Progression to third state of HIV infection	$R_{30,k,i} = \gamma_2 Z^3_{k,i}(t)$
31	Progression to AIDS	$R_{31,k,i} = \gamma_3 Z^4_{k,i}(t)$
32	Loss of vaccine protection (waning)	$R_{32,k,i} = \omega Z^1_{k,i}(t)$
33	NDR of susceptibles	$R_{33,k,i} = \mu Z^6_{k,i}(t)$
34	NDR of HIV infecteds in first disease state	$R_{34,k,i} = \mu Z^7_{k,i}(t)$
35	NDR of HIV infecteds in second disease state	$R_{35,k,i} = \mu Z^8_{k,i}(t)$
36	NDR of HIV infecteds in third disease state	$R_{36,k,i} = \mu Z^9_{k,i}(t)$
37	Death of AIDS patients	$R_{37,k,i} = (\mu + \nu) Z^{10}_{k,i}(t)$
38	HIV infection of susceptibles	$R_{38,k,i} = \lambda_{k,i}(t) Z^6_{k,i}(t)$
39	Progression to second state of HIV infection	$R_{39,k,i} = \gamma_1 Z^7_{k,i}(t)$
40	Progression to third state of HIV infection	$R_{40,k,i} = \gamma_2 Z^8_{k,i}(t)$
41	Progression to AIDS	$R_{41,k,i} = \gamma_3 Z^9_{k,i}(t)$

TABLE 2. Initial conditions and baseline values for population, trial design and biological parameters for simulating HIV infection in a sub-Saharan city.

POPULATION PARAMETERS	
Parameter	Value(s)
Duration of sexual active lifetime ($\frac{1}{\mu}$)	35 years
Annual rate of partner change ($m_{k,i}$) at $t = 0$ females (k=1) males (k=2)	Activity classes i=1-6: 0.8 1.5 100 200 300 400 1.0 2.0 5 10 15 20
Proportion of each sex per activity class at $t = 0$ females males	Activity classes i=1-6: .66 .33 .0015 .0015 .003 .003 .53 .27 .05 .05 .05 .05
Sexual mixing ($\phi_{k,i,j}(t)$)	proportional; $\phi_{k,i,j}(t) = \frac{NA_{k'j}(t)\, m_{k',j}(0)}{\sum_j NA_{k',j}(t)\, m_{k',j}(0)}$; $k = 1, 2$
Population size at $t = 0$	N=1 000 000
TRIAL DESIGN PARAMETERS	
Parameter	Value(s)
HIV incidence at sampling (λ_c) in person-years	6%
Sample size	4000
Cohort being sampled	CSW (females classes i=3 to 6), MCSC (males classes i=3 to 6)
Duration of follow-up	2 and 5 years
BIOLOGICAL PARAMETERS	
Parameter	Value(s)
Death rate due to AIDS (ν)	1 / year
Duration of infectivity phases 1 to 3 in years ($1/\gamma_1, 1/\gamma_2, 1/\gamma_3$)	$1/\gamma_1 = 0.5, 1/\gamma_2 = 6.5, 1/\gamma_3 = 1$
Per partnership probability of HIV transmission (β_{kij}) Stage I female class 1-2 to male class 1-2 female class 1-2 to male class 3-6 female class 3-6 to male class 1-6 Stage II female class 1-2 to male class 1-2 female class 1-2 to male class 3-6 female class 3-6 to male class 1-6 Stage III female class 1-2 to male class 1-2 female class 1-2 to male class 3-6 female class 3-6 to male class 1-6 * Values are doubled for male to female transmission	 0.16 0.087 0.05 0.0032 0.0017 0.001 0.051 0.026 0.0071

TABLE 3. Design of Simulations. The four vaccine trial scenarios investigate VE estimation with HARE under different models of vaccine action (Models 1 & 2, the Mixed and Distributional Models), and incidence settings (high and low). Sample size was 2000 per study arm. All scenarios assume no time-lag and no waning of vaccine effect.

Scenario	Efficacy	Vaccine Parameters	Incidence
(1) Model 1	25%	$\alpha = 1.0, \delta = 0.25$	high
	50%	$\alpha = 1.0, \delta = 0.50$	(CSW)
	75%	$\alpha = 1.0, \delta = 0.75$	
(2) Model 2	25%	$\alpha = 0.25, \delta = 1.0$	high
	50%	$\alpha = 0.50, \delta = 1.0$	(CSW)
	75%	$\alpha = 0.75, \delta = 1.0$	
(3) Mixed or	25%	$\alpha = 0.75, \delta = 0.333$	high
Distributional	50%	$\alpha = 0.75, \delta = 0.667$	(CSW)
	50%	$\alpha = 0.75, \mu_\delta = 0.667, \sigma_\delta = .167$	
	50%	$\alpha = 0.75, \mu_\delta = 0.667, \sigma_\delta = .250$	
	50%	$\alpha = 1.0, \mu_\delta = 0.50, \sigma_\delta = .167$	
	50%	$\alpha = 1.0, \mu_\delta = 0.50, \sigma_\delta = .250$	
(4) Model 1, 2	50%	$\alpha = 1.0, \delta = 0.50$	low
Mixed,	50%	$\alpha = 0.50, \delta = 1.0$	(MCSC)
Distributional	50%	$\alpha = 0.75, \mu_\delta = 0.667, \sigma_\delta = .250$	

2.2. Vaccine Efficacy Measures and Statistical Analysis. It can be argued that in order to fully characterize the vaccine's protective impact, it would be most informative (because of their different implications for the population-level effectiveness [**15, 22, 12, 35**]) to estimate each of the vaccine properties $\alpha, \mu_\delta, \sigma_\delta, \omega$ and ℓ. However, this is seldom done [**27, 8, 17**]. In practice, the principal aim of phase III clinical trials is to estimate the true efficacy of the candidate vaccine under investigation, where the true vaccine efficacy depends on the combination of all the vaccine properties. For example, in absence of time-lag and waning, the true vaccine efficacy (the quantity that we want to estimate) will be given by the product of the take and degree (true $VE = \delta$ x α). In a randomised, double-blind, placebo-controlled trial vaccine efficacy is measured by $VE = 1 - RR$, where RR is a ratio of risk comparing cumulative proportions of infecteds in the two arms at the end of the trial using CIR. Alternatively, RR can be based on HRR, which compares hazard rates in the two trial arms using infection time data [**27, 8, 6, 17, 40, 30, 18**]. However, it is well known that VE can vary with time due to misspecified model of vaccine action and frailty selection, resulting in biased estimates of maximal efficacy. For example, in absence of time-lag or waning, it has been shown that HRR provides valid estimates of VE only under Model 1 [**4, 22, 6, 24, 20**], while CIR estimates are valid only under Model 2 [**27, 8, 6, 17, 40, 30, 18**]. Under a misspecified model (i.e. using HRR under a Model 2, Mixed or Distributional vaccine, or CIR under a Model 1, Mixed or Distributional vaccine), the VE demonstrate increasing time-dependent bias [**12, 24, 20, 30, 21, 23**].

However, even under a properly specified model of vaccine action, VE estimates may vary over time due to frailty selection. Frailty selection results from heterogeneity between individuals enrolled in the trial, arising from differences in sexual behaviour, in immunological profiles or in other unknown factors. Frailty can introduce imbalances between trial arms in exposure to HIV undermining the benefit of randomisation [**6, 21, 23, 32**]. This is because those with higher frailty (e.g. the more sexually active) will, on average, acquire infection earlier in the trial than individuals with low frailty. Thus, as the trial progresses, the uninfected controls will tend to belong to—for example—the lower sexual activity classes, by comparison with the uninfected vaccinees (if the vaccine provides some degree of protection), eventually inducing differential exposure between control and treated groups over time.

Given unknown models of vaccine action and population heterogeneities, we assess the reliability of a new VE measure, which builds on an approach originally suggested by Brunet et al [**6, 24**]. In short, the approach consists of constructing smooth hazard curves in function of time t for vaccinees and controls based on follow-up data. Estimation of VE then consists of taking the hazard ratio at a certain t as close to $t = 0$ as possible before the effects of frailty and of model misspecification can influence estimates [**6, 24**]. We construct the hazard curves using hazard regression (HARE) and hazard estimation (HEFT), an adaptive log-spline technique for estimation of conditional hazards [**12, 29, 28, 41**]. The HARE and HEFT methodology is described in Appendix B.

CIR is calculated by the Cochran-Mantel χ^2 statistic and the HRR is determined by fitting a Cox proportional hazard model using exact infection times as endpoints at the end of follow-up [**27, 8, 17**]. Computation of CIR and HRR are described in Appendix B along with HARE.

Upon calculation of HRR, CIR, HARE or HEFT, vaccine efficacy was then estimated for each trial simulation by the relationships $VE_{CIR} = 1 - CIR, VE_{HRR} = 1 - HRR$. In the case of HARE (or HEFT) $VE_{HARE}(t) = 1 - \frac{h_v(t)}{h_c(t)}$, where $h_v(t)$ and $h_c(t)$ are the hazard functions of vaccinees and controls estimated by HARE (or HEFT). In the analysis, the $VE_{HARE}(t)$ curves are presented as well as estimates at $t = 6$ and $t = 12$ months instead of $t = 0$ to ensure sufficient endpoints to have a minimum level of precision. Estimation too close to $t = 0$ would produce very variable results.

Trial data from each repetition are analysed to produce point estimates and a confidence interval of VE based on CIR, HRR and HARE at the end of the follow-up period. Validity of HRR, CIR and HARE estimates is evaluated based on the true VE embedded in each simulation. True vaccine efficacy is defined as $VE_{TRUE} = \delta \cdot \alpha$ under Models 1,2 and Mixed, and $VE_{TRUE} = \mu_\delta \cdot \alpha$ under the Distributional Model, where μ_δ is the mean vaccine efficacy. Confidence interval estimation for HARE is based on bootstrapping (performed 200 times) [**32, 14**].

Simulations were carried out on a network of SUN stations. HRR and CIR analyses are performed with SAS Version 6.12. HARE and HEFT software are available from StatLib [`http://lib.stat.cmu`] and interfaces with S-Plus Version 3.4.

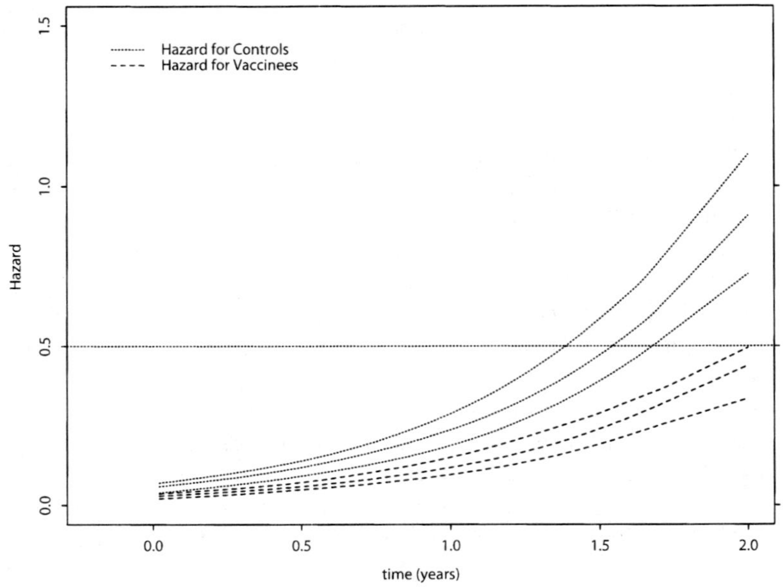

FIGURE 2. Estimation of hazard curves for controls and vaccinees using HARE in a two-year duration clinical trial in a cohort of 4000 CSW to test for a Model 1 vaccine of 50% efficacy. The average hazard curve over the 50 repetitions for controls and vaccinees are given with their 95% confidence bands.

3. Results

3.1. Validity of HARE estimates across models of vaccine action in a high incidence setting. We first consider a 2-year clinical trial for a Model 1 vaccine of 50% efficacy with instantaneous and lifelong protection (scenario 1 of Table 3). Such a vaccine reduces susceptibility of all vaccinees by 50% ($\delta = 0.50, \alpha = 1.0$). Application of HARE to the clinical trial data for this vaccine produces the hazard and VE curves displayed in Figures 2 and 3. Table 4 gives the mean and standard deviation (over the 50 repetitions) of the VE point estimates for the HRR, CIR and HARE for Model 1 vaccines of different efficacies (25%, 50% and 75%) in trials of 2 years of follow-up.

Figure 2 illustrates that HARE produces smooth continuous hazard functions over time and demonstrates a clear separation of the 2 treatment groups indicating a positive vaccine effect. The estimated VE from HARE is essentially unbiased for all $0 < t < 24$ months as indicated by the average vaccine efficacy curve (Figure 3). For this reason, the choice of t does not affect validity of HARE estimates under Model 1. HARE estimates at $t = 6$ and 12 months for a Model 1 vaccine of 50% or 75% efficacy are as valid as HRR based estimates, but at 25% efficacy HARE estimates appear to have a slight negative bias compared to the HRR under Model 1 (Table 4). CIR estimates are found to strongly underestimate particularly for low efficacy vaccines.

HARE hazard curves obtained for a 5 year long trial (Figure 4) are observed to rise initially in epidemic fashion during the first 2 to 3 years of follow-up before

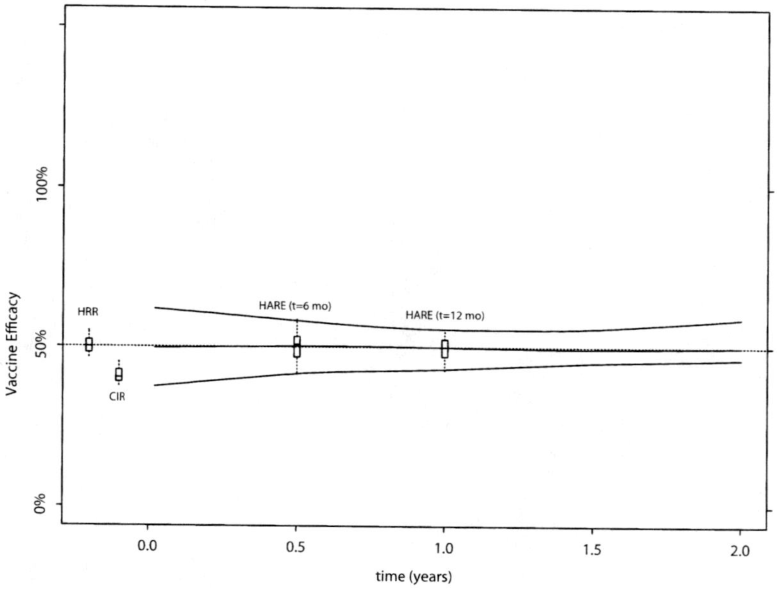

FIGURE 3. Estimation of vaccine efficacy curves using HARE in a two-year duration clinical trial in a cohort of 4000 CSW to test for a Model 1 vaccine of 50% efficacy. The average vaccine efficacy obtained with HARE over the 50 repetitions for controls and vaccinees are given with their 95% confidence bands. Boxplots of HARE vaccine estimates at $t = 6$ and $t = 12$ months are shown alongside HRR and CIR estimates. Estimates are controlled for participants sexual activity class.

reaching a plateau. These follow from the naturally occurring incidence rate of HIV in the simulation. The greater complexity of hazard curves in a 5 year follow-up requires more knots between $1\frac{1}{2}$ and $3\frac{1}{2}$ years and may produce a more variable VE curve over time (Figure 5), complicating valid estimation in some scenarios particularly for weaker vaccines. Shorter trials reduce this complexity. Comparison of Figures 2 and 3 illustrate that VE estimates based on CIR are also worse after five years' follow-up compared to two years.

Figures 6–7 illustrate the hazard and vaccine efficacy curves obtained by HARE for a Model 2 vaccine (scenario 2) of 50% efficacy in a 2 year long clinical trial. Such a vaccine confers complete protection to 50% of vaccinees, leaving the remainder unprotected ($\delta = 1.0, \alpha = 0.5$). The figure demonstrates that valid estimation is theoretically possible with HARE when $t = 0$. As expected, the HARE vaccine efficacy curve increases gradually due to the expected time-dependent over-estimation with hazard curves under Model 2. Nevertheless, when choosing $t = 6$ months, VE estimates based on HARE only incur small positive bias, as indicated in Table 4. These estimates are close to the near perfect CIR estimates at each of the efficacies considered and are better than HRR with respect to validity. When $t = 12$ months, HARE point estimates have roughly 1.5% to 4.0% absolute bias in true VE, stressing the importance of selecting t appropriately small under Model 2. As

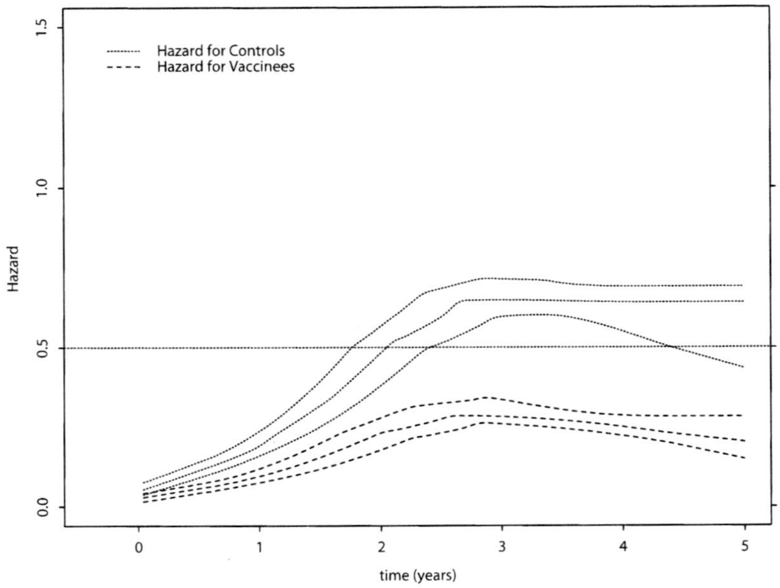

FIGURE 4. Estimation of hazard curves using HARE in a five-year duration clinical trial. Other details are as explained in Figure 2.

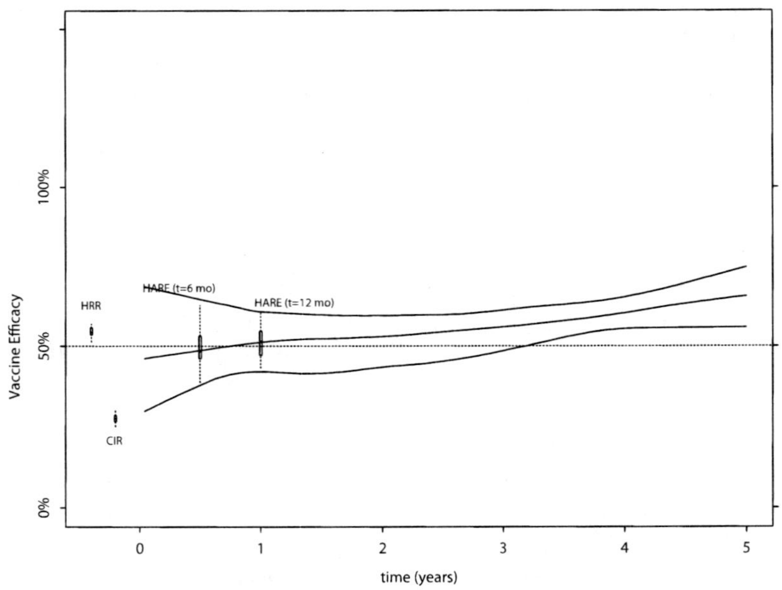

FIGURE 5. Estimation of vaccine efficacy curves using HARE in a five-year duration clinical trial. Other details are as explained in Figure 3.

under Model 1, a 5-year trial for a Model 2 vaccine does not benefit estimation with either HARE or HRR (results not shown).

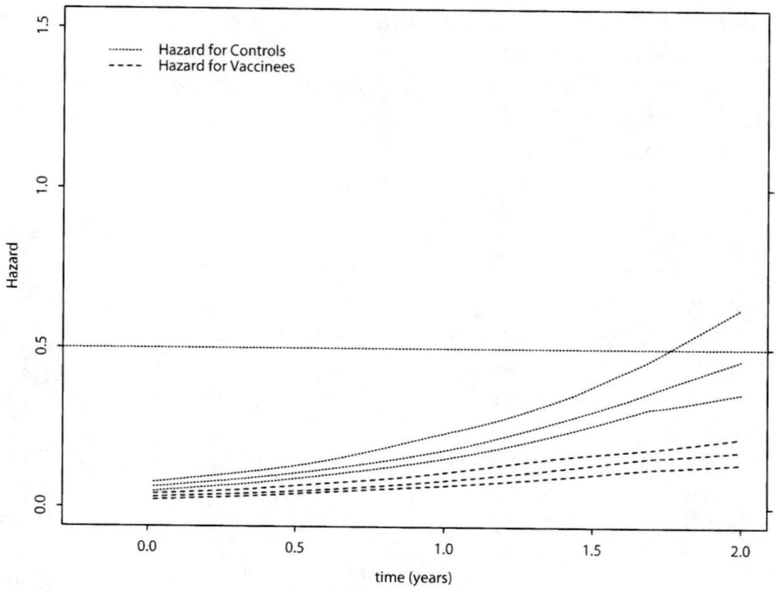

FIGURE 6. Estimation of hazard curves using HARE in a two-year duration clinical trial to test a Model 2 vaccine of 50% efficacy. Other details are as explained in Figure 2.

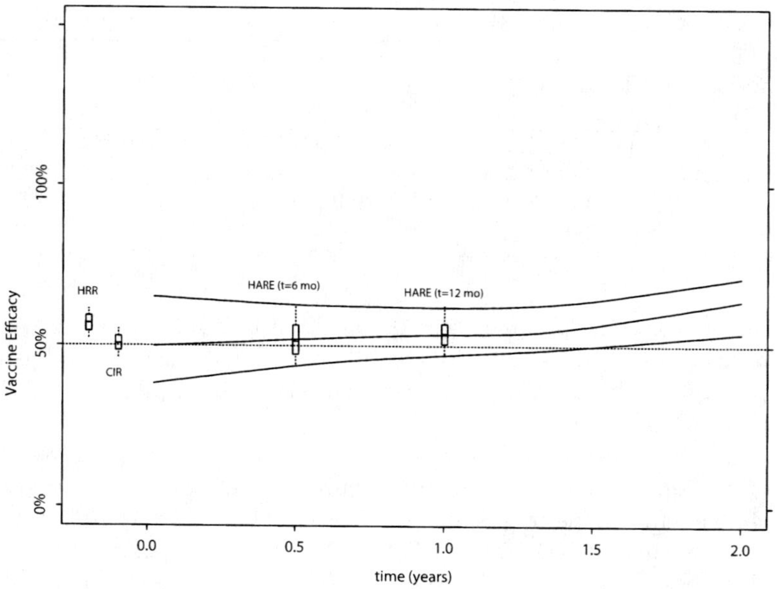

FIGURE 7. Estimation of vaccine efficacy curves using HARE in a two-year duration clinical trial to test a Model 2 vaccine of 50% efficacy. Other details are as explained in Figure 3.

Augmenting the complexity of the model of vaccine action, scenario 3 considers vaccines of 50% efficacy under the Mixed and Distributional Models with various

TABLE 4. Selected Simulation Results for Scenarios 1 to 3. Mean and standard deviations (in parentheses) for point vaccine efficacy estimates under various models of vaccine action are obtained with HRR, CIR and HARE models (at t= 6 and 12 months) over 50 repetitions of clinical trials of 2 year duration in high incidence setting.

Scenario	Selected Results		
	25% efficacy	50% efficacy	75% efficacy
Model 1	$t=6$ $t=12$	$t=6$ $t=12$	$t=6$ $t=12$
HARE	22.3(7.38) 23.6(5.18)	50.0(5.15) 49.6(4.21)	75.1(3.38) 74.8(2.63)
HRR	24.1(3.29)	50.2(2.60)	75.1(1.73)
CIR	16.0(2.50)	40.9(2.48)	70.0(2.06)
Model 2	$t=6$ $t=12$	$t=6$ $t=12$	$t=6$ $t=12$
HARE	25.7(6.67) 26.4(8.45)	51.1(6.23) 53.8(5.41)	75.9(3.42) 76.6(3.33)
HRR	31.2(4.14)	56.8(3.13)	78.8(1.99)
CIR	25.0(3.35)	50.7(3.02)	75.1(2.06)
	50% efficacy	50% efficacy	50% efficacy
Mixed and Distributional $\alpha = 100\%$	$\mu_\delta = 50\%$ $\sigma_\delta = 0\%$ $t=6$ $t=12$	$\mu_\delta = 50\%$ $\sigma_\delta = 16.7\%$ $t=6$ $t=12$	$\mu_\delta = 50\%$ $\sigma_\delta = 25\%$ $t=6$ $t=12$
HARE	50.0(5.15) 49.6(4.21)	49.4(5.36) 51.2(4.31)	51.2(6.17) 52.1(5.06)
HRR	50.2(2.60)	50.7(3.09)	51.8(3.39)
CIR	40.9(2.48) (Model 1)	44.1(3.29)	45.1(3.40)
Mixed and Distributional $\alpha = 75\%$	$\mu_\delta = 67\%$ $\sigma_\delta = 0\%$ $t=6$ $t=12$	$\mu_\delta = 67\%$ $\sigma_\delta = 16.7\%$ $t=6$ $t=12$	$\mu_\delta = 67\%$ $\sigma_\delta = 25\%$ $t=6$ $t=12$
HARE	50.0(4.95) 52.1(3.30)	50.3(5.98) 52.2(5.28)	50.8(4.39) 51.5(5.07)
HRR	52.8(2.73)	52.7(3.58)	52.8(3.02)
CIR	44.8(2.80) (Mixed Model)	46.3(3.43)	46.3(3.03)

combinations of vaccine parameters. As indicated in Table 4 for the spectrum of vaccine types considered, HARE with $t = 6$ months is at least as good as the HRR with respect to validity and outperforms when take is incomplete ($\alpha < 100\%$). CIR always underestimates true VE.

The hazard and vaccine efficacy curves obtained by HARE for 2 year follow-up for a Distributional Model vaccine ($\mu_\delta = 0.667, \sigma_\delta = 0.25, \alpha = 0.75$) are in between that of Model 1 and Model 2 (results not shown). The VE curve is found to closely follow the true value of VE with small t, while gradually rising with increasing t. Thus as in Model 2, HARE estimate at $t = 6$ months is fairly unbiased whereas that at $t = 12$ months can have slight positive bias. Application of HARE in 5 year follow-up, concur with previous conclusions that valid estimation with longer follow-up can be more complicated due to the more complex nature of the hazard curves (results not shown).

3.2. Clinical trials in a lower incidence setting. This scenario examines VE estimation with HARE under a lower incidence and prevalence setting based on

TABLE 5. Selected Simulation Results for Scenario 4. Vaccinal estimation in clinical trials with moderately low incidence (MCSC) are obtained for vaccines of true efficacy of 50%. Results are given for Model 1 and 2 plus the Distributional Model. Mean and standard deviations (in parentheses) of point estimates based on HRR, CIR, HARE at t= 6, 12 are obtained over 50 repetitions of clinical trials of 2 year duration.

Scenario	Selected Results		
MCSC	Model 1 50% efficacy ($\alpha = 1.0, \delta = 0.5$) $t = 6$ $t = 12$	Model 2 50% efficacy ($\alpha = 0.5, \delta = 1.0$) $t = 6$ $t = 12$	Distributional Model 50% efficacy ($\mu_\delta = 0.67, \alpha = 0.75,$ $\sigma_\delta = 0.25$) $t = 6$ $t = 12$
HARE	51.6(6.35) 51.2(8.96)	50.6(5.82) 50.0(6.42)	51.3(4.83) 51.1(4.65)
HRR	50.5(3.75)	51.8(3.41)	51.1(3.78)
CIR	48.2(3.73)	49.6(3.38)	48.9(3.72)

TABLE 6. Point estimates and ninety-five percent bootstrap confidence intervals for VE estimates based on HARE, HRR and CIR for a single vaccine trial with 4000 CSW. Three different vaccines, each with true efficacy of 50% are considered. Models of vaccine action are Model 1 and 2 plus the Distributional Model

Scenario	Selected Results		
CSW	Model 1 ($\alpha = 1.0, \delta = 0.5$)	Model 2 ($\alpha = 0.5, \delta = 1.0$)	Distributional Model ($\mu_\delta = 0.67, \alpha = 0.75,$ $\sigma_\delta = 0.25$)
HARE ($t = 6$)	50.7[39.9,61.4]	52.9[40.0,65.9]	49.6[33.7,65.2]
HRR	50.0[44.2,55.1]	55.2[48.9,60.9]	52.3[45.6,58.1]
CIR	40.8[35.7,45.5]	49.9[44.1,55.0]	46.8[40.7,52.3]

trials recruiting MCSC rather than CSW. Table 5 lists the VE estimates obtained with HARE, HRR and CIR for vaccines of 50% efficacy under Models 1 and 2 plus the Distributional Model ($\mu_\delta = 0.67, \alpha = 0.75, \sigma_\delta = 0.25$).

HARE with $t = 6$ months provides valid estimates of VE under each model of vaccine action. However, these are not generally better than HRR or CIR estimates even under misspecification. When the incidence in a cohort is relatively low, the traditional VE are known not to incur significant bias [**12, 6, 24**]. Thus with MCSC, HARE does not offer an advantage over traditional VE. With respect to efficacy measurement, the advantage of choosing MCSC over CSW is the diminution of the biases due to unknown vaccine models.

3.3. Variability of HARE estimates and bootstrap confidence intervals. The improved validity and stability of vaccine efficacy estimates obtained with HARE across different models of vaccine action is achieved at the cost of increased variability. In a single clinical trial (i.e. 1 repetition rather than 50), it is important to be able to determine variability of HARE estimates. Table 6 gives the 95% confidence intervals (CI) and point estimates for VE obtained by bootstrap with HARE, HRR and CIR based on the follow-up of 2000 CSWs per arm in a single clinical trial for vaccines of 50% efficacy under Models 1, 2 and Distributional ($\mu_\delta = 0.67, \alpha = 0.75, \sigma_\delta = 0.25$). Variability of HARE over the 50 repetitions does not seem influenced by different models of action. In addition to magnitude of treatment effect (vaccine efficacy) and sample size, variability also depends on the choice of t. Figures 3,5,7 indicate that standard deviation of HARE over 50 repetitions of each clinical trial was greatest at $t = 0$ months, followed by $t = 6$ months. Precision tends to be best between t =12 and 18 months. Tables 4 to 6 indicate that HARE point estimates of VE have roughly double the standard deviation when $t = 6$ months compared to HRR and CIR under the models of action, efficacies and cohorts considered. Longer follow-up (5 years, for example) improves precision in HRR and CIR estimates due to the greater number of infection endpoints, but the increase in precision is not appreciable for HARE. This is because the variability in HARE estimates is dependent on a greater number of knots and their positioning to account for the increased complexity of hazard functions over 5 years.

Not surprisingly, HARE has wider CI than HRR and CIR. Across different models of action, the lower confidence bound for the 95% CIs based on HARE is around 33-40% while the upper bound is 61-66%. This produces CIs roughly two to two and a half times as wide as that of HRR which produces a lower confidence bound around 44-49% and upper bound of 55-61% and CIR with lower and upper bounds around 35-44% and 45-55%. The standard deviations obtained for HARE by bootstrapping are similar to those obtained from the 50 repetitions of each clinical trial. For all vaccines considered, bootstrap CIs were not dramatically wider than the analytic CIs obtained for HRR and CIR.

4. Discussion

In recent years, the design and statistical analysis of clinical trials for HIV interventions has become increasingly sophisticated [**17, 33, 34, 9, 36, 7**]. For example, community randomised trials may be used to estimate not only protective efficacy of the vaccine but also the effectiveness achieved by herd immunity (the passive protection gained by non-vaccinees due to a weakened chain of infection). Also new analyses, called sieve analyses, have been developed to ascertain strain-specific efficacy against individual strains of HIV [**17, 16**]. Trials designed to test microbicides against HIV seek to estimate not only the protective efficacy against HIV but also against other bacterial sexually transmitted infections (STI). Efficacy estimation in this context is difficult because it is difficult to disentangle the potential simultaneous efficacy of the microbicide against the STI (which is also a co-factor of HIV transmission) and HIV based on interval-censored infection times for HIV and STI. Such methodological challenges have motivated the development of new study designs and statistical methods aimed at estimated complex vaccine or microbicide effects. Given our limited experience with the application of some of these methods in field conditions and the need to minimise the risk of inconclusive trial results, clinical trial simulation is an ideal framework to validate complex and expensive trial designs and analyses. This stage helps to anticipate difficulties and identify significant sources of bias and variability, allowing for correction before the conduct of the trials. Hence, the chances of making clear interpretations from trial results are maximised as is the ability to design trials confidently.

Anticipating the difficulties in statistical trial design and data analysis, one can include the potentially confounding factors into the disease transmission dynamics of the model to then assess whether statistical measures can recover the desired efficacy. As another example of using mathematical models to aid in trial design, one can introduce a level of error in data collection to examine its effect on efficacy estimation. This is relevant in the context of single-use microbicide trials where compliance data is self-reported and may compromise the validity of the efficacy estimates. Desai et al [**13, 10, 11**] are currently using the clinical trial simulation approach to inform trial design for both male circumcision trials and microbicide trials against HIV which are currently in progress in sub-Saharan Africa.

In this paper, we have illustrated how a stochastic mathematical model of HIV clinical trials can be utilised to investigate validity of traditional statistical measures of efficacy under the biasing effects of unknown model of vaccine action and frailty and to develop a new statistical measure. Since the choice of efficacy measure (or more broadly, the statistical analysis of clinical trials) will govern the power and sample size calculations for the study, it is crucial that an unbiased efficacy measure is chosen. Simulation studies illustrated here demonstrate therefore how a valid measure can be chosen or developed. Our study also demonstrated the relevance of choosing a trial duration, another trial design parameter, which is not too long to avoid potential biasing effects of frailty or misspecified vaccine models. In this way, models can also help identify when estimates are likely to be affected by different sources of biases.

In absence of waning and time-lag, we should be concerned with two main sources of biases: 1) vaccine properties and 2) population heterogeneities.

First, bias can arise due to misspecification of the model of vaccine action. This implies that use of HRR and CIR outside of Model 1 and 2 will result in increasing time-dependent biases. Under Model 2, the Mixed and Distributional models, the HRR will increasingly overestimate VE over the time course of the trial, while the CIR will increasingly underestimate under Models 1, the Mixed and Distributional, models even if vaccine protection is immediate upon vaccination and unchanging with time. This time-dependence is an undesirable property for an estimator of true efficacy (which is constant over time). Under the range of efficacies, models of vaccine action and trial designs explored, HARE with t=6 months generally produced valid estimation of reasonable variability, while not requiring any assumption on model of vaccine action. In general HARE estimates tended to be as valid or better than HRR and CIR under model misclassification. Interestingly, careful examination of HARE VE curves, and comparison of the relative magnitudes of HARE, HRR and CIR estimates, can also provide insights on the model of vaccine action when a time-lag is absent. The simplest case is Model 1 where HARE VE curves are constant and HARE estimates concur with HRR. If HARE VE curves increase and are concave-up, and HARE estimates lie between HRR and CIR, we probably have a Mixed or Distributional Model. If HARE estimates concur with CIR estimates, while HRR is greater than HARE, and the VE curves are increasing concave-up, the vaccine is probably of type Model 2. At low incidence, it may not be possible to speculate on mode of action based on relative values of HARE, HRR and CIR, since all VE are expected to converge to the same value. As seen in our MCSC scenarios, traditional VE should avoid serious misspecification bias if the baseline incidence is low (around less than 5% per year) and relatively constant over time. However, HARE has been shown to provide valid VE estimates for the range of models of vaccine action and efficacies explored even with the high incidence cohorts. HARE estimation will likely be more suitable than traditional VE for trials conducted with high incidence cohort ($> 10\%$ per year).

A second source of bias can arise due to frailty effects in heterogeneous population. Heterogeneity in sexual behaviour implies unequal exposure to HIV infection between different trial participants resulting in the most exposed placebo recipients being infected fastest. This creates an imbalance in the sexual characteristics of the remaining uninfecteds in control and vaccinated groups over time. Most often, this results in underestimation of vaccine efficacy, particularly with lengthy clinical trials. This effect will be exacerbated in population with a more assortative sexual mixing preferences than used in our simulations. On the other hand, heterogeneity in response to vaccination can cause overestimation of VE [**12**]. Here the imbalance arises because vaccinees who respond poorly will be infected more quickly than those whose immunological systems react positively, leaving the vaccine arm comprised of well-boosted patients.

Traditional measures of efficacy and HARE are unlikely to be influenced by such heterogeneities if clinical trials are reasonably short. Our simulations suggest trials of roughly 2 year duration were suitable, but it may be longer if incidence is relatively low and stable over time. Although HARE can be insensitive to such a bias if t is chosen to be too large (greater than ≈ 2 years), it proved to be robust against the frailty effects which were inherent in our simulations.

Bootstrapped CI for HARE were roughly two to two and a half times wider than the analytical calculated CI of HRR and CIR. The precision achieved in our bootstrap CIs for vaccines of 50% efficacy with 2000 participants per trial arm was sufficient to produce a lower 95% confidence bound of 33-40% in CSWs. Thus, sample size for HARE will have to be larger than for analysis based on HRR or CIR and will likely need to be greater than 2000 per study arm, if a precision greater than that observed in Table 6 is desired. Increasing follow-up duration helped precision of VE estimates based on CIR and HRR but not HARE. However, shorter trials produce greater validity in all VE measures, as this reduces biases due to heterogeneities in the population and the model of vaccine action. A complex pattern of incidence, as in the five year simulated study, may in fact complicate the interpretation of vaccine properties.

Although HARE was developed in the context of phase III trials for HIV vaccines, the results obtained can be generalized to the testing of other products where infection times are available. The HARE results and approach adopted in this study, is of particular interest for any product which may be thought to fail in some proportion of candidates while efficacy varies in the remaining proportion. Moreover, where patient heterogeneities are thought to give rise to pernicious frailty effects, HARE would again be an appropriate measure to use.

Appendix A

Force of infection: The force of HIV infection for sex k and activity class i at time t in the general population, controls, vaccinees in whom the vaccine does not take, and vaccinees who take but have not developed immunity is given by [**12**]:

$$\lambda_{k,i}(t) = m_{k,i}(t) \sum_{j=1}^{6} \beta_{k',i,j} \phi_{k,i,j}(t) \left(\frac{\sum_{h=2}^{4} \left(X_{k',j}^{h}(t) + Y_{k',j}^{h}(t) + Z_{k',j}^{h}(t) + Z_{k',j}^{h+5}(t) \right)}{NA_{k'j}(t)} \right).$$

Here $m_{k,i}(t)$ is the annual rate of partner acquisition of persons of sex k and class i, $\beta_{k',i,j}$ is the per partnership HIV transmission probability from sex k' and class j to sex k class i. $\phi_{k,i,j}(t)$ are the mixing matrix elements (probability that a person of sex k class i chooses a partner of opposite sex k' and class j), and $NA_{k',j}(t)$ is the total sexually active population of sex k' and class j. Individuals with AIDS are assumed not to contribute to the sexually active population due to the severity of their condition.

The force of HIV infection for sex k and activity class i at time t for successful vaccinees with protective immunity is given by

$$\lambda'_{k,i}(t) = (1 - \delta)\lambda_{k,i}(t),$$

where δ is defined as in main text.

Appendix B

HARE is a general framework, from the class of logspline models [**12, 29, 28, 41**], employing cubic splines and their tensor products, to model the conditional log-hazard function based on survival data. Given a possibly right-censored infection time, t, and a vector of baseline patient covariates, $\boldsymbol{x} = (x_1, \dots, x_m)$, HARE models the conditional hazard function, $\lambda(t|\mathbf{x})$, via the log-hazard function, $\alpha(t|\mathbf{x}) = \log(\lambda(t|\mathbf{x}))$, according to the model:

$$\alpha(t|\mathbf{x}) = \sum_{j=1}^{p} \beta_j B_j(t|\mathbf{x}).$$

Here $B_1, \dots, B_p$ are linear spline functions of time or covariates and the $\beta_1, \dots, \beta_p$ are the parameters estimated by maximum likelihood methods. An automatic procedure for stepwise addition and deletion of splines (in time and in the covariates) corresponds to an adaptive method for knot placement and covariate selection. Throughout this procedure, a sequence of models are considered from which the Bayes information criterion is used to select the optimal model. The HARE algorithm also evaluates covariate interactions and non-proportionalities in hazards, and accounts for them by admitting the appropriate interaction terms with time or other covariates.

The unconditional hazard function is also estimated using HEFT (hazard estimation with flexible tails) according to

$$\alpha(t) = \sum_{j=1}^{p} \beta_j B_j(t),$$

where $B_1, \ldots, B_p$ are cubic splines and the log hazard function has continuous derivative.

As explained in Kooperberg et al [**29**], the hazard curve for vaccine efficacy estimation is then $\lambda(t|\mathbf{x}) = \lambda_0(t) \cdot \lambda_1(q(t)|\mathbf{x})$, where $\lambda_0(t) = \exp(\alpha(t))$ is the hazard estimated with HEFT and $\lambda_1(q(t)|\mathbf{x})$ is the hazard estimated with HARE applied to transformed infection times $q(t) = -\log(S_0(t))$ and $S_0(t)$ is the survival function corresponding to $\lambda_0(t)$. HEFT used this way as a 'pre-processor' for HARE has 3 advantages: (i) the resulting hazard curve is a smooth continuous function of time estimated solely from possibly censored survival times and patients' baseline covariates; (ii) fewer knots are required for the HARE hazard function and fewer discontinuities in the first derivative of the HARE hazard function result; and (iii) because HARE employs linear splines, the hazard function for HARE beyond the first and last knot (including near $t = 0$) are necessarily constant. This is no longer true based on the transformation with HEFT and corresponds with Brunet's approach [**6**]. For simplicity we say HARE for the estimation of the hazard function in this method, understanding that HEFT is concurrently employed.

Computation of HRR is based on fitting a Cox proportional hazard model to the trial data. If $\lambda_o(t)$ is the baseline hazard in the trial population, then the Cox model is expressed by $\lambda(t|x_1, \cdots, x_n) = \lambda_o(t)\exp(\sum_i b_i x_i)$ where $x_1, \cdots, x_n$ are observed covariates and b_i are the corresponding parameters to estimate using maximum likelihood methods. If $\hat{b}_v$ is the parameter corresponding to vaccination status x_v then the HRR is given by HRR $= \exp(\hat{b}_v)$ and the $100(1-\alpha)\%$ confidence limits for HRR are given by $[\exp(\hat{b}_v - Z_{\alpha/2}\sqrt{V_v}), \exp(\hat{b}_v + Z_{\alpha/2}\sqrt{V_v})]$ where V_v is the vth diagonal element of the variance-covariance matrix from the likelihood estimation method.

Computation of CIR is based on the Mantel-Haenszel estimator for the relative risk in 2 by 2 tables while controlling for h strata of ordinal covariates. Let $n_{h,ij}$ denote the cell frequency in row i and column j of stratum h, $n_{h,i\cdot}$ and $n_{h,\cdot j}$ the row and column totals, and n_h the overall total for stratum h. In the case of a vaccine trial the $n_{h,11}$ corresponds to the number of HIV-positive cases among vaccinees in stratum h, $n_{h,2\cdot}$ the total number of controls, $n_{h,21}$ the number of HIV-positives among controls, $n_{h,1\cdot}$ the total number of vaccinees and $n_{h,\cdot 1}$ the number of HIV-positives in both trial arms. Then CIR is given by

$$CIR = \frac{\sum_h n_{h,11} n_{h,2\cdot}/n_h}{\sum_h n_{h,21} n_{h,1\cdot}/n_h}$$

The $100(1-\alpha)\%$ confidence limits are given by

$$[CIR\exp(-Z_{\alpha/2}\sqrt{Var}), CIR\exp(+Z_{\alpha/2}\sqrt{Var})].$$

where

$$Var = \frac{\sum_h (n_{h,1\cdot} n_{h,2\cdot} n_{h,\cdot 1} - n_{h,11} n_{h,21} n_h)/n_h^2}{\sum_h (n_{h,11} n_{h,2\cdot}/n_h)(\sum_h n_{h,21} n_{h,1\cdot}/n_h)}.$$

References

1. M Alary, CM Lowndes, and MC Boily, *Community randomized trials for HIV prevention: the past, a lesson for the future?*, AIDS **17** (2003), 2661–2663.
2. RM Anderson and RM May, *Infectious diseases of humans: dynamics and control*, Oxford University Press, Oxford, U-K, 1991.
3. MC Boily and RM Anderson, *Human immunodeficiency virus transmission and the role of other sexually transmitted diseases. measures of association and study design*, Sex Transm Dis **23** (1996), 312–32.
4. MC Boily, KN Desai, BR Mâsse, M Alary, and RM Anderson, *Some important issues in the design of phase III HIV vaccine efficacy trials*, Vaccine **17(7-8)** (1999), 989–1004.
5. MC Boily, CM Lowndes, and M Alary, *Complementary hypothesis concerning the community sexually transmitted disease mass treatment puzzle in Rakai, Uganda*, AIDS **14** (2000), 2583–92.
6. RC Brunet, CJ Struchiner, and ME Halloran, *On the distribution of vaccine protection under heterogeneous response*, Mathematical Biosciences **116(1)** (1993), 111–25.
7. H Cao, P Kanki, and JL Sankale et al, *Cytotoxic T-lymphocyte cross-reactivity among different human immunodeficiency virus type 1 clades: implications for vaccine development*, Journal of Virology **71** (1997), 8615–8623.
8. D Collett, *Infectious diseases of humans: dynamics and control*, Chapman and Hall, London, U-K, 1992.
9. S Datta, EM Halloran, and IM Longini, *Augmented HIV vaccine trial design for estimating reduction in infectiousness and protective efficacy*, Statistics in Medicine **17** (1998), 185–200.
10. K Desai, MC Boily, and GP Garnett, *Ensuring phase III microbicide trials against HIV adequately estimate treatment efficacy: Guidance from dynamical models*, Meeting of the International Society of Sexually Transmitted Diseases Research (ISSTDR) (Ottawa Canada), July 2003.
11. K Desai, MC Boily, GP Garnett, and BR Mâsse, *The use of mathematical modeling to validate statistical power and protective efficacy of circumcision against HIV and STI in a current phase III study in Kisumu, Kenya*, 3rd Joint International Conference of ISCB and SCT (London (U-K)), July 2003.
12. K Desai, MC Boily, BR Mâsse, M Alary, and RM Anderson, *Simulation studies of phase III clinical trials to test the efficacy of a candidate HIV-1 vaccine*, Epidemiology and Infection **123** (1999), 65–88.
13. K Desai and GP Garnett, *How reliable does self-reported sex behaviour need to be for valid microbicide efficacy estimation?*, Microbicides 2004 Conference (London, U-K), March 2004.
14. B Efron and RJ Tibshirani, *An introduction to the bootstrap*, Chapman and Hall, London, U-K, 1993.
15. A Ghani and MC Boily, *The epidemiology of HIV/AIDS: Contributions to infectious diseases epidemiology*, pp. 59–88, Cambridge University Press, 2003.
16. P Gilbert, S Self, M Rao, A Naficy, and J Clemens, *Sieve analysis: methods for assessing from vaccine trial data how vaccine efficacy varies with genotypic and phenotypic pathogen variation*, J Clin Epidemiol **54(1)** (2001), 68–85.
17. PB Gilbert, SG Self, and MA Ashby, *Statistical methods for assessing differential vaccine protection against human immunodeficiency virus types*, Biometrics **54** (1998), 799–814.
18. S Greenland and RR Frerichs, *On measures and models for the effectiveness of vaccines and vaccination programmes*, Int J Epidemiol **17** (1988), 456–63.
19. H Grosskurth, R Gray, R Hayes, D Mabey, and M Wawer, *Control of sexually transmitted diseases for HIV-1 prevention: understanding the implications of the Mwanza and Rakai trials*, Lancet **355** (2000), 1981–7.
20. M Haber, E Halloran, IM Longini, and L Watelet, *Estimation of vaccine efficacy in non-randomly mixing populations*, Biom J **37(1)** (1995), 25–38.
21. EM Halloran, IM Longini, and CJ Struchiner, *Estimability and interpretation of vaccine efficacy using frailty mixing models*, American Journal of Epidemiology **144(1)** (1996), 83–97.
22. ME Halloran, *Statistical issues in phase III vaccine trial design*, J R Statist Soc A **161** (1998).
23. ME Halloran, M Haber, and IM Longini, *Interpretation and estimation of vaccine efficacy under heterogeneity*, Am J Epidemiol **136** (1992), 328–43.

24. ME Halloran, IM Longini Jr, MJ Haber, CJ Struchiner, and RC Brunet, *Exposure efficacy and change in contact rates in evaluating prophylactic HIV vaccines in the field*, Statistics in Medicine **13(4)** (1994), 357–77.
25. R Hayes, *Can RCTs measure the endpoints in which we are interested?*, Int J STD and AIDS **12 (suppl 2)** (2001), 13.
26. A Kamali, M Quigley, J Nakiyingi, J Kinsman, Kengeya-Kayondo, R Gopal, and et al., *Syndromic management of sexually-transmitted infections and behaviour change interventions on transmission of HIV-1 in rural Uganda: a community randomised trial*, Lancet **361** (2003), 645–52.
27. DG Kleinbaum, LL Kupper, and H Morgenstern, *Epidemiologic research*, Van Nostrand Reinhold, New-York, NY, 1992.
28. C Kooperberg and DB Clarkson, *Hazard regression with interval-censored data*, Biometrics **53** (1997), 1485–1494.
29. C Kooperberg, CJ Stone, and YK Truong, *Hazard regression*, Journal of the American Statistical Association **90(429)** (1995), 48–94.
30. JS Koopman and RJ Little, *Assessing HIV vaccine effects*, Am J Epidemiol **142(10)** (1995), 1113–20.
31. EL Korenromp, C Van Vliet, H Grosskurth, A Gavyole, CP Van der Ploeg, L Fransen, and et al., *Model-based evaluation of single-round mass treatment of sexually transmitted diseases for HIV control in a rural African population*, AIDS **14** (2000), 573–93.
32. JF Lawless, *Statistical models and methods for lifetime data*, Wiley, New-York, NY, 1982.
33. IM Longini, MG Hudgens, EM Halloran, and K Sagatelian, *A markov model for measuring vaccine efficacy for both susceptibility to infection and reduction in infectiousness for prophylactic HIV vaccines*, Statistics in Medicine **18** (1999), 53–68.
34. IM Longini, K Sagatelian, WN Rida, and EM Halloran, *Optimal vaccine trial design when estimating vaccine efficacy for susceptibility and infectiousness from multiple populations*, Statistics in Medicine **17** (1998), 1121–1136.
35. AR McLean and SM Blower, *Imperfect vaccines and herd immunity to HIV*, Phil Trans R Soc Lond B **253** (1993), 9–13.
36. P Peduzzi, S Donta, and M Iwane, *A review of the design of vaccine efficacy trials and a proposal for the design of the VA cooperative study of active immunotherapy of HIV infection*, Controlled Clinical Trials **18(5)** (1997), 397–419.
37. WH Press, SA Teukolsky, WT Vetterling, and BF Flannery, *Numerical recipes in fortran*, Cambridge University Press, Cambridge, U-K, 1986.
38. WN Rida and DN Lawrence, *Some statistical issues in HIV vaccine trials*, Statistics in Medicine **13** (1994), 2155–77.
39. NJ Robinson, D Mulder, B Auvert, J Whitworth, and R Hayes, *Type of partnership and heterosexual spread of HIV infection in rural Uganda: results from simulation modelling*, Int J STD and AIDS **10** (1999), 718–25.
40. PG Smith, LC Rodrigues, and PEM Fine, *Assessment of the protective efficacy of vaccines against common diseases using case-control and cohort studies*, Int J Epidemiol **13** (1984), 87–93.
41. CJ Stone, M Hansen, C Kooperberg, and YK Truong, *The use of polynomial splines and their tensor products in extended linear modeling*, Annals of Statistics **25** (1997), 1371–1470.
42. MJ Wawer, NK Sewankambo, D Serwadda, TC Quinn, LA Paxton, N Kiwanuka, and et al, *Control of sexually transmitted diseases for AIDS prevention in Uganda: a randomised community trial. Rakai project study group*, Lancet **353** (1999), 525–35.
43. IAVI Website.

(Kamal Desai, Marie-Claude Boily and Roy M. Anderson) Dept of Infectious Disease Epidemiology, Imperial College London, St-Mary's Hospital, Norfolk Place, London, W2 1PG United-Kingdom

E-mail address: `kamal.desai@imperial.ac.uk`

E-mail address: `mc.boily@imperial.ac.uk`

E-mail address: `roy.anderson@imperial.ac.uk`

(Benoît Mâsse) SCHARP - FHCRC, 1100 Fairview Avenue North, M2-A200 P.O. Box 19024 Seattle, WA 98109

E-mail address: bmasse@scharp.org

DIMACS Series in Discrete Mathematics
and Theoretical Computer Science
Volume **70**, 2006

Causal tree of disease transmission and the spreading of infectious diseases

Alexei Vázquez

ABSTRACT. We represent an epidemic outbreak by its causal tree of infection transmission, where nodes represent infected agents and arcs represent the disease transmission from an agent to another. The tree structure allows us to calculate different magnitudes quantifying the epidemic outbreak using iterative approaches. We focus on the expected outbreak size, and analyze its temporal evolution for different reproductive number and generation time distributions. We show that when the expected reproductive number is unbounded the outbreak size is proportional to agent population size and the temporal evolution is slower than exponential. The proposed framework can be used to model epidemic outbreaks using both empirical data obtained from previous outbreaks or by characterizing the contact process responsible for the disease transmission.

1. Introduction

A general framework for the mathematical modeling of epidemic spreading should allow us to understand the main features of the spreading dynamics, as well as being able to accommodate realistic spreading mechanisms and statistical properties obtained from empirical data. Mathematical approaches based on the mixed population hypothesis have been quite successful in this direction, determining the temporal evolution of the expected number of infected individuals with the estimation of a few parameters [**2, 10**]. These models have also been extended to include different transmission rates in a heterogeneous population [**21, 23**] and realistic distributions of infectious periods [**20**].

More recently, the partial mapping of several contact networks underlying the transmission of biological and computer viruses is making possible the development of network modeling frameworks. [**29, 22, 26, 3, 24, 12, 34**]. We can now perform numerical experiments modeling the possible outbreak scenarios of an infectious disease in a real environment, such as the spreading of an airborne virus within an urban settlement [**12, 24**] or a computer virus via email [**3, 34**]. Some analytical frameworks have also been developed to characterize the spreading dynamics on networks, explaining some features observed in the numerical simulations, such as

2000 *Mathematics Subject Classification.* 60J80,60J85,92B05,92D30.
Key words and phrases. infectious diseases, spreading dynamics, causal tree.

the existence or absence of an epidemic threshold [**29, 28, 22, 5**], the final outbreak size [**25, 26, 24**], and the spreading velocity [**4**].

Yet, we are still lacking a general network approach that allows us to incorporate empirical distributions of disease transmission times and reproductive numbers. Some hints in this direction can be obtained from the Belmman-Harris age-dependent branching process [**15**]. Further work is, however, required to extend their results to the case of an unbounded expected reproductive number. This last point is of particular importance since it has been recently noted that several graph representations of real systems are characterized by a degree distribution with a power law tail [**1**], and in this case the expected reproductive number may be unbounded [**7, 29**].

In this work we study the spreading of an infectious diseases within an agent population. We use the generic term agent to identify the entity that can host and transmit the disease. In turn we use the generic term disease to identify the entity that can be hosted by an agent and transmitted from an agent to another. Obvious examples are the transmission of infectious diseases, such as SARS or AIDS, among humans. Less obvious examples are the spreading of ideas and rumors ("infections of the mind") among humans. Other examples are found within electronic communications, such as the spreading of computer viruses, chain letters and hoaxes among computer users [**14**].

We represent the spreading process by the causal tree of disease transmission. The causal tree is a rooted and weighted tree containing all the disease transmissions instances: agent A infected agent B, and their generation times, the time elapsed between the infection of B by A. Each individual in the causal tree is characterized by its reproductive number, giving how many other agents it infects, and the generation times. In Section 2 we characterize the statistical properties of the reproductive numbers and generation times, focusing on two different scenarios: 1- the disease spreading on a graph, such as the spreading of a virus on the Internet, and 2- the disease spreading through a contact process, such as sexual contacts. We emphasize that in several communication systems the expected reproductive number is unbounded, meaning that it diverges with increasing the system size. Next, in Section 3 we characterize the statistical properties of an epidemic outbreak exploiting the recursive iteration of the local spreading properties studied in Section 2. In particular, we determine the temporal evolution of the expected number of infected agents, leaving the calculation of higher moments for future work. For the case of a bounded expected reproductive number we reproduce some results obtained for the Bellman-Harris age-dependent branching process [**15**]. We also characterize the case of an unbounded expected reproductive number, which exhibit some new features. In this case the outbreak is extensive once it starts, meaning that the expected number of infected agents is proportional to the agent population size, while the temporal evolution of the initial epidemic growth is slower than exponential. The implications of these results to the disease spreading among humans and computers are discussed.

2. Local disease transmission

Consider the spreading of an infectious disease on a population of N_0 susceptible agents and, within that population, consider a probe agent i that became infected and potentially could transmit the disease to other agents (see inset of Figure 1).

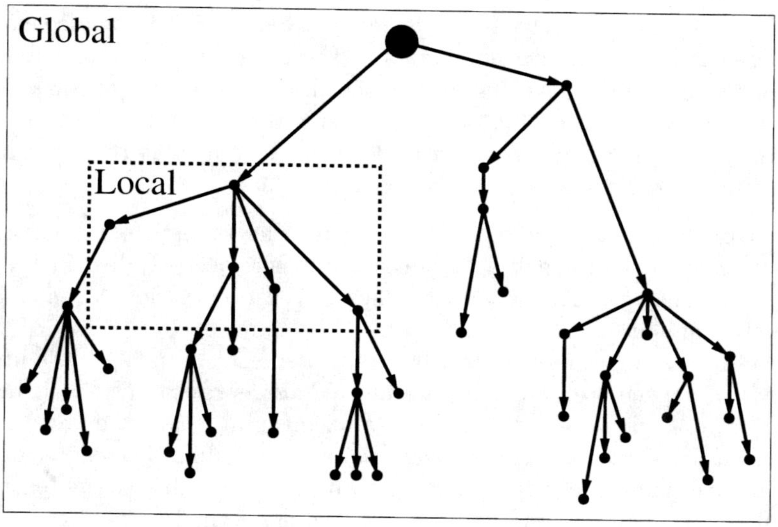

FIGURE 1. **Causal tree of disease transmission:** Schematic representation of a causal tree of disease transmission. Each node in the tree represents an infected agent and each arc represents the disease transmission from one agent to another: primary case $\rightarrow$ secondary case. We explicitly distinguish between patient zero (big circle) and other infected agents (smaller circles). Within the dashed square we consider a probe node, its out-degree giving its reproductive number and the arc's lengths giving the generation times.

We make an explicit distinction between the first infected agent ($i = 0$), or patient zero, and infected agents other than patient zero ($i = 1, \ldots, N_0 - 1$). The infection of patient zero comes from an exogenous source, such as an animal host in the case of human diseases or a hacker in the case of computer viruses. The infection of other agents, however, come from another agent that was infected at some previous time. Thus, we could imagine patient zero as any patient selected at random, while the disease transmission introduces some biases in the statistical properties of the agents being subsequently infected [**23, 2, 29**].

The probe agent will be characterized by the reproductive number and the generation time:

DEFINITION 2.1. The *reproductive number* $\mathcal{R}_i$ is the number of secondary infectious generated by agent i, given it is infected.

DEFINITION 2.2. The *generation time* $\mathcal{G}_{ij}$, is the time elapsed from the infection of a primary case i to the infection of a secondary case j.

We assume that the agent's reproductive numbers are independent random variables prescribed by the probability distributions $r_k = \mathbf{P}\{\mathcal{R}_0 = k\}$ and $\tilde{r}_k = \mathbf{P}\{\mathcal{R}_i = k|i > 0\}$, with expected reproductive number $R = \sum_k r_k k$ and $\tilde{R} = \sum_k \tilde{r}_k k$, respectively. We also assume that the generation times are independent random variables with the distribution functions $G(\tau) = \mathbf{P}\{\mathcal{G}_{0j} \leq \tau|j > 0\}$ and $\tilde{G}(\tau) = \mathbf{P}\{\mathcal{G}_{ij} \leq \tau|i,j > 0\}$, with probability density functions (pdf) $g(\tau) = dG(\tau)/d\tau$ and

$\tilde{g}(\tau) = d\tilde{G}(\tau)/d\tau$, respectively. In the following we are going to deduce expressions for the expected reproductive numbers and the generation time distributions for two different scenarios. The first one is the disease transmission on an existing structure, such as the spreading of a computer virus on the Internet. The second is the disease transmission through a contact process, such as the transmission of sexually transmitted diseases through sexual contacts.

2.1. Spreading on an existing graph. The statistical properties of the reproductive number of agents lying on a graph has been studied in [**7, 27, 26, 29, 28**]. We analyze then here to emphasize the observation of an unbounded reproductive number.

Consider a population of susceptible agents represented by a simple undirected graph, where vertices represent agents and edges represent disease transmission channels. The graph is assumed to be static, meaning that its adjacency matrix remain invariable during the course of the disease spreading. The degree of a vertex is given by the number of edges incident to it and represents the potential reproductive number of the corresponding agent. We make the following assumptions:

(*i*) The graph is a random graph with a given degree distribution p_s.
(*ii*) Given an infected vertex i and one of its neighbors j, the infection is transmitted from i to j with probability b, independently of the time when it happens.
(*iii*) Patient zero is any vertex selected at random.
(*iv*) The timing of the disease transmission from an infected vertex to its susceptible neighbors is independent of the graph topology.

Under these approximations we obtain that

THEOREM 2.3. *If (i)-(iv) are satisfied then*

$$R = b\sum_{s=1}^{\infty} p_s s \tag{2.1}$$

$$\tilde{R} = b\frac{\sum_{s=1}^{\infty} s(s-1)p_s}{\sum_{s=1}^{\infty} sp_s} \ . \tag{2.2}$$

PROOF. If the probe agent is represented by a vertex with degree s then from (*ii*) it follows that it infects k, $k = 1, \ldots, s$, of its neighbors with probability

$$v_k(s) = \binom{s}{k} b^k (1-b)^{s-k} \ . \tag{2.3}$$

If the probe agent is patient zero then from (*iii*) it follows that it has degree s with probability p_s, resulting in

$$r_k = \sum_{s=k}^{\infty} p_s v_k(s) \ . \tag{2.4}$$

From this equation we obtain the expected reproductive number in (2.1).

If the probe agent is an infected agent other than patient zero, represented by a vertex with degree s, then it can infect at most $s-1$ other agents, the remaining agent being the one from where it received the infection. Furthermore, this probe

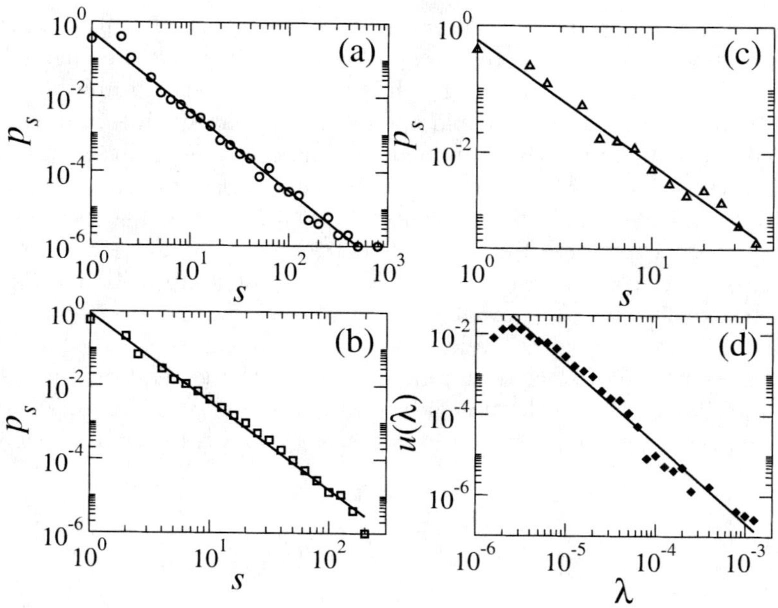

FIGURE 2. (a),(b),(c) Degree distribution of three graphs representing different communication networks. (a) Autonomous system representation of the Internet. (b) Router representation of the Internet. (c) Gnutella peer-to-peer network. For more information about the statistical properties of these graphs see [**33, 30**]. The continuous lines represent power law tails $p_s \sim s^{-\gamma}$ with $\gamma = 2.1$ (a), 2.4 (b) and 2.0 (c). (d) Probability density function $u(\lambda)$ of the rate λ at which email users send emails, as obtained from the dataset reported in [**11**]. The continuous line represents a power law tail $u(\lambda) \sim \lambda^{-\gamma}$ with $\gamma = 2.0$.

agent is not a vertex selected at random, but a vertex at the end of an edge selected at random. In the case of random graphs with a fixed degree distribution the vertex at the other end has degree s with probability $sp_s / \sum_{l=1}^{\infty} sp_s$ [**27**], resulting in

$$\tilde{r}_k = \sum_{s=k+1}^{\infty} \frac{sp_s}{\sum_{l=1}^{\infty} lp_l} v_k(s-1) \; . \tag{2.5}$$

From this equation we obtain the expected reproductive number in (2.2).

□

The degree distribution of many real graphs has the power law tail $p_s \sim s^{-\gamma}$, with $2 < \gamma < 3$ [**1**]. Some representative examples of electronic communication networks are shown in Figure 2(a),(b),(c). When $2 < \gamma < 3$ from (2.2) we obtain that $\tilde{R}$ is unbounded, where by unbounded we mean that $\tilde{R}_0 \to \infty$ when the agent population size tends to infinity. This fact has dramatic consequences on the global spreading of the disease (see Section 3).

EXAMPLE 2.4 (Email based computer worms). An email based computer worm is a "malicious" code that arrives to an email user (agent) via an infected email and, when activated by the email user, self-broadcast to all the email addresses on its address book. In this case b represents the probability that the infected email is opened by the email user, and the graph is the address book graph [**3**]. An email user receiving an infected email could open it during one email access session. The duration of an email access session is generally much smaller than the time between to email access sessions and, therefore, each email access session can be considered as instantaneous. We model the sequence of $l = 1, 2, \ldots$ email access sessions as a renewal process [**13**], where the times $\mathcal{A}_l$ between the l and $l+1$ access sessions are independent random variables with a common distribution $A(\tau) = \mathbf{P}\{\mathcal{A}_l \leq \tau\}$, with expected value $\mu_{\rm A}$. The event of receiving an email is uncorrelated with the event having an email access session, implying that the time at which an email is received is any time selected at random. Thus, the generation time, the time elapsed until its opening, is the time interval till the next email access session. This time is the residual waiting time in renewal theory, and is distributed according to [**13**]

$$G(\tau) = \tilde{G}(\tau) = \frac{1}{\mu_{\rm A}} \int_0^\tau d\tau' \left[1 - A(\tau')\right] \ . \tag{2.6}$$

Hence, to model the spreading of an email based computer worm we need to collect empirical data about the email users' address books and the timing of their email access sessions.

2.2. Spreading through a contact process. Consider a population of N_0 susceptible agents and a contact process among them responsible for the disease transmission. A typical example is the spread, through sexual contact, of a sexually transmitted disease on a population of sexually active individuals. To model the disease spread we assume that:

- (*i*) Given an agent i, $i = 1, \ldots, N_0$, the sequence of times when it establishes a contact is modeled by a renewal process [**13**], with the inter-contact time distribution function $C_i(\tau)$, pdf $c_i(\tau) = dC_i(\tau)/d\tau$, and expected value Λ_i.
- (*ii*) Λ_i are independent random variables with the distribution function $U(\lambda) = \mathbf{P}\{\Lambda_i \leq \lambda\}$, pdf $u(\lambda) = dU(\lambda)/d\lambda$ and expected value μ_U.
- (*iii*) On each contact m, $m = 1, 2, \ldots$, other agents are simultaneously contacted with probability q_m, with expected value $M = \sum_{m=1}^\infty q_m m$.
- (*iv*) The agent's population is homogeneous regarding the disease transmission probability upon contact, characterized by the probability $b(t)$ that the disease is transmitted at time t given a contact is established and the agent became infected at time $t = 0$.
- (*v*) Patient zero is any agent selected at random.

The agent distinction in (*i*) and (*ii*) allows us to consider heterogeneous populations where different agents may establish contacts with different rates [**21, 23, 2**]. The fact that more than one agent can be contacted simultaneously (*iii*) allows us to consider contact processes with concurrency. This is the case of sexually transmitted diseases, where a sexually active individual may maintain sexual relations with more than one sexually active individual during a certain period of time [**2**], and of email contacts, where an email may be sent to more than one recipient. Under these approximations we obtain

THEOREM 2.5. *If (i)-(v) are satisfied then*

$$R = \int_0^\infty dt\beta(t) \tag{2.7}$$

$$G(\tau) = \frac{1}{R}\int_0^\tau dt\beta(t) \ , \tag{2.8}$$

where

$$\beta(t) = Mb(t)\frac{1}{N_0}\sum_{i=1}^{N_0}\sum_{l=1}^{\infty} c_i^{l\star}(t) \ ; \tag{2.9}$$

and

$$\tilde{R} = \int_0^\infty dt\tilde{\beta}(t) \tag{2.10}$$

$$\tilde{G}(\tau) = \frac{1}{\tilde{R}}\int_0^\tau dt\tilde{\beta}(t) \ , \tag{2.11}$$

where

$$\tilde{\beta}(t) = Mb(t)\frac{1}{N_0\mu_U}\sum_{i=1}^{N_0}\Lambda_i\sum_{l=1}^{\infty} c_i^{l\star}(t) \ . \tag{2.12}$$

where $\star$ *denotes the convolution operation:* $f\star g(t) = \int_0^\infty df(\tau)g(t-\tau)$ *and* $f^{l\star}(t)$ *is the l-th order convolution of* $f(t)$.

PROOF. Consider a probe agent i that became infected at $t = 0$. This agent establishes contacts at later times t_{i1}, t_{i2}, ... potentially infecting the contacted agents. Following (i) the contacting times are given by

$$t_{il} = \sum_{n=1}^{l}\tau_{in} \ , \tag{2.13}$$

where τ_{in} are independent random variables with the identical distribution $C_i(\tau)$. Let $\mathcal{R}_{il}$ be the number agents it actually infects on the l-th contact, resulting in the reproductive number

$$\mathcal{R}_i = \sum_{l=1}^{\infty}\mathcal{R}_{il} \ . \tag{2.14}$$

The number of agents infected on each contact is determined by q_m and $b(t)$, and therefore it is independent of i. Thus, in the following we drop the subscript i when writing $\mathcal{R}_{il}$. We obtain that

$$\mathbf{P}\{\mathcal{R}_l = s\}(t) = \sum_{m=s}^{\infty} q_m\binom{m}{s}b(t)^l[1-b(t)]^{m-s} \ . \tag{2.15}$$

If the probe agent is patient zero then from (v), (2.14) and (2.15) it follows that

$$(2.16)\qquad r_k = \frac{1}{N_0}\sum_{i=1}^{N_0}\prod_{n=1}^{\infty}\int_0^{\infty} dC_i(\tau_n)\sum_{s_l=0}^{\infty}\delta_{k,\sum_{l=1}^{\infty}s_l}\prod_{l=0}^{\infty}\mathbf{P}\{\mathcal{R}_l = s_l\}\left(\sum_{n=1}^{l}\tau_n\right),$$

where δ_{ij} is the delta Kronecker symbol ($\delta_{ii} = 1$ and $\delta_{ij} = 0$ for all $i \neq j$). From (2.16) we obtain the expected reproductive number in (2.7), where $\beta(t)$ is the expected number of agents that patient zero infects between time t and $t + dt$. Finally, by definition $G(\tau) = \int_0^\tau dt\beta(t)/\int_0^\infty dt\beta(t)$ resulting in (2.8).

If the probe agent is an infected agent other than patient zero then it is not an agent selected at random, but an agent that has already established a contact with an infected agent. In this case we take into account that agents with frequent contacts are more susceptible to become infected, and subsequently will transmit the disease at higher rates. To be more precise, the probability that agent i establishes a contact between time t and $t + dt$ is given by Λ_i. In turn the total number of agents establishing a contact between time t and $t + dt$ is given by $N_0\mu_U dt$. Thus, if an infected agent establishes a contact between time t and $t + dt$ with another agent then this other agent is i with probability $\Lambda_i/N_0\mu_U$. The rest of the proof is similar to that for patient zero after replacing $(N_0)^{-1}\sum_i$ by $(N_0\mu_U)^{-1}\sum_i\Lambda_i$. □

EXAMPLE 2.6 (Poisson contact process). If agent i establishes contacts at a constant rate Λ_i then $C_i(\tau) = 1 - e^{\Lambda_i\tau}$ [**13**]. In this case from (2.7)-(2.11) we obtain

$$(2.17)\qquad R = \mu_U M\int_0^\infty b(t)\ ,$$

$$(2.18)\qquad \tilde{R} = \frac{\mu_{2U}}{\mu_U}M\int_0^\infty b(t)\ ,$$

$$(2.19)\qquad G(\tau) = \tilde{G}(\tau) = \frac{\int_0^\tau b(t)}{\int_0^\infty b(t)}\ ,$$

where $\mu_{2U} = \int_0^\infty dU(\lambda)\lambda^2$ is the second moment of the contact rate distribution. Note that the generation time distributions are only determined by the transmission probability $b(t)$. Indeed, when the contacts are established at a constant rate the distribution of the time when an actual disease transmission takes place will only depend on $b(t)$. It is also worth noticing that in the long time limit a renewal process with renewal time distribution $C_i(\tau)$ can be approximated by a Poisson process with rate [**13**]

$$(2.20)\qquad \Lambda_i = \frac{1}{\int_0^\infty dC_i(\tau)\tau}\ .$$

Hence, (2.17)-(2.19) may be a good approximation even when the contact process underlying the disease transmission is not a Poisson process.

When analyzing sexually transmitted diseases $u(\lambda)$ represents the pdf of the rate λ at which sexually active individuals acquires new sexual partners. Empirical data collected for several countries reveals that $u(\lambda)$ is characterized by a power law tail $u(\lambda) \sim \lambda^{-\gamma}$ [**18, 17, 31**]. The exponent γ resulting from the fit to the empirical data has values close to but larger than three. These observations should be considered with caution since γ is close to three and further refined measurements may reveal that γ is smaller than three, resulting in an unbounded $\tilde{R}_0$ in (2.18).

As sexually transmitted diseases spread via sexual contacts email viruses spread via email contacts, requiring us to investigate the contact rate distribution for the case of email contacts. The contact rate of an email user is given by the inverse of the average time between two consecutive email sent by that user. We have computed the distribution of this magnitude using a dataset containing the email history of 3180 email users within an university environment [**11**]. In Figure 2 we show that the distribution of email contact rate has also a power law tail, with exponent $\gamma \approx 2$, indicating that $\tilde{R}$ (2.18) is unbounded.

3. Global disease transmission

The recursive disease transmission, from one infected agent to some susceptible agents, from the new infected agents to other susceptible agents, and so on, may result in an outbreak with several infected agents (see Figure 1). We assume that to each infected agent, other than patient zero, we can assign one and only one infected agent from who he received the infection. In this case, we can represent an epidemic outbreak by an oriented weighted tree, where the root node $i = 0$ represents patient zero, nodes $i > 0$ represents infected agents other than patient zero, and each arc (i, j) represents the transmission of the disease from i to j. The number of arcs emanating from a node gives its out-degree and in turn the agent's reproductive number $\mathcal{R}_i$. Furthermore, to each arc (i, j) we assign a nonnegative real number $\mathcal{G}_{ij}$ giving the length of the time interval from the infection of i to the infection of j, *i.e.* the generation time. Since the out-degrees and arc's weights are random variables we thus obtain a set of random oriented weighted trees. More precisely:

DEFINITION 3.1. A *random causal tree* is a rooted and weighted tree where:

(1) The node's out-degrees are independent random variables prescribed by the probability distributions $r_k = \mathbf{P}\{\mathcal{R}_0 = k\}$ and $\tilde{r}_k = \mathbf{P}\{\mathcal{R}_i = k | i > 0\}$.
(2) The arc's weights are independent random variables with the distribution functions $G(\tau) = \mathbf{P}\{\mathcal{G}_{0j} \leq \tau | j > 0\}$ and $\tilde{G}(\tau) = \mathbf{P}\{\mathcal{G}_{ij} \leq \tau | i, j > 0\}$.
(3) The tree has a diameter D.

The last hypothesis is introduced to take into account that the agent population is finite and, therefore, the causal tree diameter could be at most equal to the total number of agents. Furthermore, for the case of a disease spreading on a graph (2.1) D is given by the graph diameter.

Consider a random causal tree and one of its nodes i. There is one and only one path from the root to i. We say that node i belongs to generation d if there are d arcs in the path from the root to i, and we denote by Γ_d the set of all nodes in the d-th generation. In turn, focusing on the tree branch rooted at i, there is only and only one path from i to nodes j in that branch. The sum of the arc's weights in the path from i to j gives the infection time t_{ij} of j given i was infected at time $t_{ii} = 0$. We then say that a node j is infected at time t if $t_{ij} \leq t$. Let $\mathcal{N}_i(t)$ be the number of infected nodes at time t in the branch rooted at i and $P_N^{(d)}(t) = \mathbf{P}\{\mathcal{N}_i(t) = N|i \in \Gamma_d\}$ be the probability distribution of $\mathcal{N}_i(t)$ given $i \in \mathcal{G}_d$. We introduce the generating functions

$$F^{(d)}(x,t) = \sum_{N=0}^{\infty} P_N^{(d)}(t)x^N \tag{3.1}$$

$$H(x) = \sum_{k=0}^{\infty} r_k x^k \tag{3.2}$$

$$\tilde{H}(x) = \sum_{k=0}^{\infty} \tilde{r}_k x^k \ . \tag{3.3}$$

We can exploit the recursive structure of a random causal tree to derive recursive relations for the generating function $F^{(d)}(x,t)$. More precisely

THEOREM 3.2. *$F^{(d)}(x,t)$ satisfies the recursive relations:*

$$F^{(d)}(x,t) = \begin{cases} xH\left(\int_0^t dG(\tau)F^{(d+1)}(x,t-\tau) + 1 - G(t)\right) \ , & d = 0 \\ x\tilde{H}\left(\int_0^t d\tilde{G}(\tau)F^{(d+1)}(x,t-\tau) + 1 - \tilde{G}(t)\right) \ , & 1 < d < D \\ x \ , d = D \ . \end{cases} \tag{3.4}$$

PROOF. Consider a node $i \in \Gamma_d$, with reproductive number $\mathcal{R}_i$, and let us denote by j, $j \in \{1, 2, \ldots, \mathcal{R}_i\}$, its neighbors in the $d+1$ generation. Thus

$$\mathcal{N}_i(t) = 1 + \sum_{j=1}^{\mathcal{R}_i} \mathcal{N}_j(t - \mathcal{G}_{ij}) \ . \tag{3.5}$$

$N_j(t - \mathcal{G}_{ij})$ are independent random variables with the distribution

$$\mathbf{P}\{\mathcal{N}_j(t-\mathcal{G}_{ij}) = N|j \in \Gamma_1\} = \int_0^t dG(\tau)P_N^{(1)}(t-\tau) + \delta_{N,0}\left(1 - G(t)\right) \tag{3.6}$$

for $d = 0$, and

$$\mathbf{P}\{\mathcal{N}_j(t-\mathcal{G}_{ij}) = N|j \in \Gamma_{d+1}\} = \int_0^t d\tilde{G}(\tau)P_N^{(d+1)}(t-\tau) + \delta_{N,0}\left(1 - \tilde{G}(t)\right) \tag{3.7}$$

for $d > 0$. From (3.5)- (3.7) we obtain

$$\begin{aligned} P_N^{(0)}(t) &= \sum_{k=0}^{\infty} r_k \sum_{N_1=0}^{\infty} \cdots \sum_{N_k=0}^{\infty} \delta_{\sum_{j=1}^k N_j + 1, N} \\ &\times \prod_{j=1}^{k} \left[\int_0^t dG(\tau)P_{N_j}^{(1)}(t-\tau) + \delta_{N_j,0}\left(1 - G(t)\right)\right] \end{aligned} \tag{3.8}$$

for $d = 0$, and

$$P_N^{(d)}(t) = \sum_{k=0}^{\infty} \tilde{r}_k \sum_{N_1=0}^{\infty} \cdots \sum_{N_k=0}^{\infty} \delta_{\sum_{j=1}^{k} N_j+1,N} \times \prod_{j=1}^{k} \left[\int_0^t d\tilde{G}(\tau) P_{N_j}^{(d+1)}(t-\tau) + \delta_{N_j,0} \left(1 - \tilde{G}(t)\right) \right] \quad (3.9)$$

for $0 < d < D-1$. Since the causal tree ends at generation D we obtain the boundary condition.

$$P_N^{(D)}(t) = \delta_{N,1} \quad (3.10)$$

for $d = D$. Finally, substituting (3.8), (3.9) and (3.10) into the generating function (3.1) we obtain the recursive equations in (3.4).

□

This is a good point to mention the differences between our formalism and the Bellman-Harris age-dependent branching process [**15**]. First, in the Bellman-Harris process all the secondary cases are generated simultaneously, while in a random causal tree each secondary case has its own generation time. Second, in the Bellman-Harris process the number of generations is unbounded ($D \to \infty$) while we explicitly assume that there is a maximum number of generations D. Third, and final, Bellman and Harris obtain a self-consistent equation for the generating function of the number of new descendants generated between time t and $t + dt$, while we obtain recursive relations for the generating function of the total number of descendants up to time t.

3.1. Expected outbreak size. From the recursive relations (3.4) we can obtain recursive relations for the moments of $P_N^d(t)$. We focus our attention in the first moment (the expected outbreak size) leaving the calculation of higher moments for later work. Let $N(t)$ be the expected total number of infected nodes up to time, and $n(t)$ the expected number of nodes that are infected between time t and $t + dt$, which in turn satisfy

$$n(t) = \frac{dN(t)}{dt} . \quad (3.11)$$

We obtain the following result

THEOREM 3.3.

$$n(t) = \sum_{d=1}^{D} R\tilde{R}^{d-1} g \star \tilde{g}^{(d-1)\star}(t) . \quad (3.12)$$

PROOF. The expected number of infected agents in the branch rooted at $i \in \Gamma_d$, given that i became infected at $t = 0$, is given by

$$N^{(d)}(t) = \frac{\partial F^{(d)}(1,t)}{\partial x} . \quad (3.13)$$

Making use of the recursive relations (3.4) we obtain

$$
(3.14) \qquad N^{(d)}(t) = \begin{cases} 1 + R\int_0^t dG(\tau)N^{(1)}(t-\tau)\ , & d=0 \\ 1 + \tilde{R}\int_0^t d\tilde{G}(\tau)N^{(d+1)}(t-\tau)\ , & 1<d<D \\ 1\ , d=D\ . \end{cases}
$$

Iterating these recursive relations from $d = D$ to $d = 0$ we obtain an expression for $N(t) = N^{(0)}(t)$. Finally, substituting this expression in (3.11) we obtain (3.12). □

3.2. Large population size. A fundamental concern in epidemiology is to determine whether an outbreak can result in an epidemic, infecting a significant number of susceptible agents in a short time. The final size of the outbreak is given by the expected value of the total number of infected agents, denoted by N_0. From (3.12) we obtain

$$
(3.15) \qquad N_0 = 1 + \int_0^\infty dt n(t) = 1 + R\frac{\tilde{R}^{D-1} - 1}{\tilde{R} - 1}\ .
$$

If D, R and $\tilde{R}$ are finite then N_0 is finite. Yet, if one of these magnitudes becomes infinitely large then N_0 may also become infinitely large. We consider two possible scenarios:

3.2.1. *$R < \infty$, $\tilde{R} < \infty$ and $D \to \infty$:* First we focus in the case where it takes a large number of generations before the outbreak reaches all the susceptible agents. In this case we obtain the following series representation for the expected outbreak size:

COROLLARY 3.4. If $R < \infty$, $\tilde{R} < \infty$ and $D \to \infty$ then

$$
(3.16) \qquad n(t) = \sum_{d=1}^{\infty} R\tilde{R}^{d-1} g \star \tilde{g}^{(d-1)\star}(t)\ .
$$

PROOF. Setting $D \to \infty$ in (3.12) we obtain (3.16). The question is whether this series converges and, therefore, it is a series representation of $n(t)$. Let $\hat{n}(\omega) = \int_0^\infty dt e^{-\omega t} n(t)$ be the Laplace transform of $n(t)$. In turn we denote by $\hat{g}(\omega)$ and $\hat{\tilde{g}}(\omega)$ the Laplace transforms of $g(\tau)$ and $\tilde{g}(\tau)$. From (3.16) we obtain

$$
(3.17) \qquad \hat{n}(\omega) = \frac{R\hat{g}(\omega)}{1 - \tilde{R}\hat{\tilde{g}}(\omega)}\ .
$$

Since $g(\tau)$ and $\tilde{g}(\tau)$ are probability densities then $\hat{g}(\omega)$ and $\hat{\tilde{g}}(\omega)$ are defined and continuous for all $\omega \geq 0$. Yet, if the denominator in the *r.h.s.* of (3.17) equals zero then $\hat{n}(\omega)$ is not defined. Let α be the positive solution, if there is any, of the equation

$$
(3.18) \qquad \tilde{R}\hat{\tilde{g}}(\alpha) = 1\ .
$$

If $\tilde{R} < 1$ then (3.18) has no positive solution and, therefore, $\hat{n}(\omega)$ in (3.17) is defined for all $\omega \geq 0$. If $\tilde{R} > 1$ then (3.18) has a positive solution and, therefore, $\hat{n}(\omega)$ in (3.17) is defined for all $\omega > \alpha$. In either case we can compute the inverse Laplace transform

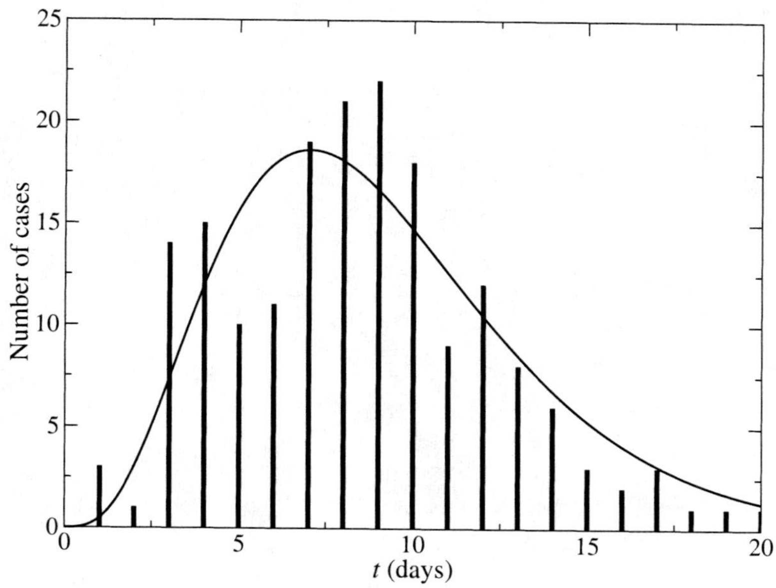

FIGURE 3. **Gamma distribution of generation times:** Number of secondary cases generated by a primary case for a SARS outbreak in Singapore, as reported in [**19**] (bars). The solid line is the best fit to the gamma pdf (3.20) times a pre-factor, resulting in $\theta \approx 4.3$.

$$n(t) = \frac{1}{2\pi\imath} \int_{\omega_0 - \imath\infty}^{\omega_0 + \imath\infty} e^{\omega t} \hat{n}(\omega) \ , \tag{3.19}$$

where $\omega_0 > 0$ for $\tilde{R} < 1$ and $\omega_0 > \alpha$ for $\tilde{R} > 1$. Since (3.19) is defined for all $t > 0$ then (3.16) converges for all $t > 0$ and it is a series representation of $n(t)$.

□

REMARK 3.5. (3.12) has two different long time asymptotic behaviors depending on the value of $\tilde{R}$:

- When $\tilde{R} < 1$ the Laplace transform of $n(t)$ is defined for all $\omega \geq 0$. Hence, $\int_0^\infty dt n(t) < \infty$ and, therefore, $n(t) = \mathcal{O}(1/t)$ when $t \to \infty$. This means that the epidemic outbreak will die out before a significant number of susceptible agents become infected.
- When $\tilde{R} > 1$ the Laplace transform of $n(t)$ is defined for $\omega > \alpha$ and, therefore, $n(t) \sim e^{\alpha t}$ when $t \to \infty$.

These two different asymptotic behaviors has already been obtained for the Hellman-Harris process [**15**].

EXAMPLE 3.6 (Gamma distribution of generation times). The empirical data often support the hypothesis of a gamma distribution of generation times [**19, 16**]. An example is shown in Figure 3 for a SARS outbreak in Singapore. Let us assume that $g(\tau) = \tilde{g}(\tau)$ and they are given by the gamma pdf

$$g(\tau) = \tilde{g}(\tau) = \frac{\theta}{\mu_G \Gamma(\theta)} \exp\left(-\frac{\theta\tau}{\mu_G}\right)\left(\frac{\theta\tau}{\mu_G}\right)^{\theta-1} , \tag{3.20}$$

where μ_G is the expected generation time and $\theta \geq 1$. Substituting (3.20) into (3.16) we obtain

$$n(t) = \frac{\theta R_0}{\mu_G \tilde{R}_0^{1-1/\theta}} \exp\left(-\frac{\theta t}{\mu_G}\right) \sum_{d=1}^{\infty} \frac{1}{\Gamma(\theta d)} \left(\frac{\tilde{R}_0^{1/\theta} \theta t}{\mu_G}\right)^{\theta d-1} . \tag{3.21}$$

In particular,

$$n(t) = \frac{R}{\mu_G} \exp\left(\frac{(\tilde{R}-1)t}{\mu_G}\right) \tag{3.22}$$

for $\theta = 1$ and

$$n(t) = \frac{2R}{\mu_G \tilde{R}^{1/2}} \exp\left(-\frac{2t}{\mu_G}\right) \sinh\left(\frac{\tilde{R}^{1/2} 2t}{\mu_G}\right) . \tag{3.23}$$

for $\theta = 2$. This example illustrate how, in some cases, we can express $n(t)$ in terms of elementary functions. Whenever this is not possible, the series representation can be used to compute $n(t)$ numerically.

3.2.2. *$R < \infty$, $D < \infty$ and $\tilde{R} \to \infty$:* When $\tilde{R} \to \infty$ it may take just a few generations such that all the susceptible agents become infected. In this case, the temporal evolution of the expected number of new infected agents will be dominated by those terms in (3.12) with higher powers of $\tilde{R}$. More precisely

COROLLARY 3.7. If $R < \infty$, $D < \infty$, $\tilde{R} \to \infty$, and $g(\tau) > 0$ and $\tilde{g}(\tau) > 0$ for all $\tau > 0$ then

$$n(t) \sim N_0 g \star \tilde{g}^{(D-1)\star}(t) \left[1 + \mathcal{O}\left(\frac{1}{\tilde{R}}\right)\right] . \tag{3.24}$$

PROOF. If $g(\tau) > 0$ and $\tilde{g}(\tau) > 0$ for all $\tau > 0$ then $g \star \tilde{g}^{(d-1)\star}(t) > 0$ for $t > 0$ and $d \geq 1$. From (3.12) and this fact it follows that

$$\frac{n(t) - R\tilde{R}^{D-1} g \star \tilde{g}^{(D-1)\star}(t)}{R\tilde{R}^{D-1} g \star \tilde{g}^{(D-1)\star}(t)} = \mathcal{O}\left(\frac{1}{\tilde{R}}\right) . \tag{3.25}$$

Furthermore, from (3.15) we obtain

$$N_0 \sim R\tilde{R}^{D-1} \left[1 + \mathcal{O}\left(\frac{1}{\tilde{R}}\right)\right] . \tag{3.26}$$

Finally, from (3.25) and (3.26) we obtain (3.24).

□

REMARK 3.8. In this case the expected number of new infected agents is of the order of N_0 for $t > 0$, indicating that the outbreak can be considered as an epidemic from its starting time. In such a case it is more appropriate to work with the expected number of new infected agents relative to the population size. Thus, we define the pdf of the new infections between time t and $t + dt$

$$\rho(t) = \frac{n(t)}{N_0} = g \star \tilde{g}^{(D-1)\star}(t) \,, \tag{3.27}$$

where the second equality follows from (3.24) and it holds in the $\tilde{R} \to \infty$ limit.

REMARK 3.9. There may be cases where both $\tilde{R}$ and D diverges. An example is the spreading of a disease on a random graph with a given degree distribution, where the degree distribution has a power law tail $p_s \sim s^{-\gamma}$ with $2 < \gamma < 3$ and a maximum degree $k_{\max} = N_0^{\delta}$, where N_0 is the graph size. From (2.2) we obtain that $\tilde{R} \sim N_0^{\delta(3-\gamma)}$ when $N_0 \to \infty$, while D scale at most as $\log N_0$ [**8, 9**]. In this case (3.24) and (3.27) are still valid up to some logarithmic corrections to D.

EXAMPLE 3.10 (Gamma distribution of generation times). If the generation times are distributed according to the gamma distribution (3.20), then from (3.27) we obtain the gamma pdf

$$\rho(t) = \frac{\theta}{\mu_G \Gamma(\theta D)} \exp\left(-\frac{\theta t}{\mu_G}\right) \left(\frac{\theta t}{\mu_G}\right)^{\theta D - 1} \,, \tag{3.28}$$

which is characterized by a polynomial growth of order $\theta D - 1$ followed by an exponential decay. This result completely departures from the exponential growth predicted by current mathematical approaches to the spreading dynamics [**35**].

4. Conclusions

The causal tree of infection transmission is a suitable object to characterize the spreading dynamics of infectious diseases. Its flexibility allow us to consider different generation time distributions, such as the gamma distribution of generation times that is often used to fit empirical data. It also allow us to extend previous studies of the Bellman-Harris age-dependent branching process to include the case when the expected reproductive number is unbounded. In this last case we obtain that the spreading dynamics is extensive from its very starting time, meaning that number of infected agents is proportional to the population size. Furthermore, the initial epidemic growth is not necessarily exponential as predicted by previous mathematical approaches, but depends on the shape of the generation time distribution. For instance, the initial epidemic growth is polynomial for a gamma distribution of generation times.

We find out contradictory evidence regarding the AIDS epidemics. While sexual network measurements suggest that $\tilde{R}$ is bounded, there is empirical evidence indicating that the AIDS epidemics exhibits a polynomial growth in certain countries [**23, 6, 32**]. Further work is required to determine whether this polynomial growth has a different origin or the sexual network data is incomplete. On the other hand, the empirical evidence indicates that $\tilde{R}$ is unbounded for several communication networks. Therefore, our predictions can be tested using empirical data for computer virus outbreaks.

While we have limited the analysis to the expected outbreak size, we can calculate higher order moments as well, and in principle the outbreak size probability distribution as a function of time. This point is extremely important to understand the initial phase of the outbreak were just a few agents are infected and the fluctuations around the expected outbreak size are significant.

References

[1] R. Albert and A.-L. Barabási. Statistical mechanics of complex networks. *Rev. Mod. Phys.*, 74:47–95, 2001.

[2] R. M. Anderson and R. M. May. *Infectious diseases of humans.* Oxford Univ. Press, New York, 1991.

[3] J. Balthrop, S. Forrest, M. E. J. Newman, and M. M. Williamson. Technological networks and the spread of computer viruses. *Science*, 304:527–529, 2004.

[4] M. Barthélemy, A. Barrat, and A. Vespignani. Velocity and hierarchical spread of epidemic outbreaks in scale-free networks. *Phys. Rev. Lett.*, 92:178701–178704, 2004.

[5] M. Boguña, R. Pastor-Satorras, and A. Vespignani. Absence of epidemic threshold in scale-free networks with connectivity correlations. *Phys. Rev. Lett.*, 90:028701–04, 2003.

[6] R. Brookmeyer and M. H. Gail. *AIDS epidemiology: a quantitative approach.* Oxford Univ. Press, New York, 1994.

[7] D. S. Callaway, M. E. J. Newman, S. H. Strogatz, and D. J. Watts. Network robustness and fragility: Percolation on random graphs. *Phys. Rev. Lett.*, 85:5468–5471, 2000.

[8] F. Chung and L. Lu. The average distances in random graphs with given expected degrees. *Proc. Natl. Acad. Sci. USA*, 99:15879–15882, 2002.

[9] R. Cohen and S. Havlin. Scale-free networks are ultrasmall. *Phys. Rev. Lett.*, 90:058701–4, 2003.

[10] D. J. Daley and J. Gani. *Epidemic modelling: an introduction.* Cambridge University Press, Cambridge, 1999.

[11] J.-P. Eckmann, E. Moses, and D. Sergi. Entropy of dialogs creates coherent structures in e-mail traffic. *Proc. Natl. Acad. Sci. USA*, 101:14333–14337, 2004.

[12] S. Eubank, H. Guclu, V. S. A. Kumar, M. Marathe, A. Srinivasan, Z. Toroczcai, and N. Wang. Modelling disease outbreaks in realistic urban social networks. *Nature*, 429:180–184, 2004.

[13] W. Feller. *An introduction to probability theory and its applications.* John Wiley & Sons, New York, 1966. Vol. II.

[14] D. Harley, R. Slade, and U. E. Gattiker. *Viruses revealed.* Osborne/McGraw-Hill, Berkeley, 2001.

[15] T. E. Harris. *The Theory of Branching Processes.* Springer-Verlag, Berlin, 2002.

[16] D. T. Haudon and *et el.* The construction and analysis of epidemic trees with reference to the 2001 UK foot-and-mouth outbreak. *Proc. R. Soc. Lond. B*, 270:121–127, 2003.

[17] J. H. Jones and M. S. Handcock. An assessment of preferential attachment as a mechanism for human sexual network formation. *Proc. R. Soc. Lond. B Biol. Sci.*, 270:1123–8, 2003.

[18] F. Liljeros, C. R. Edling, L. A. N. Amaral, H. E. Stanley, and Y. Berg. The web of human sexual contacts. *Nature*, 411:907–908, 2001.

[19] M. Lipsitch and *et al.* Transmission dynamics and control of severe acute respiratory syndrome. *Science*, 300:1966–1970, 2003.

[20] A. L. Lloyd. Realistic distributions of infectious periods in epidemic models: changing patterns of persistence and dynamics. *Theor. Pop. Biol.*, 60:59–71, 2001.

[21] R. M. May and R. M. Anderson. Transmission dynamics of HIV infection. *Nature*, 326:137–142, 1987.

[22] R. M. May and A. L. Lloyd. Infection dynamics on scale-free networks. *Phys. Rev. E*, 64:066112–066115, 2001.

[23] T. M. May and R. M. Anderson. The transmission dynamics of human immunodeficiency virus (HIV). *Phil. Trans. R. Soc. Lond. B*, 321:565–607, 1988.

[24] L. A. Meyers, B. Pourbohloul, M. E. J. Newman, D. M. Skowronski, and R. C. Brunham. Network theory and SARS: Predicting outbreak diversity. *J Theor. Biol.*, 232:71–81, 2004.

[25] Y. Moreno, R. Pastor-Satorras, and A. Vespignani. Epidemic outbreaks in complex heterogeneous networks. *Eur. Phys. J. B*, 26:521–529, 2002.

[26] M. E. J. Newman. Spread and epidemic disease on networks. *Phys. Rev. E*, 66:016128–016138, 2002.

[27] M. E. J. Newman, S. H. Strogatz, and D. J. Watts. Random graphs with arbitrary degree distribution and their applications. *Phys. Rev. E*, 64:026118–026135, 2001.

[28] R. Pastor-Satorras and A. Vespignani. Epidemic dynamics and endemic states in complex networks. *Phys. Rev. E*, 63:066117–066125, 2001.

[29] R. Pastor-Satorras and A. Vespignani. Epidemic spreading in scale-free networks. *Phys. Rev. Lett.*, 86:3200–3203, 2001.

[30] R. Pastor-Satorras and A. Vespignani. *Evolution and structure of the Internet: A Statistical Physics approach.* Cambridge University Press, Cambridge, 2004.

[31] A. Schneeberger, C. H. Mercer, S. A. Gregson, N. M. Fergurson, C. A. Nyamukapa, R. M. Anderson, A. M. Johnson, and G. P. Garnett. Scale-free networks and sexually transmitted diseases. *Sex. Transm. Dis.*, 31:380–387, 2004.

[32] B. Szendriöi and G. Csányi. Polynomial epidemics and clustering in contact networks. *Proc. R Soc. Lond. B Biol. Sci.*, 271:S364–6, 2004.

[33] A. Vázquez. *Degree correlations and clustering hierarchy in networks: measures, origin and consequences.* PhD thesis, International School for Advanced Studies, 2002.

[34] A. Vázquez and A.-L. Barabási. Non-Poisson contact processes in virus spreading. unpublished.

[35] A. Vázquez. Polynomial growth in age-dependent branching processes with diverging reproductive number. http://xxx.lanl.gov/abs/cond-mat/0505116.

Department of Physics and center for Complex Networks Research, University of Notre Dame, IN 46556, USA

E-mail address: `avazque1@nd.edu`

DIMACS Series in Discrete Mathematics
and Theoretical Computer Science
Volume **70**, 2006

Structure of Social Contact Networks and Their Impact on Epidemics

Stephen Eubank[1], V.S. Anil Kumar[2], Madhav V. Marathe[3], Aravind Srinivasan[4], and Nan Wang[5,6]

ABSTRACT. Traditional epidemiological research has focused on rate-based differential-equation models on *completely mixing* populations. In this paper, we outline an approach based on a combination of network theory and discrete-event simulations to study epidemics in *large urban areas*. We survey some of our results published in *Nature* (2004) and the *Proc. ACM-SIAM Symposium on Discrete Algorithms* (2004), and present some new results on: (i) mathematical properties of large social contact networks, as well as (ii) simulation-based dynamic analysis of disease-spread in such networks. We identify a number of new measures that are significant for understanding epidemics and for developing new strategies in policy planning. We also perform a very detailed structural analysis of the social contact networks produced by **TRANSIMS**, a simulator for detailed transportation/traffic studies, and study two random graph models to generate realistic social networks: Chung-Lu's model and the configuration model. We also develop combinatorial formulations and approximation algorithms for quarantining, vaccination and sensor placement, as aids to decision-making.

1. Introduction

The explosive growth of urban population in the past century has led to a variety of new problems related to public health- the high density of people and their interaction lead to a significant risk of epidemics [**1**]. This was evident in the

---

[1]Part of the work was done while the author was in the Basic and Applied Simulation Science group at Los Alamos National Laboratory.

[2]Part of the work was done while the author was in the Basic and Applied Simulation Science group at Los Alamos National Laboratory and was supported by the Department of Energy under Contract W-7405-ENG-36.

[3]Part of the work was done while the author was in the Basic and Applied Simulation Science group at Los Alamos National Laboratory.

[4]This material is based upon work supported in part by the National Science Foundation under Grant No. 0208005.

[5]Part of the work was done while the author was visiting Los Alamos National Laboratory.

[6]This material is based upon work supported in part by the National Science Foundation under Grant No. 0208005.

2000 *Mathematics Subject Classification.* Primary 05C85 Graph algorithms; Secondary 68R10 Graph theory.

recent SARS epidemic, and is a testimony to the "small world" nature of today's society. Coupled with recent fears of bio-terror attacks, there has been a spurt of research on understanding epidemics and techniques to aid policy planning, e.g., for vaccination, quarantining and disease-detection strategies.

Traditional epidemiological research has focused on rate based differential equation models on completely mixing populations, i.e., all the people are allowed to interact with each other; see [**10, 22, 25**] for a comprehensive discussion on this subject. An attractive feature of this modeling approach is that it allows one to obtain analytical expressions for a number of interesting parameters such as the numbers of sick, infected and recovered individuals in a population. But such a modeling approach does not capture the complexity of human interactions that serves as a mechanism for disease transmission. In addition, typically the number of different subpopulation types considered is small (for analytical tractability) and parameters such as mixing rate and reproductive number are either unknown or hard to observe.

In this paper, we outline an approach based on a combination of network theory and discrete event simulations to study epidemics in *large urban areas* - the main idea is that a better understanding of the characteristics of the social contact network can give better insights into disease dynamics and vaccination/quarantining strategies, which can be used in the epidemic simulation. For instance, our recent work in [**16**] shows that a better understanding of the underlying network structure leads to more refined conclusions, e.g. in some cases mass vaccination might not be needed in the presence of a better disease detection strategy. Similar work by Meyers et al. [**28**] has demonstrated that new insights on the disease dynamics can be obtained by understanding the contact structure carefully. Interestingly, analysis of social networks in urban regions for effectively containing the spread of Cholera was done in the late 1800s in London [**9**]: in this outbreak, a map was used to chart the outbreak and relate it to a contaminated water pump; shutting down the pump immediately brought the outbreak to an end. The earliest formal work on use of network structure for epidemiological studies appears to be that of Elveback, Fox and Ackerman [**14**]. Recently, a number of other authors have also undertaken a similar approach [**26, 37**]. In contrast to the work of [**28, 26**], we study *realistic and large* urban social contact networks for an entire city consisting of well over a million nodes.

Recently there has been a resurgence of research in complex networks: the renewed interest is driven by a number of empirical and theoretical studies showing that network structure plays a crucial role in understanding the overall behavior of complex systems. See [**11, 3, 2, 4, 28, 33**] and the references therein for recent results in this active area. However, properties of social contact networks that are crucial for understanding epidemics have been explored only recently [**31, 33, 32, 34, 28**]. Another recent direction of research has been to determine random graph models that can generate such networks: the traditional Erdős-Rényi-like model does not capture many important features of real networks. Unfortunately, as we argue later, many of these random graph models, such as the preferential attachment model, are not suited for social network analysis.

2. Our Contributions.

In this paper, we survey our recent results in [**16, 17**] and present new results on (i) mathematical properties of large social contact networks and (ii) simulation based dynamic analysis of disease spread on such networks. The social contact networks we study are obtained by using **TRANSIMS** – a simulation based tool for urban transport planning (see Section 3 for details). We identify a number of new measures that are significant for understanding epidemics and developing new strategies for policy planning. Some of these measures, such as demographic mixing rates, can be determined only because of the very detailed and realistic nature of the networks we study. The resulting understanding of these networks is used in conjunction with a parallel discrete event simulation system called **EpiSims** [**9, 18**] - this is a tool to perform detailed simulations of disease transmission on a synthetic urban population. Our main contributions in this paper are threefold:

(1) **Analysis and random generation models of large social networks.** We perform very detailed structural analysis of the social contact networks produced by **TRANSIMS** and identify new measures that have relevance for modeling epidemics. The structural measures we survey here were first reported in [**16, 17**]. In addition, we perform the first analysis of some temporal and cultural aspects of such graphs. We also study two random graph models to generate realistic social networks: the first, based on the Chung-Lu model, was first discussed in [**17**]; the second, the *configuration model*, is introduced in this paper.

(2) **Combinatorial Models for Decision Making in Epidemiology.** We develop combinatorial formulations and approximation algorithms for quarantining, vaccination and sensor placement[1] problems, as an aid in decision making. Our formulations and results crucially use the underlying contact structure; they demonstrate the additional value of such models compared to traditional complete mixing models.

(3) **Simulation Based Empirical Evaluation.** We consider several vaccination strategies motivated by the network structure, and study their efficacy using **EpiSims**. We use the new structural measures we identify in developing the vaccination strategies.
EpiSims is then used to compute the efficacy of these vaccination strategies by taking into account the stochastic nature of disease transmission. The goal of this paper is not to develop the *optimal* vaccination strategy, but, rather to come up with several reasonable ones, and compare them by simulation; the rationale is that large scale simulation such as **EpiSims** appears to be the only reasonable computational method for this purpose.

Organization. Section 3 describes **TRANSIMS** and **EpiSims** in some detail. It also contains a description of how the social contact network is constructed. Section 4 describes the structural analysis of the Portland social contact network, and touches upon random-graph models. In Section 5, we formulate combinatorial problems that model basic policy-planning problems relevant to epidemiology and describe efficient approximation algorithms for solving these problems. Section 6

[1]The sensor placement problem was first discussed in [**17**].

describes simulation results on different vaccination schemes, motivated by the network structure. Section 7 discusses random-graph models, and Section 8 contains concluding remarks. As mentioned earlier, some of the results described in this paper appeared in [**16**] and [**17**].

3. Constructing Realistic Social Networks

In order to understand the spread of contagious diseases, we need a realistic representation of a social contact network. The Transportation Analysis and Simulation System (**TRANSIMS**) developed at Los Alamos provides a way to generate synthetic realistic social contact networks in a large urban region. It is based on the assumption that the transportation infrastructure constrains people's choices about what activities to perform and where to perform them. **TRANSIMS** produces positions of all travelers on a second-by-second basis for a large metropolitan area and it has effectively been used to construct detailed mobility patterns for the city of Portland. We refer the reader to [**6**] and the web-site `http://transims.tsasa.lanl.gov` for more extensive descriptions of this tool. **TRANSIMS** conceptually decomposes the transportation planning task using three different time scales, as follows.

(1) Creating a population and activities Data about land use and demographic information, combined with survey data from thousands of households is employed to create a synthetic population, where each person has a specific home address. A sequence of daily activities, and the locations where these activities are to be done, is determined for each person, based on the activity surveys, travel time and land use data.

(2) Assigning Routes and trip-chains Second, an intermediate time-scale consists of assigning routes and trip-chains to satisfy the activity requests. To do this, the estimated locations are fed into a routing algorithm to find minimum cost paths through the transportation infrastructure consistent with constraints on mode choice [**8, 5**]. An example constraint might be: "walk to a transit stop, take transit to work using no more than two transfers and no more than one bus". This step is coupled with the simulation of the actual movement of people on their chosen routes, and is repeated till some sort of near-equilibrium is attained.

(3) Detailed simulation Finally, the movement of people along their chosen routes is simulated. This simulation is extremely detailed: it resolves distances down to 7.5 meters and times down to one second. It provides an updated estimate of time-dependent travel times for each edge in the network, including the effects of congestion. This estimate is fed back to the Routing (step (2)) and location estimation (step (1)) algorithms, which produce new plans. This feedback process continues iteratively until it converges to a "quasi-steady state" in which no one can find a better path in the context of everyone else's decisions. The entire process estimates the demand on a transportation network using census data, land usage data, and activity surveys.

A substantial effort has been spent on calibration and validation of the output produced by **TRANSIMS**, and it has been deployed in the city of Portland (see [**6**] for details). Various microscopic and macroscopic quantities produced by **TRANSIMS** have been verified in the city of Portland; these include (i) traffic invariants

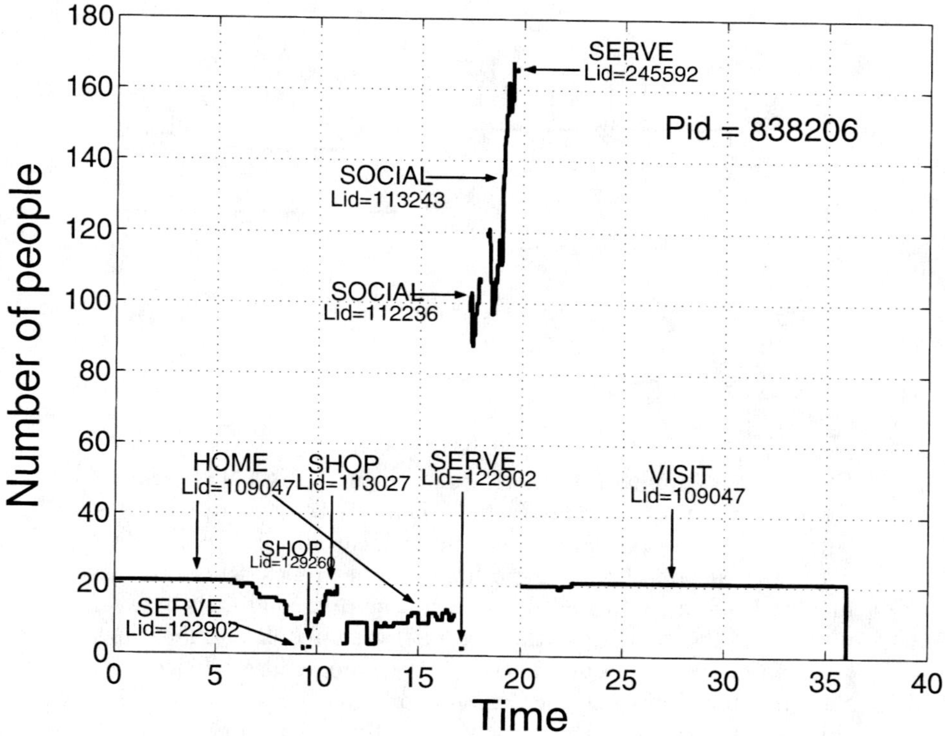

FIGURE 1. Figure showing, for a randomly chosen synthetic individual (whose person-id is pid=838206 as shown in the figure) in Portland, the activities, their locations (marked with lid's as their location-id's) and their time durations (in hour) over the course of 1.5 days. The x-axis indicates the time when an activity happens, the y-axis indicates the number of people in the same location where the activity is taken by the chosen individual. In Portland data there are nine activity types, namely `home, work, shop, visit, social, other, serve, school, college`. Each edge in the people-location bipartite graph is labeled by one of these activities.

such as flow density patterns, jam wave propagation, (ii) macroscopic quantities, such as activities and population densities in an entire city, number of people occupying various locations in a time varying fashion, time varying traffic density split by trip purpose and various modal choices over highways and other major roads, turn counts, number of trips going between zones in a city, etc. **TRANSIMS** produces a comprehensive representation of people and their activities over the course of a day. Figure 1 shows an example of this for a randomly chosen synthetic individual. It is important to note that simulations such as **TRANSIMS** appears to be the *only way* to obtain information about some of the measures discussed here.

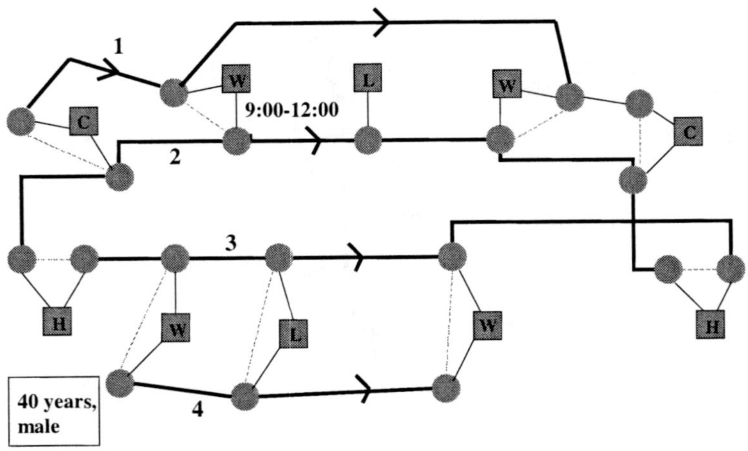

FIGURE 2. An illustration of various steps in **TRANSIMS**, and the networks that are constructed. The squares denote locations, with the letters specifying the type of locations (H - home, W - work, C - carpool, L - place for lunch). The circles denote people, moving from one location to another. The thin solid lines between people and locations show the edges between people and locations, i.e., the edges of the graph G_{PL} - these edges are labeled with the time duration when the person is present at the location. The thick solid lines (with the arrows) show the "trajectory" of a person (4 persons in this figure), as they move from one location to another; this also illustrates the temporal aspects of the network - for instance, person 1 moves from home to a carpool (viewed as a location), to a work location, and so on. At a location, all people who are at that location at the same time are connected by dashed edges - these are the edges of the graph G_P. The people also have labels - one such label (40 year, male) is shown in the figure.

3.1. Network Representations. In summary, **TRANSIMS** generates the following information for a city - demographic information for each person and location, and a minute-by-minute schedule of each person's activities and the locations where these activities take place. This information can be abstractly represented by a (vertex and edge) labeled bipartite graph G_{PL}, where P is the set of people and L is the set of locations. If a person $p \in P$ visits a location $\ell \in L$, there is an edge $(p, \ell, label) \in E(G_{PL})$ between them, where *label* is a record of the type of activity of the visit and its start and end points. Each vertex (person and location) can also have labels. The person labels correspond to his/her demographic attributes such as age, income, etc. The labels attached to locations specify the location's attributes such as its x and y coordinates, the type of activity performed, maximum capacity, etc. Note that, there can be multiple edges between a person and a location recording different visits. When studying the topological structure of contact networks, we will sometimes consider and sometimes ignore the labels and the multiplicity of the edges; see [**16**] for a discussion of why the time-labels can be ignored for various diseases. We use the term *people-location* graph to refer to the above bipartite graph, wherein multiple edges are discarded and time labels are omitted.

We also consider another graph G_P induced on the set of people: $(p_1, p_2) \in E(G_P)$ if there is a location $\ell \in L$ such that $(p_1, \ell), (p_2, \ell) \in E(G_{PL})$, and the time intervals during which p_1 and p_2 are present at ℓ overlap, i.e., there is a common location at which the two people p_1, p_2 are present at the same time. This graph will be referred to as the *people-people* graph.

In this paper, all the data is for the city of Portland, Oregon, USA; our ongoing research is studying the (broadly similar) structures of other urban areas such as Chicago.

3.2. EpiSims: Simulating the Spread of Disease. **EpiSims** is a tool for simulating the spread of disease on a social contact network. We now provide a brief overview of this tool; further details can be found in [**18, 15**]. Using the information generated by **TRANSIMS**, the simulation maintains a parameterized model for the state of the health of each person, and updates this continuously based on interaction with other people, and transmission of the disease through these contacts. This enables us to get estimates of both the geographic and demographic distribution of disease as a function of time; it also allows us to evaluate the impact of different vaccination/quarantining policies. Different aspects of this tool are discussed below.

Disease Model within each Host: **EpiSims** uses a single parameter, the *disease load*, to represent the effect of a disease upon a host. The load in **EpiSims** is intended to be analogous to viral titre in a throat swab, number of spores or bacteria present, concentration of toxin, etc. However, it need not reproduce such clinical aspects of these loads as distribution throughout the body. It is merely a parameter that is used to determine whether a person is infected, symptomatic, too sick for normal activities, infectious, or dead - the higher the disease load, the sicker the person. Each individual in the simulation who is exposed (either through exposure to an initial release or through contact with an infected and infectious person) will progress through a series of disease stages. An exposed individual will either become infected or not with a probability based upon the disease model and the individual's demographics. Individuals who become infected either develop a clinical case of the disease or not. For instance, some fraction of those infected with smallpox never develop a fever or symptoms of the disease. As above, the probability of developing clinical symptoms depends upon victim characteristics. An isolated contaminated person's or location's load grows or shrinks at predetermined rates, depending on the characteristics of the person and location. All locations share a single common exponential growth or decay rate, depending on the disease. For example, the amount of virus present in the environment would decay exponentially if there were no sources (infected people); the amount of bacteria might grow exponentially; while the number of spores would remain fixed. The disease model also specifies a set of threshold values for determining the effect of the load on an individual; these thresholds determine whether an individual is infected, symptomatic, infectious, dead, etc.

Disease transmission and progression: In **EpiSims**, an infectious person contaminates his or her environment, in a process analogous to sneezing or coughing. The contamination may be restricted to a small region near the infected person, and/or it may spread to an entire location, which is roughly the size of an apartment building, office building, or shopping mall. Transmission occurs as uninfected people absorb virus (or bacteria, spores, etc.) from a contaminated location.

Geographical locations, as well as people, have a disease load associated with them, representing the level of contamination of the location. Disease load in a location has an associated exponential growth rate, which may be positive, negative, or zero. This allows **EpiSims** to model non-infectious diseases, transmission of disease between people who are never in direct contact, or diseases with non-human vectors. The simulation can be initialized by contaminating a specific location at a specific time and/or by assigning a non-zero load to one or more people.

There are two corresponding parameters controlling the interaction of each person with his or her local environment: the *shedding rate*, the fraction of the individual's load that is shed to the environment per hour, and the *absorption rate*, the fraction of the environment's load that is absorbed by an individual per hour. These parameters are specific to the individual, and can be set from an estimate of how long a person must be in close contact with an infectious person before becoming infected.

4. Structural and Cultural Measures of the Social Network, and their Implications

In this section we study basic structural and cultural properties of the social contact network for Portland. By cultural properties, we primarily mean demographic analysis of locations and people, especially as it is constrained by their interaction. To our knowledge an integrated structural and cultural analysis of large social contact networks has not been done before.

We begin with the structural analysis of the G_{PL} and G_P networks for Portland. In addition to standard measures, such as degree and clustering coefficient distributions, we identify new measures which are more relevant to disease dynamics: overlap ratios, expansion, shattering, temporal degrees and demographic mixing rates. As we argue later, the overlap ratio is a more useful measure than the clustering coefficient. We also explain the significance of expansion and shattering for network epidemiology. The temporal degrees and demographic mixing rates have not been studied at this level of detail (due to the lack of sufficient data), and can be used for developing new vaccination policies.

Degree Distribution and Clustering Coefficient. In the bipartite graph G_{PL} for Portland, we have 1615860 (1.6 million) people, 181230 (181K) locations, and 6060679 (6.1 million) edges. Figure 3 shows the degree distributions of the locations and people in the bipartite graph, G_{PL} for the Portland data. A large part of the degree sequence of locations follows a Power-law distribution, i.e., $n_k \propto k^{-\beta}$, where n_k denotes the number of locations of degree k; for the Portland data, $\beta \approx 2.8$. The degree sequence of people is roughly Poissonian.

The degree sequence of people in G_P is shown in Figure 4, and looks quite different than the degree sequence of G_{PL}. The graph G_P for Portland is not fully connected, but has a giant component with 1615813 people. We also determine the numbers of length-2 paths and triangles: a length-2 path is an unordered pair of edges $((a,b),(b,c))$ that share one vertex and a triangle is an unordered triple of vertices (a,b,c) such that each of the three pairs is an edge. Let Δ denote the

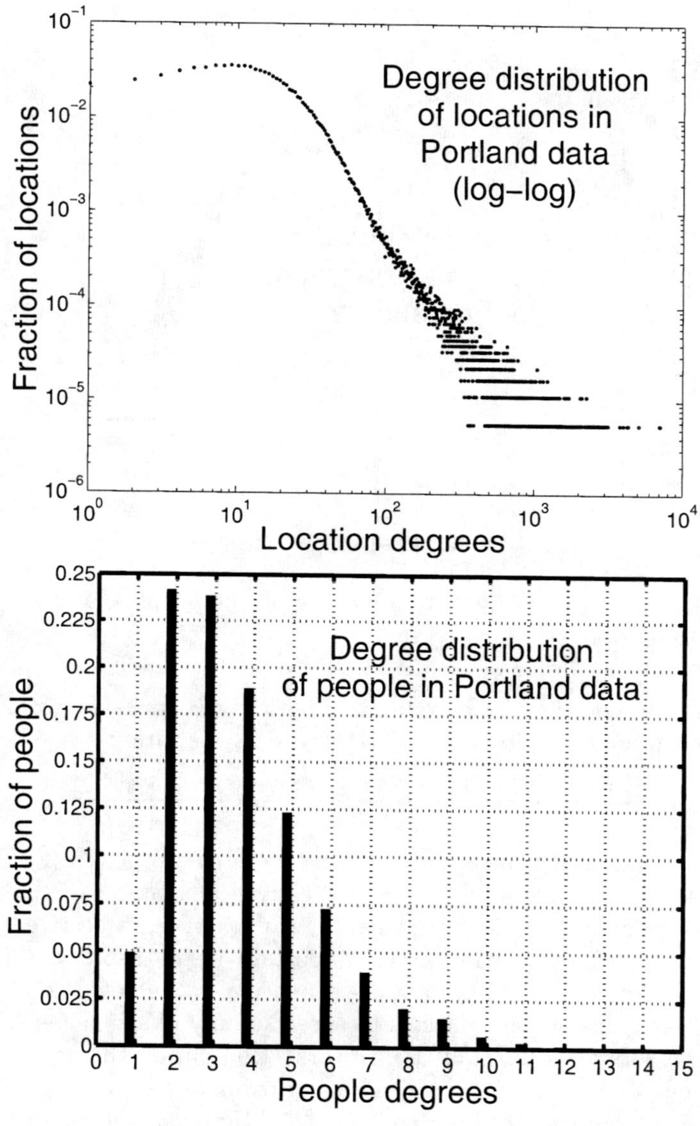

FIGURE 3. Degree distributions of locations and people in the bipartite graph G_{PL} for Portland data. The location degrees range from 1 to 7091, people degrees range from 1 to 15.

number of triangles, L_2 the number of length-2 paths, then the (overall) clustering coefficient is defined as $3\Delta/L_2$. As shown in Table 1 (in Section 7), for G_P for Portland data, $\Delta \simeq 6.3117 \times 10^{11}$ and $L_2 \simeq 3.349 \times 10^{12}$; the clustering coefficient for the Portland data is about 0.565268. Recent literature on social networks (see e.g. [**4, 32**]) has given a lot of importance to this measure, suggesting that a large clustering coefficient implies a more "tight-knit" interaction; however, we argue later that the overlap ratios and expansion are much better measures in this regard.

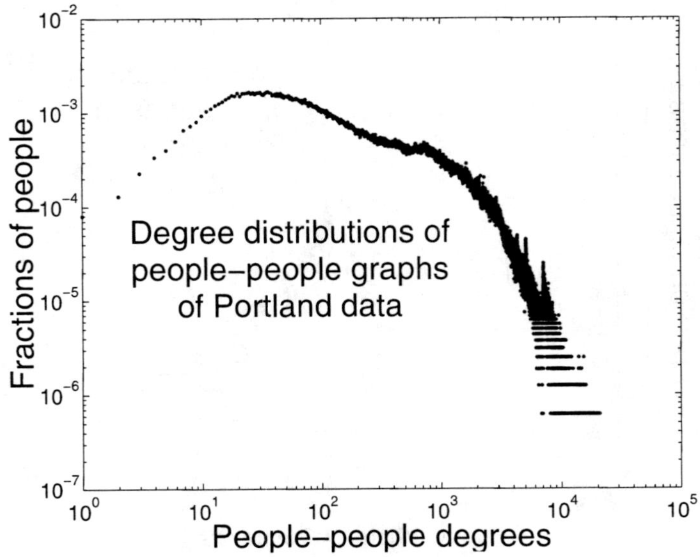

FIGURE 4. Degree distribution in the people-people graph for the Portland data.

Expansion. We consider the two standard notions of expansion in the graph G_P. The edge expansion of a subset $S \subseteq P$ is defined as the ratio

$$\frac{|\{e = (u, v) : \ (u, v) \text{ is an edge and } u \in S, v \notin S\}|}{|S|}.$$

The vertex expansion of a subset $S \subseteq P$ is defined as the ratio $|\{u \notin S : (u, v)$ is an edge and $v \in S\}|/|S|$. The edge (vertex, respectively) expansion of G_P is the minimum, taken over all $S \subset P, |S| \leq |P|/2$, of the edge (vertex, respectively) expansion of S. The vertex and edge expansions are important graph-theoretic properties that capture fault-tolerance, speed of data dissemination in the network, etc. Roughly, the higher the expansion, the quicker the spread of any phenomenon (disease, gossip, data etc.) along the links of the network. Computing the expansion exactly is computationally intractable, but can be approximated within a polylogarithmic factor using the results of Leighton and Rao [**27**]. However, the algorithm of [**27**] is currently unsuitable due to its high computational cost for analyzing large graphs such as the ones studied here; hence we use random sampling to estimate the vertex and edge expansions.[2] We collected approximately $500,000$ random samples of different sizes and calculated the smallest vertex and edge expansion, among all samples. Figure 5 summarizes the results. The Y-axis plots the smallest expansion value found among the $500,000$ independent samples; the X-axis plots the set size S as a percentage of the total number of vertices in the graph (the sampling probability). The plots labeled "Vertex expansion-2" and "Edge expansion-2" in Figure 5 show the expansion in the graph G_P, while the plots marked "Vertex expansion-1" and "Edge expansion-1" show the same quantity on a sparser people-people graph

[2]Random walk based methods have been used in property-testing type of algorithms for determining expansion (see e.g. [**21**])

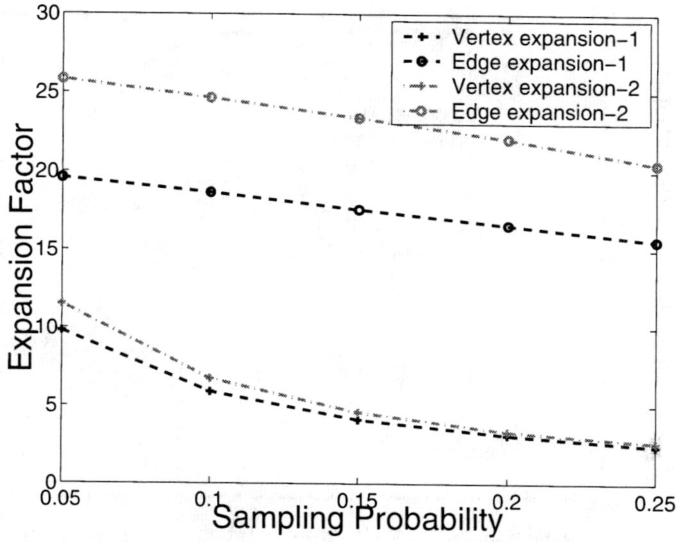

FIGURE 5. Expansion of the people-people graph: the plots marked "Vertex expansion-2" and "Edge expansion-2" show the vertex and edge expansion for the graph G_P, while "Vertex expansion-1" and "Edge expansion-1" show the corresponding quantities in the graph obtained by retaining only those edges that involve an interaction of at least 1 hour. This leads to a much sparser graph and correspondingly lower values of vertex and edge expansions.

- the graph is made sparser by only retaining edges between individuals who came in contact for at least one hour. It is evident that the expansion rate does go down in the sparser graph; nevertheless, both the plots show a very high expansion rate. *Significance of High Expansion.* The high expansion implies that contagious diseases would spread very fast, and makes early detection imperative, in order to control the disease. We discuss detection strategies later. Recent papers, such as [**11, 2, 13, 34**], have proposed strategies such as vaccination of high-degree people. In the light of the high expansion, such strategies are unlikely to be very effective. To quantify the effectiveness of such a vaccination policy, we study a natural measure called **shattering** - given a parameter $\alpha > 0$, this corresponds to the minimum size of the largest connected component, over all possible ways of removing up to αn nodes. Vaccinating an individual can be viewed as removing all incident edges on this node (since the individual will no longer contract the disease and further transmit it). A vaccination scheme (corresponding to node deletions) that leads to small connected components implies that the disease would not spread beyond any component. Therefore, the size of the largest connected component in the graph resulting from the deletion of all "vaccinated" nodes is a measure of the effectiveness of the vaccination scheme. In other words, vaccination should *shatter the graph* into small components. Figure 6 shows the largest component size after the "high degree node" heuristic is implemented - the largest component remains very stable, and continues to remain unique until all nodes of degree 11 are deleted,

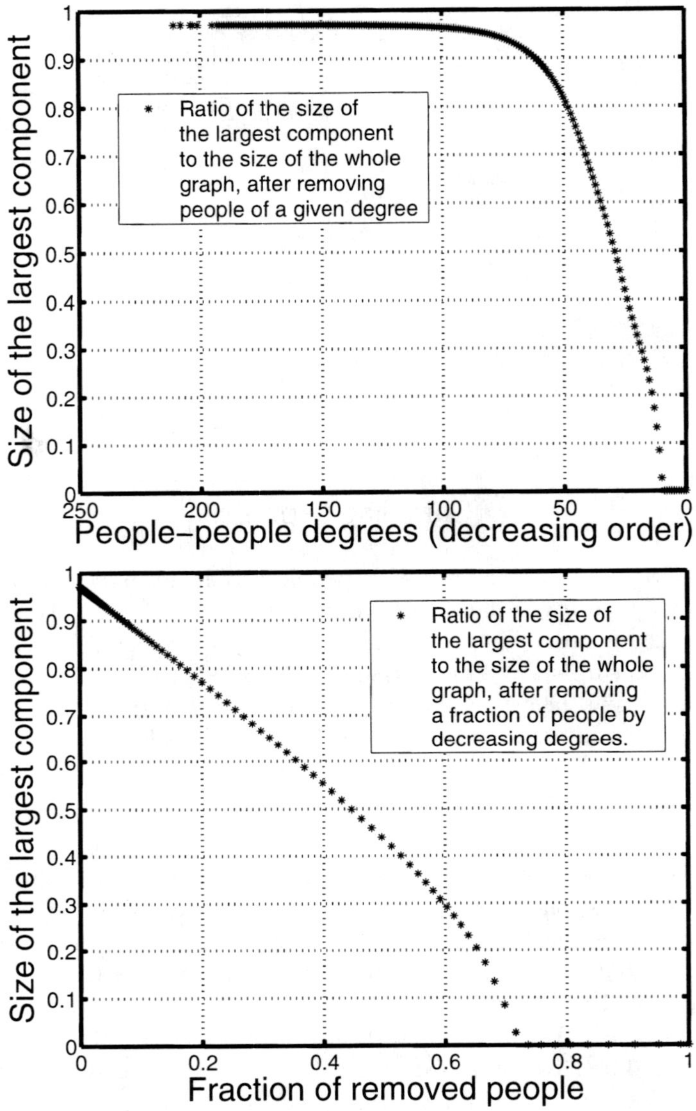

FIGURE 6. Size of the giant connected component after each iteration.

which requires deleting a large fraction (0.698) of the nodes. This suggests that for contagious diseases, the "high degree node" heuristic is in practice no different than mass vaccination.

Overlap Ratio. For a set $L' \subseteq L$ of locations, let $N(L')$ be the set of individuals visiting at least one of the locations in L', i.e., $N(L') = \{p \in P : (p, l) \in E(G_{PL}) \text{ and } l \in L'\}$. Then the overlap ratio of L' is defined by $\frac{|N(L')|}{\sum_{l \in L'} deg(l)}$. For a given integer d, the Point-Overlap-Ratio(d) is the overlap ratio defined for the set of locations of degree d, and the Cumulative-Overlap-Ratio(d) is the overlap ratio of the set of all locations having degree at least d. The plots in Figure 7 show the overlap ratios (of Portland data and data generated by random models (see Sections 7.2) and 7.3), for locations considered in decreasing order of degree. The plots show that high-degree vertices are visited by *almost-disjoint* sets of individuals. In other words, most pairs of distinct high-degree locations are visited by (almost) disjoint sets of individuals during a day. This is an important structural property of the social network under investigation and is likely to be true for many other such social networks. This has important implications from the standpoint of designing effective strategies for monitoring the onset of an epidemic and is discussed further in Section 5.3.

Significance of High Overlap ratio. As shown in [**17**], the high value of overlap ratio implies that (approximate) dominating sets in the bipartite graph G_{PL} are small; we discuss in section 5.3 how a dominating set can be used for disease monitoring. Also, the overlap ratio is a more refined measure of the tight-knit nature of social interaction than the clustering coefficient - a graph could have a specific clustering coefficient even though different subgraphs look very different.

Temporal degree distributions. Network analysis has typically only dealt with static graphs, but real graphs are dynamic- even simple measures such as degree distributions are temporal functions. Figures 9, 10, and 11 show the temporal variation in degrees for six different location types in Portland; for each location type, the distribution of four randomly chosen locations is shown. The degree distributions reflect the basic trend that one expects; for example, the number of individuals at home is high in the early morning hours, decreases during the day and then shows an increase during evening hours. Work locations, in contrast, show a complementary behavior. Instead of "high degree" type of vaccination strategies, one can propose much more refined schemes by using the temporal degrees.

Cultural Measures Next, we discuss cultural measures, which consist of demographic and temporal analysis. We study the following measures: (i) Temporal degree distributions, (ii) activity statistics, and (iii) demographic mixing. Such a study necessarily requires having a detailed representation, such as the one from **TRANSIMS**.

Activity Durations. As described earlier in Section 3, the data from **TRANSIMS** also contain information related to the type of activity a person does at a location; the types of activities range from `home` and `work` to `school`- this describes the kind of activity done at the location. Figures 12 and 13 show the distributions of lengths of some activities, obtained from the temporal G_{PL} graph, and shows some interesting features. For instance, consider the uppermost graph in Figure 12, which corresponds to the activity type `work`. There are two peaks in the distribution: the first peak is around 4 hours and the second is around 8 hours; these peaks correspond well with our intuition of half and full work days. Activity length information could also be useful for decision making: for instance, in contact tracing, it might suffice to ignore activities that had much smaller duration.

Demographic mixing. Unlike in uniform mixing models, contacts between people are very non-uniform, and depend on a host of demographic factors. For instance, teens have more contacts with other teens and with some 30-40 year olds (probably parents, teachers) than with people of other age groups, as Figure 14

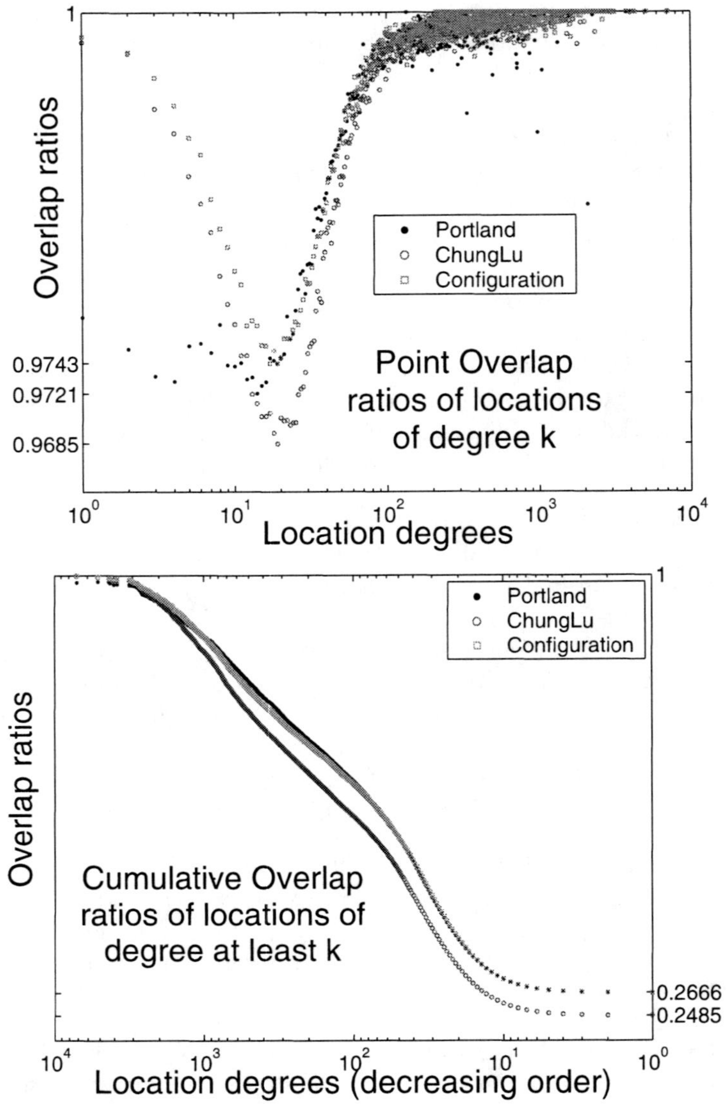

FIGURE 7. Overlap ratios (Section 4) for the dominating set problem – comparison between Portland data and data generated by Chung-Lu's model (Section 7.3) and the configuration model (Section 7.2).

shows. To capture this inhomogeneity in the contacts, we consider people of different age-groups, and determine the average number of contacts with people of other ages; Figures 14 ands 15 shows the distributions for three specific age-groups of 16, 30 and 60 (see [**16**] for more details). Such demographic mixing information can be used in determining refined vaccination policies.

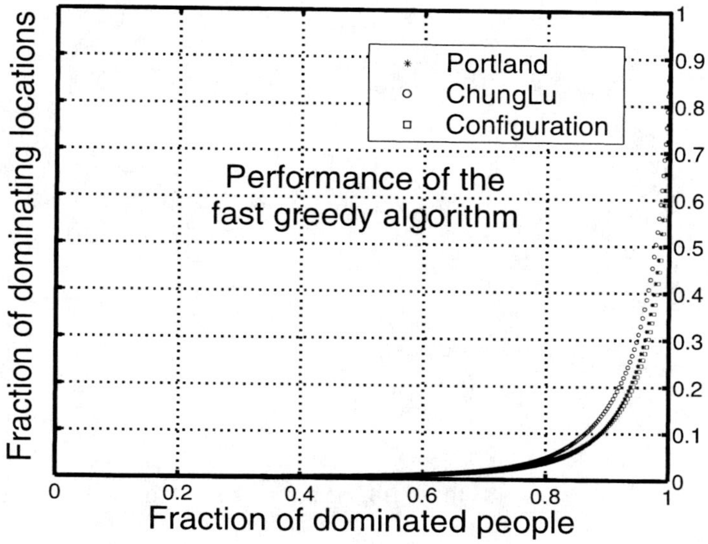

FIGURE 8. Performance of the fast greedy algorithm (Section 5.3) for the dominating set problem – comparison between Portland data and data generated by Chung-Lu's model (Section 7.3) and the configuration model (Section 7.2).

5. Using Network Structure for Policy Planning

A significant part of epidemiology deals with understanding vaccination and quarantining policies, and answering questions such as whom to vaccinate. The potential for answering such questions is greatly reduced if we stick to uniform mixing models. In this section we show how three policy planning problems can be formulated in terms of the network structure, and, in some cases, can be solved efficiently.

5.1. Modeling the efficacy of Vaccination Policies. The problem is to formulate a simple model for determining the efficiency of a vaccination scheme. Using the network structure, one way to model this problem is to consider the shattering problem defined in section 4 - the vaccination is effective if the giant component size goes down. In this model, the discussion in Section 4 shows that the policy of vaccinating all people of degree larger than some threshold is not very effective. Another model could be to look at the diameter of the giant component, or the average distance between a pair of nodes.

In the first model above, the best vaccination strategy would be to choose a set of nodes to vaccinate (and remove from the network), so that each component in the remaining graph becomes small. If we are given a parameter $\rho \in (0, 1)$, and require each component to have at most ρ fraction of the nodes, then this reduces to the ρ-separator problem [**27**]. This problem is **NP**-hard, and [**27**] gives a polylogarithmic approximation to the optimum. Unfortunately, this algorithm is unlikely to scale for such large graphs, and an interesting problem is to find a faster approximation algorithm.

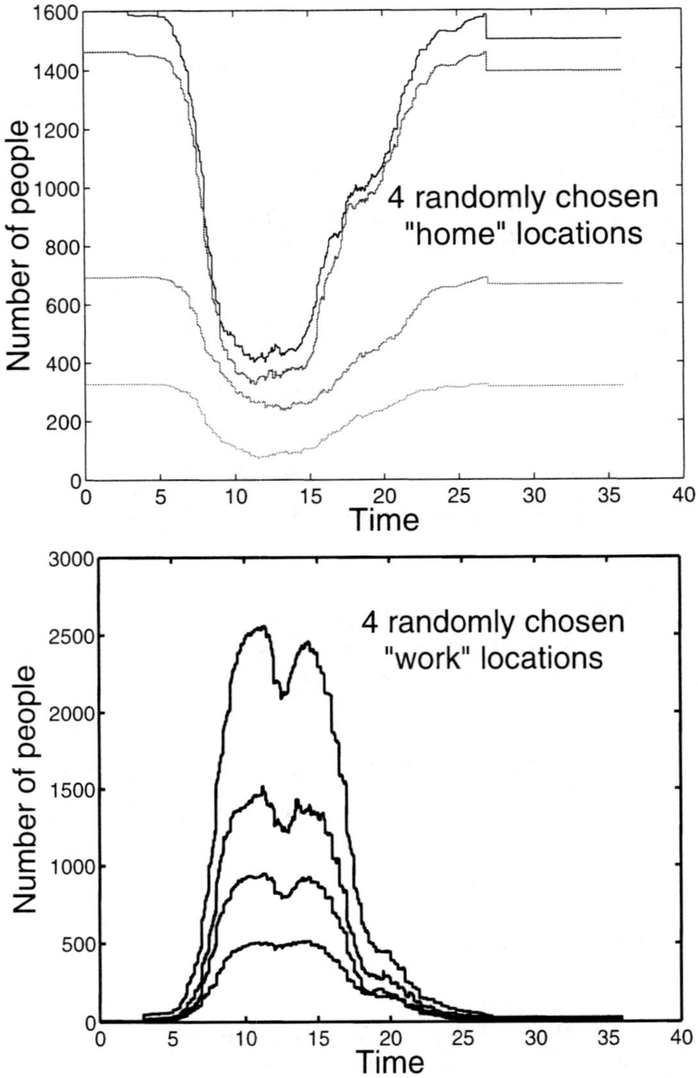

FIGURE 9. Temporal degree distributions for different types of activity locations. The types of activity locations are: `home` and `work`. Each plot contains the temporal degree of four randomly chosen activity locations of a given type, where the x-axis shows the time in hours, and the y-axis shows the number of people at that time (x) and that location (doing the specific activity). For example, the top plot shows the temporal degree distribution for four randomly chosen home locations. The home location is really a block of homes, and that accounts for the large sizes.

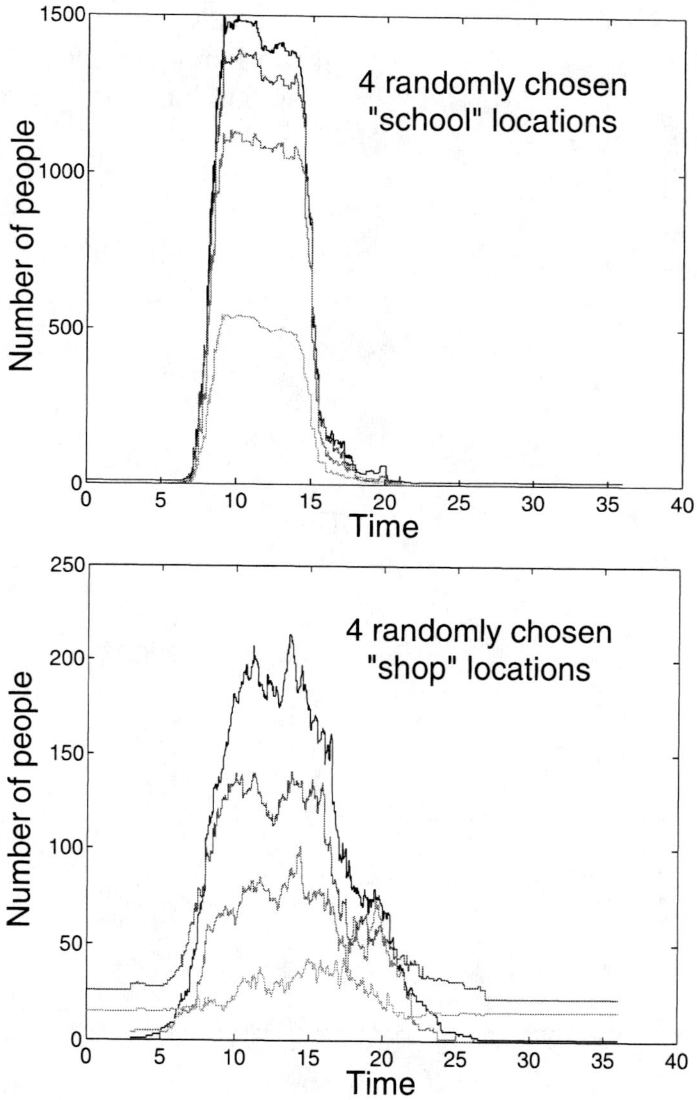

FIGURE 10. Temporal degree distributions for different types of activity locations. The types of activity locations are: `school` and `shop`. Each plot contains the temporal degree of four randomly chosen activity locations of a given type, where the x-axis shows the time in hours, and the y-axis shows the number of people at that time (x) and that location (doing the specific activity).

5.2. The Quarantining/Vaccination Problems. A basic problem for public health workers that we consider next is: given a set $I \subset P$ of infected nodes in the graph G_P, what is the optimal set of nodes to vaccinate or quarantine? There are two aspects of cost here: one is the number (or total cost) of people to vaccinate or quarantine, and the other is the set of people who are reachable from I after

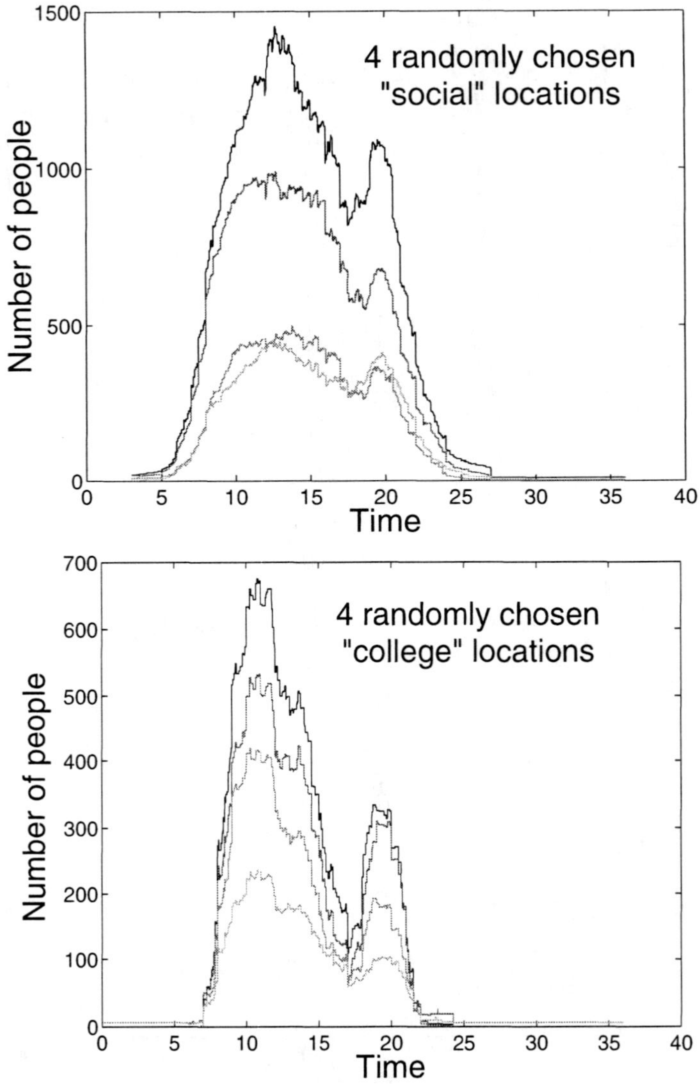

FIGURE 11. Temporal degree distributions for different types of activity locations. The types of activity locations are: `social` and `college`. Each plot contains the temporal degree of four randomly chosen activity locations of a given type, where the x-axis shows the time in hours, and the y-axis shows the number of people at that time (x) and that location (doing the specific activity).

deleting the nodes that get vaccinated (this models a highly infectious disease). We describe two formulations of this problem here.
(a) The VACCINATION PROBLEM (VP): given a graph $G(V, E)$, an initial infected set I, a parameter C, and cost $c(v)$ for each node v, choose a set of nodes $S \subseteq V \setminus I$

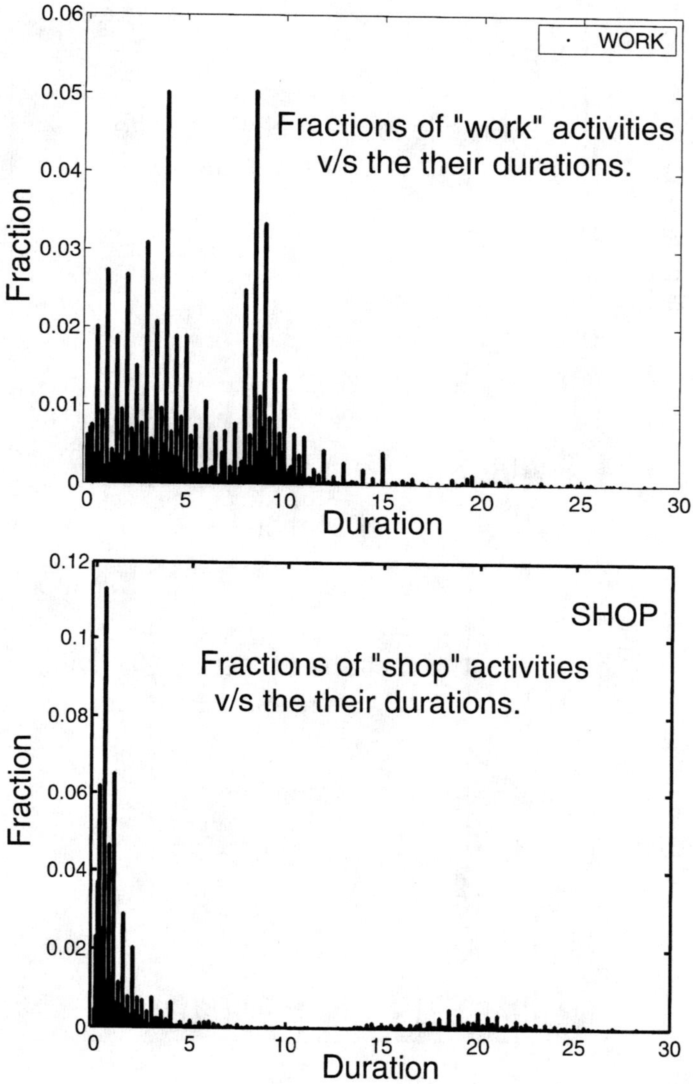

FIGURE 12. Distribution of activity lengths for `work` and `shop` activities. For each activity type, and for each possible duration of times d, the plot shows the fraction of this activity lasted for d time units.

having cost $c(S) = \sum_{v \in S} c(v) \leq C$, such that the size of the set

$$A_G(I, S) = \{v \mid v \text{ has a path from some } w \in I \text{ in } G(V \setminus S)\}$$

is minimized. The set S is the people who are vaccinated, and the set $A_G(I, S)$ models the set of people that could get infected by a highly infectious disease.
(b) The QUARANTINING PROBLEM (QP): given a graph $G(V, E)$, an initial infected set I, a parameter B, and cost $c(e)$ for each edge e, choose a cut $(S, \bar{S})$ such that $I \subseteq S$, $|S| \leq B$, and the cost of the cut is minimized. Unlike vaccination,

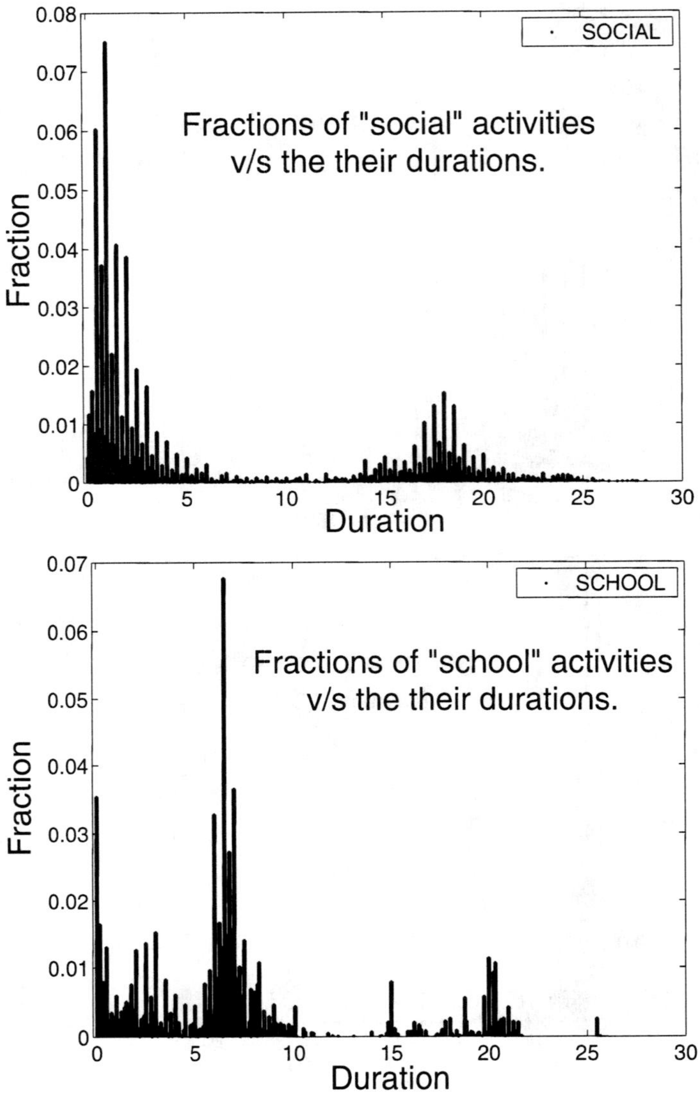

FIGURE 13. Distribution of activity lengths for `social` and `school` activities. For each activity type, and for each possible duration of times d, the plot shows the fraction of this activity lasted for d time units.

quarantining involves cutting down some of the contacts - this is captured by the edge deletions in this model.

We show that the VP and QP problems are **NP**-complete and give a bicriteria approximation for them, using network flows.

LEMMA 1. *The VP and QP problems are* **NP**-*hard.*

PROOF. We will show that the decision versions of these problems, with a bound C on the (edge/vertex) cut size and bound B on the number of nodes that

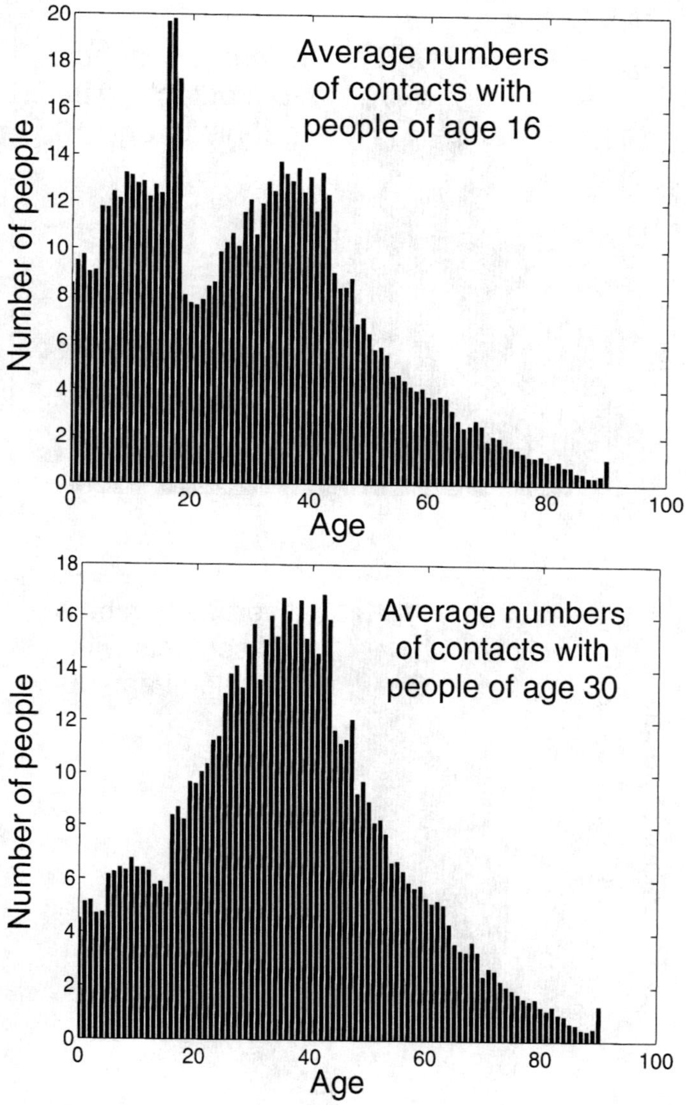

FIGURE 14. Contacts with each age-group, for people of ages 16 and 30. For each of these age groups (say A), and for each possible age-group (say B) on the X-axis, the plot shows the average number of contacts that group A makes with group B in the Y-axis. The average for a given age is computed by computing a distribution for each person p of that age and then summing up these distributions and dividing the resulting values by the total number of individuals of that age.

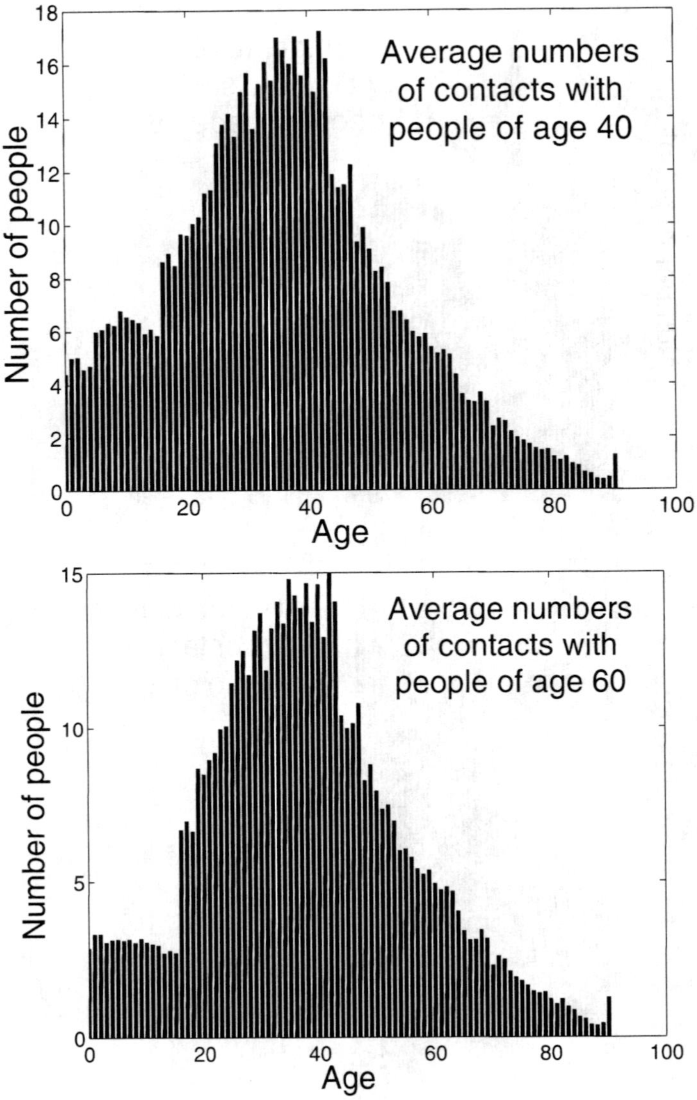

FIGURE 15. Contacts with each age-group, for people of ages 40 and 60. For each of these age groups (say A), and for each possible age-group (say B) on the X-axis, the plot shows the average number of contacts that group A makes with group B in the Y-axis. The average for a given age is computed by computing a distribution for each person p of that age and then summing up these distributions and dividing the resulting values by the total number of individuals of that age.

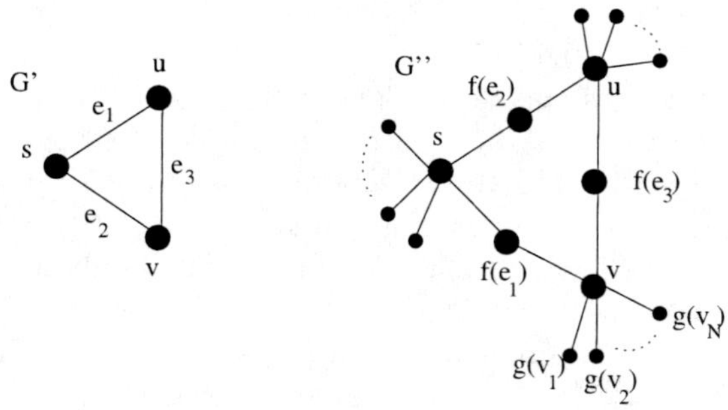

FIGURE 16. The transformations done in the reduction for VP.

get infected, are **NP**-complete. These decision problems are clearly in **NP**. The hardness is by reduction from the **NP**-complete Bipartition problem [**20**].

An instance of Bipartition involves a graph $G(V, E)$, with cost $c(e)$ on each edge e, and bound C; the problem is to decide whether there is a partition (V_1, V_2) such that $|V_1| = \lfloor n/2 \rfloor, |V_2| = \lceil n/2 \rceil$ and $c(V_1, V_2) \leq C$. We will always assume w.l.o.g. that $C \leq \sum_{e \in E} c(e)$. We first describe the reduction from Bipartition to QP. Given an instance $G(V, E)$ of Bipartition, we construct a new graph G' in the following manner. Add a new vertex s to G, with an edge from s to each vertex in V. Each edge $(s, v), v \in V$ has cost $c(s, v) = \alpha = \sum_{e \in E(G)} c(e) + 1$. Now we consider the QP problem on graph G' with $I = \{s\}$ (the infected set), with bounds $C' = C + \lceil n/2 \rceil \alpha$ and $B' = \lfloor n/2 \rfloor + 1$. We show that this instance is feasible if and only if the given Bipartition instance is. Suppose there is a solution $(S, \bar{S})$ to the QP problem with bounds C' and B' with $s \in S$. We first claim that $|S| = B'$. For, if $|S| < B'$, the cost of the cut $(S, \bar{S})$ would be at least

$$(n + 1 - |S|)\alpha \geq (n + 1 - \lfloor n/2 \rfloor)\alpha = \lceil n/2 \rceil \alpha + \alpha > \lceil n/2 \rceil \alpha + C = C'.$$

On the other hand, given that $|S| = B'$ and the cost of the cut $(S, \bar{S})$ is at most C', we claim that the *bipartition* $(V_1 = S \setminus \{s\}, V_2 = V \setminus S)$ is a solution with cost at most C to the Bipartition problem on $G(V, E)$. This is because in the QP problem, the cost of the cut $(S, \bar{S})$ contributed by $\{s\}$ is exactly $\lceil n/2 \rceil \alpha$, thus the cost of the cut contributed by $V_1 = S \setminus \{s\}$ is at most $C' - \lceil n/2 \rceil \alpha = C$. Conversely, if (V_1, V_2) is a solution to the Bipartition problem such that $|V_1| = \lfloor n/2 \rfloor$, it is easy to verify that $(S = V_1 \cup \{s\}, V_2)$ is a solution to the QP problem; thus QP is NP-complete.

For the VP problem, the reduction needs to be modified, since we are dealing with vertex cuts. ¿From the graph G' constructed above, we construct another graph G'' in the following manner. $V(G'') = V_A \cup V_B \cup V_C$, where $V_A = V(G')$, $V_B = \{f(e) : e \in E(G')\}$, and $V_C = \{g(v, 1), \ldots, g(v, N) : v \in V_A\}$, for $N = n^4$ being a large number; Figure 16 illustrates the reduction on a small example. Here, f and g are just one-to-one indexing functions. V_B is partitioned into two sets $V_B = V_{B1} \cup V_{B2}$, where $V_{B1} = \{f(e) : e = (s, v) \in E(G')\}$ and $V_{B2} = \{f(e) : e = (v, w) \in E(G'), v, w \neq s\}$. The vertex costs are defined in the following manner: (i) for each $v = f(e) \in V_{B1}, c(v) = \alpha = \sum_{e' \in E(G')} c(e') + 1$; (ii) for each $v = f(e) \in V_{B2}, c(v) = c(e)$; and (iii) letting M be the sum of the costs of all vertices in V_B, we define, for each $v \in (V_A \cup V_C)$, $c(v) = M$. The edges $E(G'')$

are defined in the following manner: (i) for each edge $e = (s, v) \in E(G')$, we have the edges $(s, f(e))$ and $(f(e), v)$ that go between V_A and V_B; (ii) for each edge $e = (v, w) \in E(G'), v, w \neq s$, we have the edges $(v, f(e))$ and $(f(e), w)$ that go between V_A and V_B; and (iii) we have the edges $(v, g(v, i))$ for each $v \in V_A, i = 1, \ldots, N$ (these edges go between V_A and V_C). We now consider the VP problem on G'' with $I = \{s\}$ and bounds $C' = C + \lceil n/2 \rceil \alpha$ and $B' = (N+2)\lfloor n/2 \rfloor + n^2$. We argue below that the Bipartition instance has a solution if and only if the VP instance on G'' has a solution with the given B', C'.

Suppose the above VP problem is feasible, and $S \subseteq V(G'')$ is a solution, with $c(S) \leq C', |A_{G''}(I, S)| \leq B'$. Then, we argue now that $(V_1 = A_{G''}(I, S) \cap V_A, V_2 = V \setminus V_1)$ is a solution to the Bipartition problem with cost C. Since each vertex $w \in V_A \cup V_C$ has cost $c(w) = M > C'$, $S \subseteq V_B$. Also, since for each vertex $v \in V_{B1}$, $c(v) = \alpha > \sum_{v' \in V_{B2}} c(v')$, it follows that $|V_{B1} \cap S| \leq \lceil n/2 \rceil$. Every vertex in V_{B1} must lie either in $A_{G''}(I, S)$ or in S, and, therefore, $|V_{B1} \cap A_{G''}(I, S)| \geq \lfloor n/2 \rfloor$; this, in turn, implies that $|V_A \cap A_{G''}(I, S)| \geq \lfloor n/2 \rfloor$. Also, for each $v \in A_{G''}(I, S) \cap V_A$, we have for all i that $g(v, i) \in A_{G''}(I, S)$, because $S \cap V_C = \phi$; therefore, the bound $|A_{G''}(I, S)| \leq B'$ shows that $|V_A \cap A_{G''}(I, S)| \leq \lfloor n/2 \rfloor$, for that $N = n^4 \gg n^2$. The above statements together imply $|V_1 = A_{G''}(I, S) \cap V_A| = \lfloor n/2 \rfloor$, and this further implies $V_{B1} \cap S = \lceil n/2 \rceil$. Since $c(S) = \sum_{v \in S \cap V_{B1}} c(v) + \sum_{v \in S \cap V_{B2}} c(v)$, it follows that $\sum_{v \in S \cap V_{B2}} c(v) \leq C$, and, therefore, the cut (V_1, V_2) has cost at most C in G. Conversely, suppose (V_1, V_2) is a solution to the Bipartition problem of cost C. Then, it can be verified easily that $S = \{f(e) : e \in \text{cut}(V_1, V_2)\} \cup \{f(e) : e = (s, v) \in E(G'), v \in V_2\}$ is a solution to the VP problem: $c(S) = C + |V_2|\alpha = C'$, and $A_{G''}(I, S) = (|V_1 \cup \{s\}|)(N+2) + |\{e \in V_{B2} : e \in V_1 \times V_1\}| \leq B'$. Together, these imply that the VP problem is also NP-complete. □

To simplify the discussion, we first describe an approximation for QP, and later describe how this can be modified to work for the VP problem. In our discussion, we will assume that the graph is directed - an undirected graph can be made directed by putting edges in both directions.

Bicriteria Results for QP. We describe a $(1 + 2\epsilon, 1 + 2/\epsilon)$ approximation algorithm for QP, for any given $\epsilon \in (0, 1)$. That is, if the least number of newly-infected people in an instance of QP with bound C is denoted by OPT, our approximation algorithm produces a solution with the cost of the cut at most $(1 + 2\epsilon)C$ and at most $(1 + 2/\epsilon)OPT$ newly-infected people.

Let $G(V, E)$ be an instance of QP, with $I \subseteq V$ being the infected set, and C being the bound on the cost of the cut. The algorithm is outlined in Figure 17.

LEMMA 2. *For any given $\epsilon > 0$, the Algorithm in Figure 17 produces a solution with cut cost at most $(1 + 2\epsilon)C$ and at most $(1 + 2/\epsilon)OPT$ infected nodes, where OPT is the number of infected people in the optimal solution with cut cost C.*

PROOF. We will first show that if $\beta = \epsilon C/OPT$, the solution obtained by solving the minimum cut is an $(1 + \epsilon, 1 + 1/\epsilon)$ approximation. Let $(X, \bar{X})$ be the optimal solution with $c(X, \bar{X}) \leq C$, $I \subseteq X$ and $|X \setminus I| = OPT$. Then the solution $(X \cup \{s\}, \bar{X} \cup \{t\})$ has cut cost of $C + \beta \cdot OPT$. Now suppose the minimum cut in G' is $(S \cup \{s\}, \bar{S} \cup \{t\})$, for $S \subseteq V(G)$. Clearly, $I \subseteq S$ (else the edges of cost ∞ have to cross the cut). Let C' be the cost of the cut $(S, \bar{S})$ in G. Then,

Input: Graph G, cost $c(e)$ on each edge e, the infected set I and $\epsilon > 0$.
Repeat the following steps for $\beta = (1+\epsilon^2)^i$ for $i = -\log_{(1+\epsilon^2)}(n/(C\epsilon)), \ldots, -1, 0, 1, \ldots, \log_{(1+\epsilon^2)}(C\epsilon)$ and choose the best solution:

(1) Construct a new graph G': Add a source s and sink t to G. Add edges $(s, v), \forall v \in I$ with cost ∞ and edges $(v, t), \forall v \notin I$ with cost β. All edges of G retain their old costs.
(2) Compute the minimum s-t cut, $(S, \bar{S})$ for the current value of β. The candidate solution is $(S \setminus \{s\}, \bar{S} \setminus \{t\})$.

FIGURE 17. A Bicriteria Algorithm for QP

Input: Graph G, cost $c(v)$ on each vertex v, the infected set I and $\epsilon > 0$.
Repeat the following steps for $\beta = (1+\epsilon^2)^i$ for $i = -\log_{(1+\epsilon^2)}(n/(C\epsilon)), \ldots, -1, 0, 1, \ldots, \log_{(1+\epsilon^2)}(C\epsilon)$ and choose the best solution:

(1) Construct a new edge weighted graph G': For each vertex v, we split it into two vertices v_{in} and v_{out}, and add the edge $e = (v_{in}, v_{out})$ having cost $c(e) = c(v)$ for $v \in V \setminus I$, and $c(e) = \infty$ for $v \in I$. In addition, for each edge (v, w) in the original graph, we add the edges $e = (v_{out}, w_{in})$ having cost $c(e) = \infty$.
(2) Add a source s and sink t to G'. For each vertex $v \in I$, add edges $e = (s, v_{in})$ with $c(e) = \infty$. For each vertex $v \in V \setminus I$, add edges $e = (v_{out}, t)$ with $c(e) = \beta$.
(3) Compute the minimum s-t cut, $(X, \bar{X})$, $s \in X$, for the current value of β. The candidate solution is $S = \{v : (v_{in}, v_{out}) \text{ lies in the cut}\}$, and $A(I, S) = \{v : v_{out} \in X\}$.

FIGURE 18. A Bicriteria Algorithm for VP

$C' + (|S| - |I|)\beta \leq C + \beta \cdot OPT$. Setting $\beta = \epsilon C/OPT$, this inequality implies that $C' \leq (1+\epsilon)C$ and $|S| - |I| \leq (1 + 1/\epsilon)OPT$.

Since we do not know the value of OPT, we cannot try out this exact value of β. By trying out all the powers of ϵ, given that $1 \leq OPT \leq n$, we can approximate this ratio. Suppose, the best solution is obtained for $\beta \in [\beta_0/(1+\delta), \beta_0(1+\delta)]$, where $\beta_0 = \epsilon C/OPT$ and $\delta = \epsilon^2$, and let this solution be the cut $(S, \bar{S})$ in G. As above, we have $c(S, \bar{S}) + (|S| - |I|)\beta \leq C + OPT\beta$. Since $\beta \leq \beta_0(1+\delta)$, we have $c(S, \bar{S}) \leq C(1 + \epsilon(1+\delta)) \leq C(1+2\epsilon)$, since $\epsilon < 1$. Similarly, $|S| - |I| \leq OPT(1 + 2/\epsilon)$. □

A Bicriteria approximation for VP. Figure 18 shows the bicriteria algorithm for VP, and is a modification of the algorithm in Figure 17. This algorithm assumes that the graph is directed; if G is undirected, we just put in edges directed both ways before calling the algorithm in Figure 18. The following lemma shows its correctness.

LEMMA 3. *For any given* $\epsilon > 0$*, the Algorithm in Figure 18 produces a solution with cut cost (i.e., the number of people vaccinated) at most* $(1+2\epsilon)C$ *and at most* $(1+2/\epsilon)OPT$ *infected nodes, where* OPT *is the number of infected people in the optimal solution with* C *vaccinations.*

PROOF. We firstly argue that the algorithm produces a feasible solution to the VP problem. Note that there is a finite $s-t$ cut - deleting all edges of the form (v_{in}, v_{out}), where $v \in V \setminus I$, has cost $c(S) = \sum_{v \in V \setminus I} c(v)$, and $|A(I,S)| = 0$. This corresponds to the trivial solution of vaccinating all people in $V \setminus I$, and thus no one will be infected. Another trivial solution of vaccinating no people and thus all will be infected corresponds to a finite $s-t$ cut of deleting all edges of the form (v_{out}, t), where $v \in V \setminus I$. In this finite $s-t$ cut solution, $c(S) = \beta|V \setminus I|$ and $S = \emptyset$. The two trivial finite cuts are not necessary the minimum cuts, but their existence implies that our argument will not be vacuous.

Next, note that any edge of the form $e = (s, v_{in})$, or $e = (v_{in}, v_{out})$ for $v \in I$, or $e = (v_{out}, w_{in})$ for some v, w has $c(e) = \infty$; therefore, no such edge can be part of the minimum cut $(X, \bar{X})$ - the only edges that can be in the cut are of the form (v_{in}, v_{out}), or (v_{out}, t) for $v \in V \setminus I$. Also, there can be no vertex v such that $v_{out} \in X, v_{in} \in \bar{X}$ - this would require some edge of cost ∞ to be in the cut. This implies that the set S separates the set $A(I,S)$ from $V \setminus (S \cup A(I,S))$ in the original graph G. Also, $c(X, \bar{X}) = c(S) + \beta|A(I,S)|$, where $c(S) = \sum_{v \in S} c(v)$.

As in the proof of Lemma 2, we will first show that if $\beta = \epsilon C/OPT$, the solution is an $(1+\epsilon, 1+1/\epsilon)$ approximation. Let S' be the optimal solution to VP, with $c(S') \leq C$, and $|A(I,S')| = OPT$. Since $(X, \bar{X})$ is the minimum $s-t$ cut, it must be the case that $c(S) + \beta|A(I,S)| \leq c(S') + \beta OPT$. Setting $\beta = \epsilon C/OPT$, this inequality implies that $C' \leq (1+\epsilon)C$ and $|A(I,S)| \leq (1+1/\epsilon)OPT$.

The rest of the argument, to take care of the fact that the "optimal" value of β is not known, is the same as in the proof of Lemma 2. □

5.3. Disease Detection: Sensor Placement. As discussed earlier in Section 4, the expansion of the social network is very high, leading to high rates of spread of diseases, and making simple targeted vaccination schemes infeasible. This makes the problem of early detection even more important. One way of detecting certain kinds of diseases (such as small pox and anthrax) is to place sensors in some public places. This leads to the following problem: choose a subset $S \subseteq L$ of locations to place the sensors, so that all or most people visit at least one of these locations; the goal is to choose set S of the smallest size.

We note that the sensor placement problem has been discussed elsewhere; for example, in studying municipal water networks [**7**]. In our situation, the sensor problem reduces to the classical dominating set problem. It is **NP**-hard, and a greedy algorithm gives an $O(\log |L|)$ approximation. For the G_{PL} graph, it turns out that a much simpler algorithm, called *fastgreedy* works fairly well- choose the highest degree locations so that the required fraction of people are dominated (i.e., they visit one of the chosen locations); Figures 7 and 8 show that the *fastgreedy* heuristic works very well in practice. The effectiveness of *fastgreedy* is, intuitively, due to the high overlap ratios (as explained in Section 4). In [**17**], we show that for the Chung-Lu model (discussed in Section 7), *fastgreedy* provably works very well.

6. EpiSims Based Dynamic Analysis

We now turn to simulation based analysis of the disease dynamics. Our results show that graph theoretic analysis can provide useful insights and guide the simulation based dynamic analysis. Much of the discussion in this section is from our recent article [**16**], which focused on smallpox. As noted below, many quantitative results such as total number of cases depend on details of the disease model. We are currently investigating how qualitative results can be generalized across diseases.

Our results on high expansion suggest that the disease is likely to spread quickly if it is not controlled at an early stage. However, exactly how the number of casualties depends on response delay and what constitutes *early enough* depend on disease-specific factors such as incubation period and probability of transmission, as well as scenario-specific factors such as the means of introduction. Because these dependencies cannot be easily determined from analysis of the static social network, we turn to simulation. See [**38**] for details about the particular disease model used in the simulation experiments. At present, there is no consensus on models of smallpox. The model used in our study captures many features on which there is widespread agreement and allows us to vary poorly understood properties through reasonable ranges [**16**]. Our model includes the following features (see [**16**] for definitions of some of the terms below):

- the incubation period is a truncated Gaussian distribution,
- the prodromal period is 3-5 days,
- the infectious period is 4 days, during which infectivity decreases exponentially,
- death occurs 10-16 days after the rash develops in 30% of normal cases. 95% of susceptibles exposed for three hours to a person at minimum infectivity for three hours will become infected. The (the remaining 5% have extremely high or low susceptibilities, mimicking some anecdotal transmission incidents),
- vaccination is assumed to be 100% effective pre-exposure, and its effectiveness is less if it is administered some time after the exposure.

The model also includes hemorrhagic variants with a shorter incubation period that are ten times as infectious and invariably fatal. Importantly, **EpiSims** does not specify a value for R_0, the basic reproductive number. This parameter reflects how many people in a susceptible population are directly infected by the introduction of a single infective individual. R_0 is a convolution of transmission rates and contact patterns, and **EpiSims** carries out the convolution for us. The implied value of R_0 is the ratio of numbers of people in the first and original cohorts; these estimates obviously include the effects of the simulated response strategy. For the set of experiments reported below, R_0 ranges from 0.4 to 3.4. In these scenarios, aerosolized smallpox was distributed indoors at busy locations over several hours, infecting on the order of 1000 people. We assumed that the presence of smallpox was detected on the tenth day after the attack. We studied the sensitivity of the number of casualties to three factors: *mitigation efforts, delay in implementing mitigation efforts, and whether people move about while infectious.* We simulated a passive (do nothing) *baseline* and three active responses:

- mass vaccination covering 100% of the population in four days ("mass"),

- targeted vaccination and quarantine with unlimited resources ("targeted"),
- the same targeted response, using only half as many contact tracers and vaccinators ("limited").

The choice of individuals for targeted vaccination and quarantining is based on our graph theoretic analysis and uses two heuristic methods: (i) individuals in the first neighborhood of the infected people are candidates for vaccination or quarantine based on high expansion of the network suggesting early action, and (ii) individuals with higher degrees (contacts) are more likely to be chosen from this subset. A more detailed experimental design that uses cultural measures and sophisticated graph theoretic measures is currently being conducted.

Results For a movie showing the spatial spread of disease under two different response strategies, see [**38**]. Figure 19 compares the efficacy of these strategies. For each strategy, we plot (on a logarithmic scale) the ratio of the cumulative number of deaths by day 100 to the number initially infected. The absolute numbers are less important than the rank and relative sizes of gaps between the points. Also shown are the effects of 4, 7, or 10 day delays in implementing the response. For each of the responses including the baseline, we allowed infected people to isolate themselves by withdrawing to the home. This could be due to either the natural history of the disease, which incapacitates its victims, or actions taken by public health officials encouraging people to stay home. The results are grouped according to time of withdrawal to the home:

(1) EARLY: people withdraw before they become infectious, producing the lowest estimates for R_0;
(2) LATE: people withdraw roughly 24 hours after they have become infectious; and
(3) NEVER people carry on their daily activities unless they die. The extreme cases are unrealistic, but are shown here because they demonstrate the existence of a clear transition.

The study shows that time of withdrawal to the home is by far the most important factor, followed by delay in response. This indicates that targeted vaccination is feasible when combined with fast detection. Ironically, the actual strategy used is much less important than either of these factors. Overall, these results suggest a much greater efficacy for targeted strategies than suggested by the results of Kaplan, Craft, and Wein [**25**]. It is not clear what accounts for the difference. Possibilities include: differences in mixing rates, differences in the distribution of incubation periods, and differences in transmissivity.

7. Random Graph Models

Random graph models provide an analytic framework for calculating (asymptotically) structural properties of networks, such as typical path lengths or distribution of sizes of connected components. Random graphs generated by these models also form a useful substrate for studying the behavior of phenomena that take place on networks [**32**]. The classical $G(n, p)$ random graph model of Erdős and Rényi does not capture even basic properties of real networks, such as degree distribution - this has spurred research into new models for capturing different aspects of real

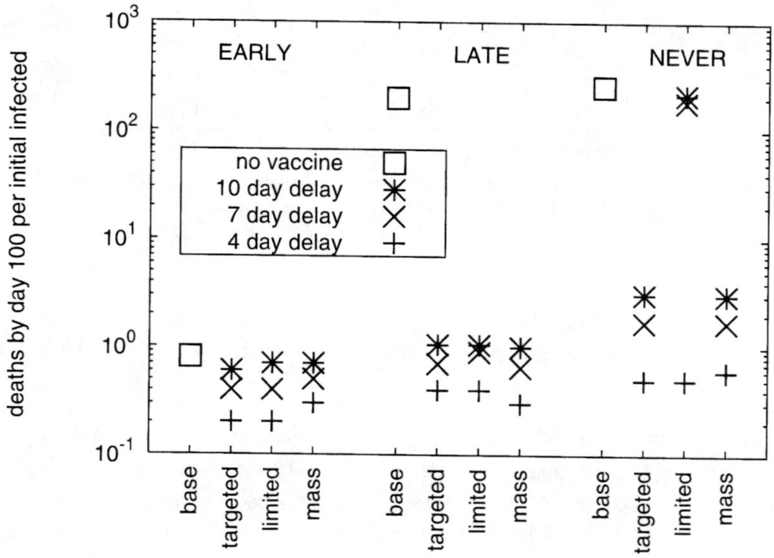

FIGURE 19. Cumulative number of deaths per number of initial infected, in case of a smallpox outbreak in downtown Portland, under a number of different response strategies.

networks. There are two lines of modeling the structures and behavior of real networks. One starts from observed structures of certain networks and constructs a model that generates networks encapsulating these structures. Through a random graph model, one can examine these structures and predict other structures over an ensemble of graphs. Instead of encapsulating given structures, another line is to explain the formation of these structures. That is, starting from some assumptions and rules, build networks in which certain structures will appear asymptotically. Although important and interesting, explaining the formation of these structures is not our purpose in this work, and we only briefly describe a representation of them, i.e., the preferential attachment model in Section 7.1. Also, due to the abundance of different models in encapsulating given structures, we only describe two of them that are relevant to our interests in Section 7.2 and 7.3.

7.1. Preferential Attachment Models. The first model trying to explain the formation of scale-free degree distribution is the preferential attachment model [**4**]. This is an evolutionary model, where nodes come in sequentially, and each node chooses some edges to nodes that are already present; the edges are not chosen uniformly, but with a higher preference for nodes that already have a higher degree. These models have been shown to be very useful for modeling the Internet web graph, but are not very promising for social networks for the following two reasons. The first is that social networks do not have very strict power laws- in the Portland data, only the location degree in G_{PL} is a power law in some range, but the people degree sequence in G_{PL} or in G_P is not a power law. But the preferential attachment models are only able to generate specific power law degree distributions. The second reason is that preferential attachment models are not defined for bipartite

	Edges	Triangles	Len.-2 paths	Clust. coef.
Portland	1077247259	631174770092	3349781340086	0.565268
Configuration	1080704055	629038069416	3308711641941	0.570347
Chung-Lu	1087038876	636683653469	3731989178759	0.511805

TABLE 1. Numbers of edges, triangles, and length-2 paths, and clustering coefficients in the people-people graph (1615860 people) in the Portland data and the Chung-Lu model.

graphs, and it is not clear whether they can be modified for G_{PL} type of graphs. Generating instances of graphs is also fairly slow in this model, and therefore, we do not consider it further.

7.2. Configuration Model. In the configuration model, initially make k copies for each vertex of degree k, then randomly pair two copies of the collection of all copies into an edge, remove these two copies and repeat the pairing process until no copies are left. Since the sum of degrees must be even, the above process is valid. At the end, if the resulting graph is a simple graph then output it, otherwise repeat and generate another graph. Obviously the configuration model uniformly generates a random graph *exactly* matching the given degree sequence. The structural properties of graphs generated by the configuration model for a fixed given degree sequence were first studied in [**30, 29**].

Although elegant and efficient, the probability of occurrence of multi-edges or self-loops is large when the degrees are large. For example, in Portland data G_{PL}, the maximum location degree is 7091, the maximum people degree is 15, and the number of edges between people and locations is 6060679. In our simulation all graphs among thousands generated by (the bipartite version of) the configuration model are non-simple, although multi-edges are few (between 500 and 700). To test the efficacy of the configuration model, we just discard those multi-edges and output the graph. Thus the degree sequence is not a perfect match but close enough. As in Portland data, the generated graph has a giant connected component composed of almost all people. Other properties also match Portland data very well, i.e., degree distribution of the people-people graph G_P (Figure 21); overlap ratios and performance of the fast greedy (Figures 7 and 8) in G_{PL}; numbers of edges, triangles, and length-2 paths, and the clustering coefficient in G_P.

7.3. Chung-Lu's model. Despite the good simulation results from the configuration model, the combinatorics of this model are awkward [**36**] and rigorous analysis is hard on this model [**12**]. Chung and Lu have proposed an alternative model [**12**] that is in many ways more convenient. In the model of Chung and Lu [**12**] one specifies the desired degree k_v of vertex v and then places edges between vertex pairs (v, w) independently with probability $P_{vw} = \frac{k_v k_w}{\sigma}$, where $\sigma = \sum_v k_v$ is twice the desired number of edges in the graph. It is easy to verify that the expected degree of each vertex is equal to its desired degree. Since each single edge has an explicit probability of appearing, many rigorous analyses can be carried through on the random graphs generated by this model. The result about dominating set in [**17**] was proved in this model. However this approach is still not entirely satisfactory. For some degree distributions the probability P_{vw} can exceed one, and

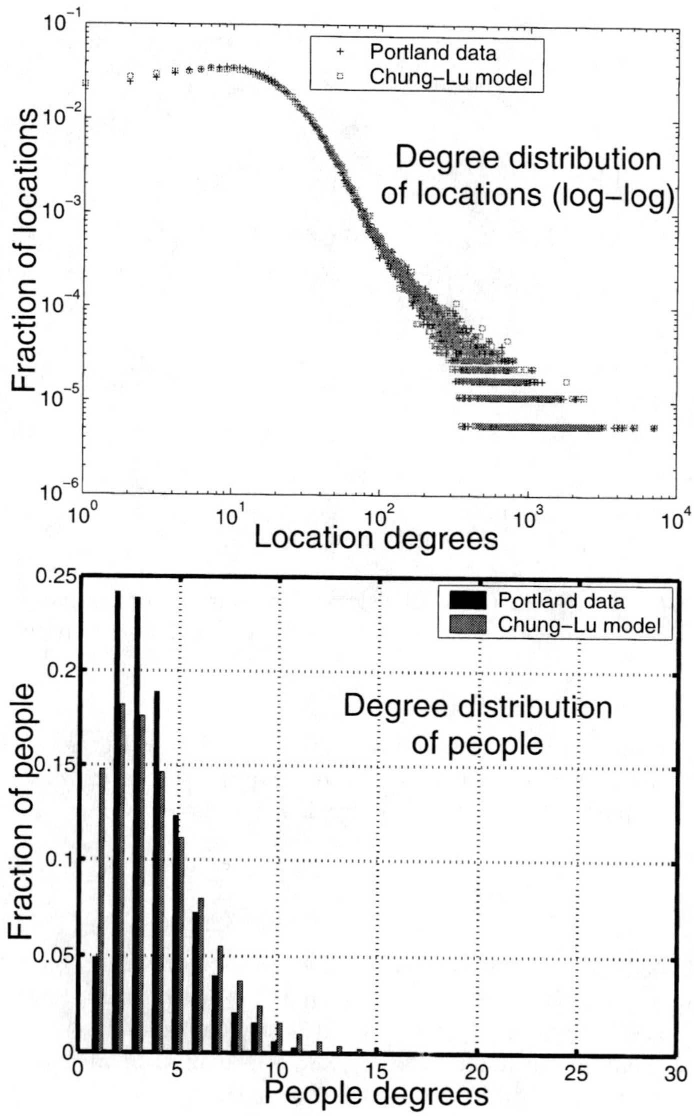

FIGURE 20. Degree distributions of locations and people in the bipartite graph G_{PL} for Portland data and the Chung-Lu model (described in Section 7). The location degrees range from 1 to 7091, people degrees range from 1 to 15.

hence the addition constraint on the desired degree distribution is $\max_v\{k_v^2\} \leq \sigma$. Translated in the G_{PL} bipartite graphs, one needs $\max_{p\in P,\ell\in L} k_p k_\ell \leq \sigma$, where $\sigma = \sum_{p\in P} k_p = \sum_{\ell\in L} k_\ell$. Fortunately Portland data satisfies this requirement. Unlike the configuration model, the degree sequence in the generated graph may not match exactly the given degree sequence. We also compare the same properties for Chung-Lu's model as we did for the configuration model (Section 7.2). The results are satisfactory, but not as good as in the configuration model.

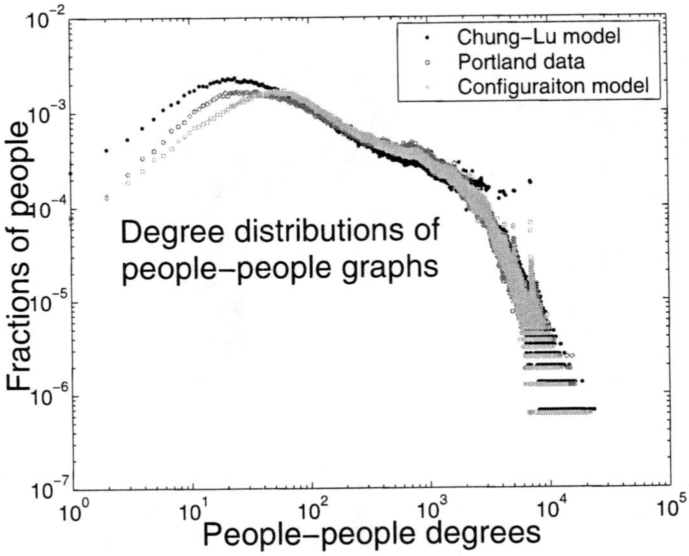

FIGURE 21. Comparison of degree distributions of people-people graphs of Chung-Lu's model, Portland data, and the configuration model.

Figures 20 and 21 show the comparison between the degree distributions for these models and the Portland data. Table 1 compares the number of edges, triangles, length 2 paths and clustering coefficient for these models and the Portland data.

8. Conclusions

In this paper, we studied epidemiology through a concrete, realistic, and full-featured social network representing Portland data, from three perspectives: (1) structural (i.e., topological, demographical, and temporal) measures of the contact networks, combinatorial formulations and approximation algorithms for certain problems in epidemiology and empirically evaluating these algorithms and structures via different random graph models; (2) methodology for generating contact networks of large urban areas starting from survey/census/transportation data; (3) several vaccination strategies motivated by the network structure, and their efficacy as determined the EpiSims simulation tool.

Acknowledgments We are very grateful to the members of the **TRANSIMS** and **EpiSims** teams at the Los Alamos National Laboratory, and to Sweta Bansal, Mac Hyman, Ira Longini, Cris Moore, Lauren Meyers, Azhar Nizam, and Zoltan Toroczkai for valuable discussions. Cris Moore suggested that we take another look at the configuration model for random graph generation. Thanks also to Lauren Meyers for sharing the slides of her talk on Network Epidemiology. Thanks to the referees of this article for their helpful comments. This work was supported in part by the National Institute of General Medical Sciences MIDAS grant U01-GM070694.

References

1. E. Zwingle. Cities. *Natl. Geo. Mag.* **202** 70-99 (2002).
2. R. Albert, A. Jeong, and A.L. Barabási. Attack and error tolerance of complex networks. *Nature*, 406:378–382, 2000.
3. R. Albert and A. Barabási, Statistical Mechanics of Complex Networks, *Rev. Mod. Phys.* 74, 47-97 (2002).
4. A.-L. Barabási and R. Albert. Emergence of scaling in random networks. *Science*, 286, 1999.
5. C. Barrett, K. Bisset, R. Jacob, G. Konjevod, and M. Marathe. An experimental analysis of a routing algorithm for realistic transportation networks. In *Proc. European Symposium on Algorithms (ESA)*, 2002.
6. C. L. Barrett, R. J. Beckman, K. P. Berkbigler, K. R. Bisset, B. W. Bush, K. Campbell, S. Eubank, K. M. Henson, J. M. Hurford, D. A. Kubicek, M. V. Marathe, O. Ramos, Jr., S. Ree, P. R. Romero, J. P. Smith, L. L. Smith, P. L. Speckman, P. E. Stretz, G. L. Thayer, E. Van Eeckhout, and M. D. Williams TRANSIMS 2.0: Transportation Analysis Simulation System: Volume 1 – Volume 6 Technical Report LA-UR-00-1723 – LA-UR-00-1767 , Los Alamos National Laboratory, 2000.
7. J. Berry and L. Fleischer and W. E. Hart and C. Phillips. Sensor Placement in Municipal Water Networks. *Proc. World Water and Environmental Resources Conference*, 2003.
8. C. Barrett, R. Jacob, and M. Marathe. Formal language constrained path problems. *SIAM J. Computing*, 30(3):809–837, 2001.
9. C. Barrett, J.P. Smith and S. Eubank. Modern Epidemiology Modeling, LANL Technical Report LA-UR-04-4176.
10. N. Bailey. *The Mathematical Theory of Infectious Diseases and its Applications.* Hafner Press, (1975).
11. A. Broder, R. Kumar, F. Maghoul, P. Raghavan, S. Rajagopalan, R. Stata, A. Tomkins, and J. Wiener. Graph structure in the web. *Computer Networks*, 33, 2000.
12. F. Chung and L. Lu. Connected components in a random graph with given degree sequences. *Annals of Combinatorics*, 6:125–145, 2002.
13. D.S. Callaway, M.E.J. Newman, S. Strogatz, and D.J. Watts. Network robustness and fragility: Percolation on random graphs. *Phys. Rev. Lett.*, 85:5468–5471, 2000.
14. K. Elveback, J. Fox and E. Ackerman. An Influenza Simulation Model for Immunization Studies *American J. Empidemiology*, 103, pp. 152-165, 1976.
15. S. Eubank and et al. Episims assessment of responses to smallpox attack (report to the office of homeland security). Technical Report LA-CP-02-254, Los Alamos National Laboratory, 2002.
16. S. Eubank, H. Guclu, V. S. Anil Kumar, M. Marathe, A. Srinivasan, Z. Toroczkai and N. Wang. Modeling disease outbreaks in realistic urban social networks. *Nature*, 429:180–184, 2004.
17. S. Eubank, V. S. Anil Kumar, M. Marathe, A. Srinivasan, and N. Wang. Structural and algorithmic aspects of massive social networks. In *Proceedings of the 15th ACM-SIAM Symposium on Discrete Algorithms (SODA)*, pages 711–720, 2004.
18. S. Eubank and J. Smith. Scalable, efficient epidemiological simulation. In *Proceedings of Symposium on Applied Computing*, 2002.
19. C. Faloutsos, P. Faloutsos, and M. Faloutsos. *On Power-Law Relationships of the Internet Topology.* Proceedings of the ACM SIGCOMM (1999).
20. M.R. Garey and D.S. Johnson. *Computers and Intractability. A Guide to the Theory of NP-Completeness*, Freeman, San Francisco CA, 1979.
21. O. Goldreich and D. Ron. On Testing Expansion in Bounded Degree Graphs. Manuscript, 2000. Available from `http://www.wisdom.weizmann.ac.il/~oded/papers.html`.
22. H. Hethcote. The Mathematics of Infectious Diseases. *SIAM Review*, **42**(4), pp. 599-653, (2000).
23. H. Halloran, I. Longini Jr, A. Nizam, & Y. Yang. Possible Containment of Bio-terrorist Smallpox. *Science*, **298**, pp. 1428-1432, (2002).

24. E. Halloran, I. Longini, D. Cowert, et.al. Community trials of Vaccination and the Epidemic Prevention Potential, *Vaccine*, 20, pp. 3254-3262, 2002.
25. E.H. Kaplan, D.L. Craft, and L.M. Wein. Emergency response to a smallpox attack: the case for mass vaccination. *Proc. Natl. Acad. Sci. USA*, 99:10935–10940, 2002.
26. I. Longini, E. Halloran, A. Nizam and Y. Yang. Containing Pandemic Influenza with Antiviral Agents *American J. Epidemiology*, 159(1), pp. 623-633, 2004.
27. T. Leighton and S. Rao. An approximate max-flow min-cut theorem for multicommodity flow problems with applications to approximation algorithms. *Journal of the ACM*, 46(6):787–832, 1999.
28. L. Meyers, M. E. J. Newman, M. Martin, and S. Schrag. Applying network theory to epidemics: Control measures for outbreaks of mycoplasma pneumonia. *Emerging Infectious Diseases*, pages 204–210, 2003.
29. M. Molloy and B. Reed. A critical point for random graphs with a given degree sequence. *Random Structures and Algorithms*, 6:161–180, 1995.
30. M. Molloy and B. Reed. The size of the largest component of a random graph on a fixed degree sequence. *Combinatorics, Probability and Computing*, 7:295–306, 1998.
31. M. E. J. Newman and J. Park. *Why social networks are different from other types of networks.* Phys. Rev. E **68**, 036122 (2003).
32. M. Newman. Random graphs as models of networks. In S. Bornholdt and H. G. Schuster, editors, *Handbook of Graphs and Networks.* Wiley-VCH, Berlin, 2003.
33. M. E. J. Newman. *The structure and function of complex networks.* SIAM Review **45**, 167–256 (2003).
34. M. Newman, S. Forrest, and J. Balthrop. Email networks and the spread of computer viruses. *Phys. Rev. E*, 66(035101), 2002.
35. M. Newman, S. Strogatz, & D. Watts. Random graphs with arbitrary degree distributions and their applications. *Phys.Rev.E* **64** 026118 (2001).
36. J. Park and M. E. J. Newman. The origin of degree correlations in the Internet and other networks. *Phys. Rev. E.*, 68(026112), 2003.
37. R. Patel, I. Longini and E. Halloran. Finding Optimal Vaccination Strategies for Pandemic Influenza Using Genetic Algorithms Technical Report,04-07, Dept. of Biostatistics, Rollins School of Public Health, Emory University, Atlanta, 2004.
38. `http://www.nature.com/nature/journal/v429/n6988/extref/nature02541-s1.htm`

Virginia Bio-Informatics Institute, Virginia Tech, Blacksburg, VA 24061.
E-mail address: `eubank@vt.edu`

Virginia Bio-Informatics Institute and Dept. of Computer Science, Virginia Tech, Blacksburg, VA 24061.
E-mail address: `akumar@vbi.vt.edu`

Virginia Bio-Informatics Institute and Dept. of Computer Science, Virginia Tech, Blacksburg, VA 24061.
E-mail address: `marathe@vt.edu`

Department of Computer Science and Institute for Advanced Computer Studies, University of Maryland, College Park, MD 20742.
E-mail address: `srin@cs.umd.edu`

Department of Computer Science, University of Maryland, College Park, MD 20742.
E-mail address: `nwang@cs.umd.edu`

DIMACS Series in Discrete Mathematics
and Theoretical Computer Science
Volume **70**, 2006

Random Graphs (and the Spread of Infections in a Social Network)

James Abello and Michael Capalbo

ABSTRACT. We say that a probability space $\mathcal{F}$ on a collection of graphs on a set of vertices is *unbiased* if, for every two vertices u and v, the probability of the event $A_{u,v}$ that u and v form an edge, is proportional to the product of their expected degrees. We say that $\mathcal{F}$ is *independent* if the $A_{u,v}$'s are mutually independent events. The collection $\mathcal{P}$ of unbiased independent probability spaces of graphs on a set N vertices contains $\{\mathcal{G}(N,p); p \in [0,1]\}$ (where every pair of vertices form an edge with probability p, and these are mutually independent events), but is much richer, for each $\mathcal{F} \in \mathcal{P}$ is parameterized by a function on N points, instead of merely by one real number in $p \in [0,1]$.

Making a few (fairly) reasonable simplifying assumptions, we first relate how far a contagious infection is likely to spread through a social network to the expected size of the largest component in a graph chosen from an independent, unbiased probability space. Then we establish a graph-theoretic result that almost completely characterizes which $\mathcal{F} \in \mathcal{P}$ are such that a graph drawn from $\mathcal{F}$ almost surely has a giant component, and which $\mathcal{F} \in \mathcal{P}$ are such that a graph drawn from $\mathcal{F}$ almost surely does not. This generalizes a theorem by Erdős and Rényi on the size of the largest component on a graph chosen from $\mathcal{G}(N,p)$.

1. Introduction

If a contagious infection starts at a single person in a social network, how far will it spread? The answer to that question of course depends on the probability of the infection spreading from one person to another. Is it possible to accurately predict with high probability the answer? Researchers [**4**], [**7**], [**10**], [**5**], [**8**] are trying to answer questions such as these, using not only simulation but also tools from graph theory. As collaboration between researchers in Epidemiology and Mathematics continues, the models used are becoming more realistic.

In this paper, we approach the question posed above, making the following simplifying assumptions. Before we state these, we present two definitions. First, for any two people in the social network, define the *transmission probability from u to v* to be the probability of the event $A_{u,v}$ that u passes on the infection to v, given that u is infected and v is not. Second, for each person v, define the *local exposure* $f(v)$ of v as $\sum_u P[A_{u,v}]$, where we write as $P[A]$ the probability of event

2000 *Mathematics Subject Classification.* 05C80.

A. So having presented the two relevant definitions, we now state the simplifying assumptions of our model. We first assume that the transmission probability from u to v is the same as the transmission probability from v to u, for each pair $\{u, v\}$ of people. We also assume that the transmission probability from u to v is proportional to the product of the local exposures of u and v. (This assumption is based on the premise that if two people have high local exposure, then their paths likely cross often.) We also assume that the events $A_{u,v}$ are mutually independent. Finally, we assume that the only way for a person to become infected is to catch it from someone already infected.

We next draw a connection between our epidemiological model and graph theory. Let $\mathcal{H}$ be a probability space of graphs on a set Y of vertices. We say that $\mathcal{H}$ is *unbiased* if the probability of the event $E_{u,v}$ = {the pair $\{u, v\}$ of vertices form an edge} is $\frac{f(u)f(v)}{M}$, where $f(y)$ is the expected degree of the vertex y, and M is the expected number of edges. We say that $\mathcal{H}$ is *independent* if the $E_{u,v}$'s are mutually independent events. First, let $\mathcal{F}$ be an unbiased, independent probability space on the set of graphs on V, the set of people in the social network, such that the expected degree of each $v \in V$ is v's local exposure $f(v)$. Then the expected number of people who will become infected if the infection starts from v is the expected size of the component in G that contains v, where G is a graph drawn from $\mathcal{F}$. Thus, if such a graph G has no giant components, then an infection can start at any vertex, and almost surely, it will be restricted to a small subset of the people in the community. On the other hand, if G almost surely does have a giant component, then it is at least quite possible (depending on where the infection starts from) that the infection will spread to a large fraction of the social network. With this in mind, the main results of this paper are Theorems 1.1 and 1.2.

THEOREM 1.1. *Let $\mathcal{F}$ be an unbiased, independent probability space on the graphs on a set V of vertices, such that every vertex v has expected degree $f(v)$ no larger than* $\min\{\sqrt{\frac{M}{16}}, \sqrt{\frac{N}{16}}\}$, *where* $N = |V|$ *and* $M = \sum_{v \in V} f(v)$. *Also, let us set* $\hat{f} = \max_{v \in V} \lceil f(v) \rceil$.

(i) Suppose the $f(v)$'s satisfy (a): $\sum_{v \in V} f^2(v) \le (1 - \varepsilon)M$ *for some* $\varepsilon \in \Omega(1)$. *Then almost every component of a graph G drawn from $\mathcal{F}$ has all components with no more than* $O(\hat{f} \log^3 N)$ *vertices.*

(ii) Suppose that the f's satisfy (b): there is a set V' of vertices such that $\sum_{y \in V \setminus V'} f^2(y)$ *is no larger than* $(1 - \varepsilon)M$ *for some* $\varepsilon \in \Omega(1)$. *Then almost surely every component of G has* $O(L \log^3 N)$ *vertices, where* $L = \max\{\sum_{v \in V'} f(v), \hat{f}\}$.

Theorem 1.1 essentially says the following. If the second-order average degree of the graphs in $\mathcal{F}$ is no larger than $1 - \varepsilon$, then a graph drawn from $\mathcal{F}$ will almost surely have only small components (i.e., at most $o(N)$ vertices in every component). (To compare, if the $f(v)$'s all take on the same value p, then they will satisfy (a) if p is no larger than $1 - \varepsilon$.) Furthermore, if there exists a small set of vertices S such that, removing S, the second-order average degree of the graphs in $\mathcal{F}$ is no larger than $1 - \varepsilon$, then a graph drawn from $\mathcal{F}$ will almost surely have only small components.

The following result is almost the converse of Theorem 1.1:

THEOREM 1.2. *Using the notation in Theorem 1.1, suppose the $f(v)$'s satisfy (a)* $\sum_{v \in V} f^2(v) \ge (1 + \varepsilon)M$ *for some* $\varepsilon \in \Omega(1)$, *and*

(b) if Y is a subset of V such that $\sum_{y\in V\setminus Y} f^2(y)$ is no larger than $(1+\frac{\varepsilon}{2})M$, then $|Y|$ is in $\Omega(N)$.
Then G drawn from $\mathcal{F}$ almost surely has a component of size $\theta(N)$.

Theorem 1.2 essentially says the following. If the average degree of the graphs in $\mathcal{F}$, even after removing any not-so-large subset of vertices, is at least $1+\frac{\varepsilon}{2}$, then a graph drawn from $\mathcal{F}$ will almost surely have a giant component (i.e., there is a component with $\theta(N)$ vertices).

If the assumptions we made above about the spread of an infection through a social network are roughly correct, and if we can estimate v's local exposure $f(v)$ well for each v, then we may use the above theorems to efficiently check how likely it is that the infection will spread to a large number of vertices in the social network. Indeed, write $V=\{v_1,\dots,v_N\}$, in decreasing order of their expected degrees, and for each integer i, let $V_i=\{v_1,\dots,v_i\}$. To use Theorem 1.1 and 1.2, it suffices to evaluate $\sum_{v\in V_i} f(v)$, $\sum_{v\in V_i} f^2(v)$, and for each integer $i\le N$, the sum $\sum_{v\in V\setminus V_i} f^2(y)$. Indeed, for example, the smallest such V' in (ii) of Theorem 1.1 would have the form $V'=V_i$ for some integer i. Having discussed the potential relevance of Theorems 1.1 and 1.2 from an epidemiological perspective, we next discuss these theorems from a graph-theoretic perspective.

First of all, both of these theorems generalize a well-known theorem by Erdős and Rényi [**6**] that establishes that the random graph drawn from the probability space $\mathcal{G}(N,\frac{c}{N})$ has only small components if c satisfies $c\le 1-\varepsilon$ for some $\varepsilon\in\Omega(1)$, and on the other hand, has a component of size $\theta(N)$ if c satisfies $c\ge 1+\varepsilon$ for some $\varepsilon\in\Omega(1)$. Secondly, Theorems 1.1 and 1.2 are related to the results presented in Aiello et. al. [**1**] and Molloy and Reed [**9**]. In both of these papers, the probability spaces $\mathcal{F}'$ considered are such that each vertex v always has degree *exactly* $f(v)$, instead of having merely *expected* degree $f(v)$. However, the size of the largest component in a graph drawn according to $\mathcal{F}'$ may be very different from the size of the largest component in a graph drawn according to $\mathcal{F}$, where each vertex v has expected degree $f(v)$. Indeed, consider the following example. Let U be a large set of vertices, and let Ω be the collection of graphs on U. Next, let f be a function on U, such that $f(v)=2$ for, say, a $\frac{1}{4}$-fraction of the vertices v, and $f(u)$ is 1 for the rest of the vertices in U. Next, let $\mathcal{F}'$ be the probability space on Ω where every graph H' in the set $\{G'|$ the degree of u in G' is $f(u)$ for each $u\in U\}$, has equal weight, and the rest have weight 0, and let G' be chosen from $\mathcal{F}'$. Then let $\mathcal{F}$ be an unbiased, independent probability space on Ω where the *expected* degree of each vertex $u\in U$ is $f(u)$, and let G be a graph chosen from $\mathcal{F}$. Then G will almost surely have a giant component, but G' almost surely will not (see [**9**]). With this in mind, it seems that the probability spaces that we are studying here are more realistic because it is difficult to enforce exact degree sequences in 'real life'.

We have very recently been informed that the techniques and results of this paper are very similar to those in [**3**].

We organize this paper in the following fashion. In §2 we present the proof to Theorem 1.1, and in §3 we present the proof to Theorem 1.2. For the rest of this paper, we use the following notation. First, for each subset S of V, write $f(S)=\sum_{s\in S} f(s)$. Next, for any random variable X, we write the expected value of X as $\mathcal{E}[X]$, and for an event A, we write the probability of event A as $P[A]$. Finally, for every two vertices u and v, we often write as $A_{u,v}$ the event that the pair form an edge in the graph drawn from $\mathcal{F}$.

2. Proof of Theorem 1.1

We now show that if $\mathcal{F}$ satisfies (a) of Theorem 1.1, then G picked according to $\mathcal{F}$ almost surely has all components no larger than $O(\hat{f}\log^3 N)$, via the following claims. (This is highly modified version of the approach presented in [**2**], pp 149–151.)

CLAIM 2.1. *Suppose that $\mathcal{F}$ satisfies (a) of Theorem 1.1. Fix a vertex $v \in V$, and pick a graph G from $\mathcal{F}$, and for each j, let S_j denote the set of vertices of distance j in G from v. For each positive integer i and for all possible $S_1, \ldots, S_i$, the following two inequalities hold.*

$$(1) \qquad \mathcal{E}[f(S_{i+1})|S_1, \ldots, S_i] \le \sum_{y\in Y_i} \frac{f(S_i)f(y)}{M} \times f(y) = \frac{f(S_i)}{M} \sum_{y \in Y_i} f^2(y).$$

$$(2) \qquad \mathcal{E}[f(S_{i+1})|S_1, \ldots, S_i] \le (1-\varepsilon) f(S_i),$$

Proof of Claim 2.1: Let us set $Y_i = V \setminus (\{v\} \cup S_1 \cup \ldots \cup S_i)$.

We first show that Inequality (1) holds. Note that $y \in Y_i$ is in S_{i+1} if and only if there is an edge in G between y and a vertex in S_i. Note that $P[A_{y,s}|S_1, \ldots, S_i]$ is $P[A_{y,s}] = \frac{f(s)f(y)}{M}$ for each $y \in Y_i$ and each $s \in S_i$, because of the mutual independence of the $A_{u,v}$'s. Then $P[y \in S_{i+1}|S_1 \ldots, S_i]$ is no larger than $\frac{f(S_i)f(y)}{M}$. From this Inequality (1) follows.

Inequality (1) and the inequality $\sum_{y\in V} f^2(y) \le (1-\varepsilon)M$, imply Inequality (2). □

CLAIM 2.2. *Let $X_1, X_2, \ldots$ be a series of nonegative random variables such that $\mathcal{E}[X_{i+1}|X_1, \ldots, X_1]$ is no larger than $(1-\varepsilon)X_i$, for some $\varepsilon \in \Omega(1)$. Then for each l, the following inequality holds.*

$$P[X_l \ge 1] \le (1-\varepsilon)^l \mathcal{E}[X_1].$$

Claim 2.2 is a corollary of the Kolmogorov-Doob Inequality, presented in [**9**], page 92 (Theorem 4.15). Indeed, the Kolmorgorov-Doob Inequality states the following: Let $X_1', X_2', \ldots$ be a series of nonegative random variables such that $\mathcal{E}[X_{i+1}'|X_1', \ldots, X_i'] = X_i'$, then for each positive λ and each l,

$$P[X_l' \ge \lambda] \le \frac{\mathcal{E}[X_l']}{\lambda}.$$

However, one can check that the equality $\mathcal{E}[X_2'] = \mathcal{E}[X_1']$ holds, and so one can use induction to show that $\mathcal{E}[X_l'] = \mathcal{E}[X_1']$. This implies the following inequality:

$$P[X_l' \ge \lambda] \le \frac{\mathcal{E}[X_1']}{\lambda}.$$

Note that Claim 2.1 (ii) implies that there exists a series $X_1', X_2', \ldots,$ of random variables that satisfy both $X_{i+1}' = (1-\varepsilon)^{-i}X_{i+1} + h(X_1, \ldots, X_i)$ for some nonnegative h, and $\mathcal{E}[X_{i+1}'|X_1', \ldots, X_i'] = X_{i+1}'$. This and the above inequality imply the following, for each positive λ:

$$P[X_l \ge \lambda(1+\varepsilon)^l] \le \frac{\mathcal{E}[X_1]}{\lambda}.$$

So pick $\lambda = (1-\varepsilon)^{-l}$, and by the above inequality, Claim 2.2 follows. □

We are now ready to prove the following claim.

CLAIM 2.3. *Suppose that $\mathcal{F}$ satisfies (a) in the statement of Theorem 1.1. Fix a vertex $v \in V$. Then with probability $1 - o(N^{-1})$, a graph G chosen from $\mathcal{F}$ satisfies the following:*

(i)If, for each i, S_i denotes the set of vertices in V of distance i from v, then S_t is empty for some $t \in O(\log N)$.

(ii) Each S_i has size no larger than $2\hat{f}\log^2 N$.

(iii) The vertex v is in a component of G that has only $O(\hat{f}\log^3 N)$ vertices.

(iv) Every component of G has $O(\hat{f}\log^3 N)$ vertices.

Proof of Claim 2.3: We first prove (i). Inequality (2) and Claim 2.2 imply that, with probability $1 - o(N^{-1})$ for $t \geq 4\varepsilon^{-1}\log N$, the set S_t indeed will be empty.

We now prove (ii). To do this, let us assume that $f(S_i)$ is no larger than $\hat{f}\log^2 N$ (this is trivially true for $i = 0$). Then $f(S_{i+1})$ and $|S_{i+1}|$ are no larger than $\hat{f}\log^2 N$ and $2\hat{f}\log^2 N$, respectively, with probability $1 - o(N^{-1})$. Indeed, note that the independence of $\mathcal{F}$ implies that $f(S_{i+1})$ and $|S_{i+1}|$ can be written as $f(S_{i+1}) = \sum_{y\in V} a_y f(y)$ and $|S_{i+1}| = \sum_{y \in V} a_y$, where each $f(y)$ has value at most $\hat{f}$, and the a_y's are 0-1 independent random variables. Furthermore, Inequality (2) above implies that $\mathcal{E}[f(S_{i+1})|S_1, \ldots, S_i]$ is no larger than $(1-\varepsilon)\hat{f}\log^2 N$. Also, note that $\mathcal{E}[|S_{i+1}||S_1 \ldots, S_i]$ is no larger than $f(S_i)$, which is no larger than $\hat{f}\log^2 N$. So these, together with Chernoff bounds, imply that $f(S_{i+1})$ and $|S_{i+1}|$ are no larger than $\hat{f}\log^2 N$ and $2\hat{f}\log^2 N$, respectively, with probability $1 - o(N^{-1})$, and so (ii) of Claim 2.3 follows.

(iii) follows immediately from (i) and (ii).

From (iii), the probability that G has more than $O(\hat{f}\log^3 N)$ vertices is at most $N \times o(N^{-1})$ which is $o(1)$, and so (iv) follows as well. □

We have just shown that if $\mathcal{F}$ satisfies Condition (a) in the statement of Theorem 1.1, then almost surely a graph G picked from $\mathcal{F}$ has no components with more than $\hat{f}\log^3 N$ vertices. So to prove the remainder of Theorem 1.1, we prove the following claim.

CLAIM 2.4. *If $\mathcal{F}$ satisfies Condition (b) in the statment of Theorem 1.1, then all components of a graph G drawn from $\mathcal{F}$ have only $O(L\log^3 N)$ vertices, where $L = \max\{f(V'), \hat{f}\}$.*

Proof of Claim 2.4: We first show that every component in $G[V \setminus V']$ has size $O(\hat{f}\log^3 N)$ with high probability. We then show that the number of vertices of V that share a component with a vertex in V' is $O(f(V')\log^3 N)$ with high probability, establishing the result.

Fix an arbitrary vertex v in $V \setminus V'$, and for each integer i, let T_i denote the set of vertices in $V \setminus V'$ of distance i in $G[V \setminus V']$ from v. Next, set $Z_i = (V \setminus V') \setminus (T_1 \cup \ldots T_i)$. Then note that

$$\mathcal{E}[f(T_{i+1})|T_1, \ldots, T_i] \leq \sum_{y \in Z_i} \frac{f(T_i)f(y)}{M} \times f(y) = \frac{f(T_i)}{M} \sum_{y\in Z_i} f^2(y).$$

However, by the assumption that $\sum_{y\in V\setminus V'} f^2(y)$ is no larger than $(1-\varepsilon)M$, it follows that

$$\mathcal{E}[f(T_{i+1})|T_1,\ldots,T_i] \leq (1-\varepsilon)[T_i]. \tag{3}$$

By using the same line of reasoning that we used to prove Claim 2.3, we can show that with probability $1-o(N^{-1})$, the component of $G[V\setminus V']$ that contains v has $O(\hat{f}\log^3 N)$ vertices with probability $1-o(N^{-1})$, and so, every component of $G[V\setminus V']$ indeed has only $O(\hat{f}\log^3 N)$ vertices with probability $1-o(1)$. To finish the proof of Claim 2.4, it suffices to show that the number of vertices of V that share a component in G with a vertex in V' is $O(L\log^3 N)$. We do this next.

For each positive integer i, let U_i denote the set of vertices u in G such that the shortest path from u to a vertex in V' has i edges. Then we can show the following inequality:

$$\mathcal{E}[f(U_{i+1})|U_1,\ldots,U_i] \leq (1-\varepsilon)f(U_i).$$

This implies that the number of vertices of V that share a component of G with a vertex in V' is indeed $O(L\log^3 N)$ with high probability, so Claim 2.4 follows. □

Theorem 1.1 follows from Claims 2.3 and 2.4. □

3. Proof of Theorem 1.2

We prove Theorem 1.2 via the following four claims.

CLAIM 3.1. *Condition (b) in the statement of Theorem 1.2 implies the following:*

If Y is a subset of V such that $\sum_{y\in V\setminus Y} f^2(y)$ is no larger than $(1+\frac{\varepsilon}{2})M$, then $f(Y)\in\Omega(M)$.

Proof of Claim 3.1: Suppose that there exists a subset Y' of V such that $\sum_{y\in V\setminus Y'} f^2(y)$ is no larger than $(1+\frac{\varepsilon}{2})M$, and $f(Y')$ is $o(M)$. First, let K be the smallest integer such that the K largest $f(v)$'s in V sum to at least $f(Y')$, and let Y be the set of K vertices $v\in V$ such that $f(v)$ is among the K largest. Then we can check that $\sum_{y\in Y} f^2(y)\geq\sum_{y\in Y'} f^2(y)$, and so $\sum_{v\in V\setminus Y} f^2(y)$ is no larger than $(1+\frac{\varepsilon}{2})M$. Furthermore, we can check that $f(Y)\leq f(Y')+\min\{\sqrt{M},\sqrt{N}\}$. This implies that $f(Y)$ is $o(M)$, and because $f(y)\geq f(w)$ for all $y\in Y$ and $w\notin Y$, this in turn implies that $K=|Y|$ is no larger than $N\times\frac{f(Y)}{M}$, which is $o(N)$ because $f(Y)$ is $o(M)$. However, this contradicts Condition (b) in the statement of Theorem 1.2, so Claim 3.1 holds. □

CLAIM 3.2. *Let S be any subset of V, and v any vertex in V not in S, and pick G from $\mathcal{F}$. Then the probability that there is an edge in G between v and at least one vertex in S is at least* $\min\{\frac{\varepsilon}{3},(1-\frac{\varepsilon}{4})\sum_{s\in S}\frac{f(s)f(v)}{M}\}$.

Claim 3.2 follows from the mutual independence on the $A_{u,v}$'s and from the following arithmetical fact: If $p_1,\ldots p_r$ are numbers in $[0,1]$, then for all $a\in[0,1]$, the quantity $1-\prod_i(1-p_i)$ is either at least a, or at least $(1-\frac{3a}{4})\sum_i p_i$. □

CLAIM 3.3. *Let V_0 be a set of $\log^2 N$ vertices such that $f(v)\geq f(w)$ for all $v\in V_0$, and all $w\notin V_0$, and let G be a graph picked from $\mathcal{F}$. Then with high probability, G satisfies the following:*

There exists an integer $t \le \log N$ such that $f(W_t)$ is at least $\hat{f}\log^4 N$, where W_t is the set of vertices w such that the shortest path in G from w to a vertex in V_{top} has t edges.

Proof of Claim 3.3: First, for each positive integer j, set $Y_j = V \backslash (V_0 \cup W_1 \cup \ldots \cup W_j)$. Next, for each j, let $F_j = \max\{f(W_1), \ldots, f(W_j)\}$, and define the event

$$E_j = \{F_{j+1} \ge \hat{f}\log^2 N\} \cup \{f(W_{j+1}) \ge (1+\frac{\varepsilon}{8})f(W_j)\}.$$

We will show that $P[E_1] \ge 1 - o(N^{-2})$, and $P[E_{j+1}|E_1, \ldots, E_j] \ge 1 - o(N^{-2})$, for each $j \ge 1$. Then Claim 3.3 will follow.

We do this in the following two subcases.

Case 1: $f(W_1 \cup \ldots \cup W_j)$ is $\Omega(M)$. Then with probability 1 there is a i such that $f(W_i)$ is at least $\hat{f}\log^2 N$, because j is $O(\log N)$, and $\hat{f}$ is $O(\sqrt{M})$, and M is $\Omega(N)$ by Condition (b) on f. So event E_{j+1} occurs with probability 1 in this subcase. This finishes Case 1.

Case 2: $f(W_1 \cup \ldots \cup W_j)$ is $o(M)$. Then let $\mathcal{W}_j$ be the set of sequences $(W_1, \ldots W_j)$, where $W_1, \ldots, W_j$ are disjoint subsets of $V \backslash V_0$ such that (i) $f(W_j)$ is at least $f(V_0)$, and (ii) $f(W_1 \cup \ldots \cup W_j)$ is $o(M)$. Note that

$$1 - P[E_{j+1}|E_1, \ldots, E_j] \le \max_{(W_1,\ldots,W_j)\in\mathcal{W}_j} P[f(W_{j+1})|W_1, \ldots, W_j \quad \le (1+\frac{\varepsilon}{8})f(W_j)].$$

Because $\mathcal{F}$ is independent, the random variable $f(W_{j+1})|W_1, \ldots, W_j$ can be written as $\sum_{y\in Y_j} a_y f(y)$, where the a_y's are mutually independent random variables whose range is $\{0,1\}$. Also observe that $f(V_0)$ is at least $\max_{y\in V\backslash V_0} f(y)\log^2 N$, so each such $f(y)$ is no larger than $\mathcal{E}[f(W_{j+1})|W_1, \ldots, W_j]\log^{-2} N$ for each $(W_1, \ldots, W_j) \in \mathcal{W}_j$. To finish the proof of Claim 3.3, it remains to show that $\mathcal{E}[f(W_{j+1})|W_1, \ldots, W_j]$ is at least $(1+\frac{\varepsilon}{4})f(W_j)$ for each $(W_1, \ldots, W_j) \in \mathcal{W}_j$. (Then one may use Chernoff bounds to show that $P[E_{j+1}|E_1, \ldots, E_j]$ is $1 - o(N^{-2})$.) So we do this next.

Claim 3.2 implies the following inequality:

$$(4) \qquad \mathcal{E}[f(W_{j+1})|W_1, \ldots, W_j] \ge \sum_{y\in Y_j} \min\left\{\frac{\varepsilon f(y)}{3}, \frac{(1-\frac{\varepsilon}{4})f(W_j)f^2(y)}{M}\right\}.$$

Next, let Y_j' be the set of vertices $y \in Y_j$ such that $\min\{\frac{\varepsilon f(y)}{3}, \frac{f(W_j)f^2(y)}{M}\}$ is $\frac{\varepsilon f(y)}{3}$. Inequality 4 implies the following inequalities.

$$(5) \qquad \mathcal{E}[f(W_{j+1})|W_1, \ldots, W_j] \ge \sum_{y\in Y_j'} \frac{\varepsilon f(y)}{3} + \sum_{y\in Y_j\backslash Y_j'} \frac{(1-\frac{\varepsilon}{4})f(W_j)f^2(y)}{M}.$$

So let us suppose that $f(Y_j')$ is $\Omega(M)$, and note that is y is in Y_j' only if $f(y)$ is $\Omega(1)$. Therefore, by Inequality (5), $\mathcal{E}[f(W_{j+1})|W_1, \ldots, W_j]$ is $\Omega(M)$, which is at least $2f(W_j)$ by the assumption that $f(W_1 \cup \ldots \cup W_j)$ is $o(M)$. So let us now suppose that $f(Y_j')$ is not $\Omega(M)$. Then Claim 3.1 implies that $\sum_{y\in Y_j\backslash Y_j'} f^2(y)$ must be at least $(1+\frac{\varepsilon}{2})M$. Thus, $\mathcal{E}[f(W_{j+1})|W_1, \ldots, W_j]$ is at least $(1+\frac{\varepsilon}{4})f(W_j)$ which implies Claim 3.3 for Case 2 as well. □

Claim 3.3 is used to prove Claim 3.4, established below, which is what we will use to finish the proof of Theorem 1.2.

CLAIM 3.4. *We define a vertex* $v \in G$ *to be* active *if there exists an integer* t *such that* $f(S_t) \geq \hat{f} \log^2 N$*, where* S_t *is the vertices in* G *of distance* t *away from* v*. With high probability, a graph* G *drawn from* $\mathcal{F}$ *has least one active vertex in* V_0*, as in Claim 3.3.*

Proof of Claim 3.4: By Claim 3.3, almost surely G is such that there is a t such that $f(W_t) \geq \hat{f} \log^5 N$. However, then G indeed would have an active vertex, because there are only $\log^5 N$ vertices in V_0, there is a vertex v in V_0 such that the set $W_{v,t}$ of vertices in $w \in W_t$ of distance t away from v satisfies $f(W_{v,t}) \geq \frac{f(W_t)}{\log^5 N}$ $\geq \hat{f} \log^2 N$. □

We now use Claims 3.3 and 3.4 to finish the rest of the proof of Theorem 1.2. Claim 3.4 establishes that G has an active vertex with probability $1 - \sigma$ for some $\sigma \in o(1)$. So let $v \in V$ be an active vertex in G, and for each integer j, let S_j be the set of vertices in G of distance j from v, and let t be the smallest integer such that $f(S_t)$ is at least $\hat{f} \log^2 N$. Then, by tracing through the line of reasoning that we used to prove Case 2 of Claim 3.3 (considering $S_{t+1}, S_{t+2}, \ldots,$) we may show that the probability that v is *not* in a component S of G where $|S| \in \Omega(N)$, is $o(N^{-1})$ (note that each vertex in each S_j is in the same component of G as v). So the probability that G is such that none of the active vertices of G are in a component S where $|S| \in \Omega(N)$, is no larger than $\sigma + N \times o(N^{-1})$, which is $o(1)$, and so Theorem 1.2 follows. □

4. Conclusion

In this paper, using a few assumptions, we have given conditions for the spread of an infection through a social network, that are close to being both necessary and sufficient. We are working on extending the mathematical techniques that we have developed here to richer models, where we may relax some of the assumptions that we have used in this paper.

References

[1] W. Aiello, F. Chung, and L. Lu. "A Random Graph Model For Power-Law Graphs", *Experimental Math* 10 (2001), no 1, 53–66.

[2] N. Alon and J. Spencer. *The Probabilistic Method.* John Wiley and Sons, Inc., 1992.

[3] F. Chung and L. Lu. "Connected components in random graphs with expected degree sequences", `http://www.math.ucsd.edu/~fan/wp/conn.pdf`.

[4] R. Cohen, S. Havlin, and D. ben-Avraham. Structural properties of scale free networks, Chapter 4 in *Handbook of Graphs and Networks*, Eds. S. Bornholdt and H. G. Schuster (Wiley-VCH, 2002).

[5] V. Eguiluz and K. Klemm. "Epidemic threshold in structured scale-free networks, *Physical Review Letters 89* (2002).

[6] P. Erdős and A. Rényi. "On the evolution of random graphs, *Publ. Math. Inst. Hung. Acad. Sci.* 5 (1960 17–61.

[7] S. Eubank, V.S. Anil Kumar, M. V. Marathe, A. Srinivasan, N. Wang, "Structure of social contact networks and their impact on epidemics", this volume.

[8] D. Kempe, J. Kleinberg, E. Tardos, "Maximizing the spread of influence through a social network".

[9] R. Motwani and P. Raghavan. *Randomized Algorithms.* Cambridge University Press, 1995.

[10] S. Hartke, "Graph-theoretic models of spread and competition", Ph.D. Thesis for Rutgers University Department of Mathematics, July 2004.

DIMACS, Rutgers University, 96 Frelinghysen Rd, Piscataway, NJ 08854

DIMACS, Rutgers University, 96 Frelinghysen Rd, Piscataway, NJ 08854

DIMACS Series in Discrete Mathematics
and Theoretical Computer Science
Volume **70**, 2006

Attempting to Narrow the Integrality Gap for the Firefighter Problem on Trees

Stephen G. Hartke

ABSTRACT. We consider a deterministic discrete-time model of a perfectly contagious disease spreading on a graph and the problem of minimizing the number of infected individuals when allowed one vaccination per time step. This model of disease spread is equivalent to a model of fire spread introduced by Hartnell [1995]. MacGillivray and Wang [2003] introduced an integer program to determine an optimal sequence of vaccinations or firefighter responses when the graph is a tree. We present additional constraints to the integer program that in practice narrow the integrality gap between the integer programming optimal and the optimal of the linear programming relaxation.

1. Introduction

Traditionally, epidemiological models assume that the population being studied is well-mixed in the sense that any pair of individuals are just as likely to come in contact and transmit a disease as any other. Some recent models [**2, 3, 10**], however, attempt to include information on which individuals come in contact. The mathematical structure of graphs are ideally suited to encode these relationships, where vertices in a graph represent individuals, and edges represent the potential for transmission of the disease between two individuals.

In this work we focus on a deterministic model of disease spread and how it behaves when interventions are occurring. We consider the most simple spread mechanism: that of a perfectly contagious disease with no cure, where vertices adjacent to infected vertices become infected at every discrete time step and, once infected, remain infected from then on. The response allowed is only a limited number of vaccinations of non-infected vertices. Specifically, let G be a connected graph where the vertices represent people and the edge uv indicates that persons u and v would transmit a disease from one person to another if one person became infected. At time $t = 0$, an outbreak of disease occurs at a root vertex. Public

2000 *Mathematics Subject Classification.* Primary 05C75 Structural characterization of types of graphs; Secondary 90C35 Programming involving graphs or networks .

Key words and phrases. firefighter, containment strategy, vaccination strategy.

The author has been supported by a National Science Foundation Graduate Research Fellowship, a National Defense Science and Engineering Graduate Fellowship, a DIMACS Graduate Research Award, and National Science Foundation grants EIA-0205116, DBI-9982983, and SBR-9709134 through DIMACS.

health officials immediately respond, vaccinating the vertices $a_{1,1}, a_{1,2}, \ldots, a_{1,c_1}$ at time $t = 1$. The disease then spreads to every non-vaccinated neighbor of an infected vertex. There is another set of vaccinations $a_{2,1}, \ldots, a_{2,c_2}$ at time $t = 2$, and the disease spreads again. This process continues until the disease can no longer spread; in other words, that all of the neighbors of infected vertices are either themselves infected or vaccinated. The main question we will investigate is finding an optimal strategy for vaccinating in order to minimize the total number of infected vertices when G is a tree and there is only one vaccination allowed per time step.

The model of disease spread just presented is equivalent to a model of fire spread introduced by Hartnell [**7**]. In this model, an outbreak of fire starts at the root vertex at time $t = 0$. In response, firefighters are placed at the vertices $a_{1,1}, a_{1,2}, \ldots, a_{1,c_1}$ at time $t = 1$, where the firefighters defend or protect each vertex from the spreading fire. The fire then spreads from burning vertices to non-defended neighbors. Firefighters are again deployed to defend the vertices $a_{2,1}, \ldots, a_{2,c_2}$ at time $t = 2$ (the vertices $a_{1,1}, a_{1,2}, \ldots, a_{1,c_1}$ remain defended), and the fire spreads again. The process continues until the fire can no longer spread. We say that the fire outbreak is *contained* after t time steps if there is some finite time t such that after the disease spreads during time t, only a finite number of vertices are burnt and the disease can no longer spread. The motivating question is again to find an optimal sequence of defended vertices that minimizes the total number of burnt vertices.

When presenting our results, we will use the terminology of firefighters. During the tth time step for $t > 0$, firefighters are deployed and then the fire spreads. A firefighter may defend neither a burnt vertex nor a previously defended vertex. Once fire has spread to a vertex v, we say that v is a *burnt* vertex. After being burnt or defended, a vertex remains in that state until the process ends. In addition to the burnt and defended vertices, we say that a vertex v is *saved* at the end of the tth time step if there is no path from v to the root consisting only of burnt and non-defended vertices at the end of the tth time step. Thus, our motivating question is equivalent to maximizing the number of saved vertices.

Several results are known about this model. Wang and Moeller [**11**], Fogarty [**6**], MacGillivray and Wang [**9**], and Develin and Hartke [**1**] studied various classes of graphs, particularly grids. Finbow, Hartnell, Li, and Schmeisser [**4**] determine the graphs that have the lowest number of expected burnt vertices when the initial root vertex where the fire outbreak begins is random.

Here we will concentrate our attention on trees. Trees form a natural class of graphs on which to consider the vaccination and firefighter problems because each defended vertex immediately saves its descendants. The low connectivity of trees means they are not as relevant in modeling the interaction of individuals. However, if each vertex represents a larger group that is internally well-connected and has few connections to other groups, then a tree structure is more reasonable. Such examples arise in disease models when considering a household as one vertex. If one individual contracts the disease, then all of the other members of his or her household are very likely to also contract the disease and become infectious. Thus it is reasonable to treat the household as a single unit.

Finbow, King, MacGillivray, and Rizzi [**5**] showed that the firefighter problem is NP-complete for trees of maximum degree three. Hence we are mainly concerned with approximations for the firefighter problem. Hartnell and Li [**8**] showed that the greedy algorithm on trees always saves at least 1/2 as many vertices as an optimal sequence of firefighter placements, and that this bound is tight. MacGillivray and Wang [**9**] presented an integer program for the firefighter problem on trees, and our focus here is the linear programming relaxation of their integer program. We present additional constraints that narrow the integrality gap between the integer programming optimal and the optimal of the linear programming relaxation.

2. Trees

We consider the firefighter problem on trees when only one vertex can be defended by a firefighter per time step. Note, however, that the results extend in a natural way to defending f vertices per time step. When a vertex v is defended, all of its descendants are immediately saved. Let $\mathrm{wt}(v)$ denote the number of vertices that are saved (including v) when v is defended.

Recall that the vertices in a tree at distance i from the root r are said to be on level i. The following is a straightforward observation.

LEMMA 2.1 (MacGillivray and Wang, Hartnell and Li). *If $a_1, a_2, \ldots$ is an optimal firefighter sequence, then a_i is on level i.*

We now present MacGillivray and Wang's integer program for finding an optimal firefighter sequence $a_1, a_2, \ldots$ for a tree. To each vertex v we associate a boolean variable $x(v)$ that indicates whether v is defended by a firefighter, and we wish to maximize the total number of vertices saved. Let the weight $\mathrm{wt}(v)$ of v denote the number of vertices saved by a firefighter defending v. Thus, $\mathrm{wt}(v)$ is equal to the number of descendants of v plus 1. To ensure that no double-counting occurs in the objective function, we require that no vertex be defended that is already saved. We enforce this requirement by adding the constraint that the sum of $x(v)$ for all ancestors v of a given vertex u and including u is at most 1. It is sufficient to add this constraint only for leaf vertices, since if u is a leaf, then the constraint for all ancestors of u is implied by the constraint for u. Lemma 2.1 gives the constraint that the sum of $x(v)$ for all of the v on a given level is at most 1. We thus have the following integer program. Here, we write $v \succ u$ or $u \prec v$ if v is an ancestor of u, and we write $v \succeq u$ or $u \preceq v$ if v is an ancestor of u or if $v = u$.

$$\text{maximize} \sum_{v \in V(G)} \mathrm{wt}(v)x(v)$$

$$\text{(1)} \qquad \text{subject to:} \sum_{v \text{ on level } \ell} x(v) \leq 1, \text{ for each level } \ell,$$

$$\text{(2)} \qquad \sum_{v \succeq u} x(v) \leq 1, \text{ for each leaf } u,$$

$$\text{(3)} \qquad x(v) \in \{0, 1\}, \text{ for each vertex } v.$$

By relaxing condition (3) that $x(v)$ is boolean we obtain a linear program. The linear programming (LP) optimal m^* provides an upper bound to the integer programming (IP) optimal m. In general, the linear program does not have an integral optimal, and so the LP optimal is strictly greater than the IP optimal.

Figure 1 shows an example where this occurs. It is an open question to bound the size of the "integrality gap," the difference between the linear programming and integer programming optimals.

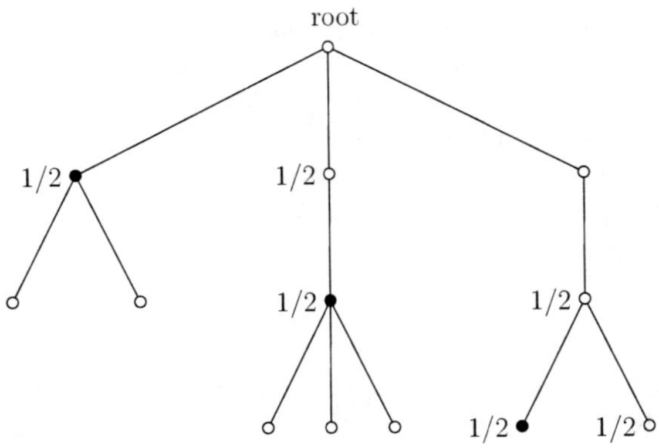

FIGURE 1. In this example on 13 vertices, the LP optimal is 8.5, whereas the IP optimal is 8. The nonzero values of $x(v)$ for the LP optimal solution appear next to the vertices, and the optimal firefighter sequence is indicated with black vertices.

MacGillivray and Wang showed that by adding the non-linear constraints $x(v)x(u) = 0$ for every non-root vertex v and every descendant u of v, then the optimal solution is integral. In general, solving such a non-linear optimization problem is hard. We take a different approach: by adding additional constraints, we will attempt to narrow the integrality gap.

The effect of the leaf constraint (2) is that if a vertex v is defended, then none of v's descendants can also be defended. It is tempting to instead use the constraint

$$x(u) + \sum_{v \prec u} x(v) \leq 1, \text{ for each vertex } u. \tag{4}$$

However, constraint (4) is too restrictive, since it also forbids two descendants on different levels being defended when v is not defended. A weaker approach is to only include in the constraint descendants that are themselves mutually exclusive. All of v's descendants on a given level is one such set. Thus, we add the constraint

$$x(u) + \sum_{\substack{v \preceq u \\ v \text{ on level } i}} x(v) \leq 1, \text{ for each vertex } u \text{ and each level } i \text{ below } u. \tag{5}$$

Note that with this constraint, we still need the leaf constraint. When using constraint (5) on the tree shown in Figure 1, the LP optimal is the same as the IP optimal.

However, Figure 2 shows an example where there is still an integrality gap using constraint (5). The tree shown in Figure 2 does suggest adding u's ancestors into the summation as well. Thus, we have the constraint

$$\sum_{v \succeq u} x(v) + \sum_{\substack{v \preceq u \\ v \text{ on level } i}} x(v) \leq 1, \text{ for each vertex } u \text{ and each level } i \text{ below } u. \tag{6}$$

When using constraint (6) on the tree in Figure 2, the LP optimal is the same as the IP optimal.

However, Figure 3 shows an example where there is still an integrality gap using constraint (6).

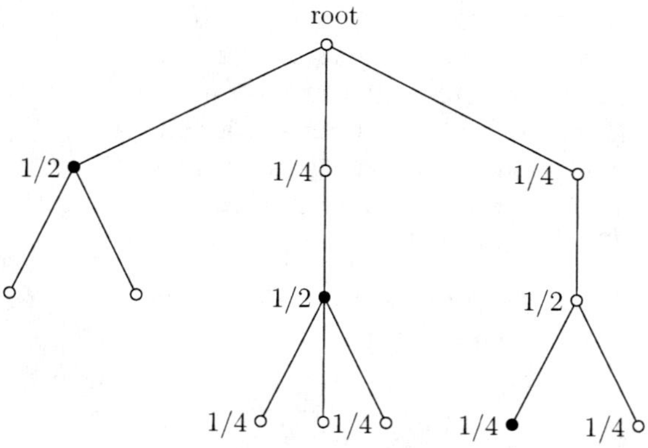

FIGURE 2. In this example on 12 vertices, the LP optimal when using constraint (5) is 7.5, whereas the IP optimal is 7. The nonzero values of $x(v)$ for the LP optimal solution appear next to the vertices, and the optimal vaccination sequence is indicated with black vertices.

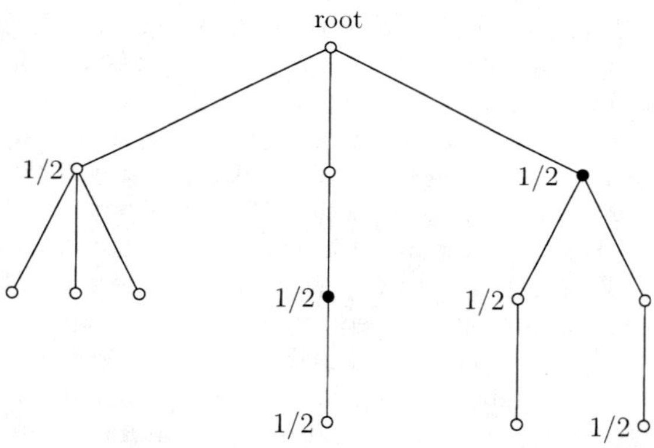

FIGURE 3. In this example on 13 vertices, the LP optimal when using constraint (6) is 7.5, whereas the IP optimal is 7. The nonzero values of $x(v)$ for the LP optimal solution appear next to the vertices, and the optimal vaccination sequence is indicated with black vertices.

For small trees, the LP optimal when using constraint (6) is the IP optimal. In fact, we have verified this by computer for trees with up to 11 vertices. We are thus led to

CONJECTURE 2.2. *The tree in Figure 3 is the smallest tree such that the LP optimal when using constraint (6) is not the IP optimal.*

To verify the conjecture, only trees with 12 vertices still need to be examined.

For large trees, the LP optimal is very often the IP optimal, and when different is very close. This observation is based on computer experimentation. Approximately 1.68 million trees with 100 vertices were randomly generated, and the LP optimal of MacGillivray and Wang's program, the LP optimal with constraint (6), and the IP optimal were calculated. A random tree is generated by starting with the root vertex and adding vertices one at a time, where a vertex is connected to a vertex in the existing tree chosen uniformly at random. Of these trees, 5.22% had the LP optimal of MacGillivray and Wang's program greater than the IP optimal, and the difference was at most 6.34% of the IP optimal. When using constraint (6), 0.70% had the LP optimal greater than the IP optimal, and the difference was at most 3.73% of the IP optimal. This data leads us to

CONJECTURE 2.3. *The ratio of the LP optimal to the IP optimal, with or without constraint (6), is bounded for all trees.*

3. Conclusion

Linear programming provides an upper bound in the firefighter problem on trees, and hence on the number of people that can be saved in the vaccination problem on trees. As mentioned in the introduction, trees are not as relevant in modeling the interaction of individuals because of their low connectivity. However, if each vertex represents a larger group that is internally well-connected and has few connections to other groups, then a tree structure is more reasonable. Although we do not have provable bounds on how close the LP optimal is to the IP optimal, the LP optimal does still provide an upper bound on the number of people that can be saved and experimental data suggests that this estimate is usually quite close. Such information is certainly of interest to public health officials who are interested in the number of people who become infected despite an optimal vaccination response.

One of the two main challenges in using this method is that the social network must be a tree. However, insights into the LP and IP optimals on trees may give insights on how to formulate and solve the vaccination problem on general graphs. The other main challenge is that the optimal solution to the linear program gives little information about the optimal solution for the integer program. Different methods of rounding can be used to convert the linear programming solution to an integral solution, but the produced integral solution may not be optimal and experimentally is usually quite poor. Devising a rounding scheme that produces a provably good integral solution would be one way to prove bounds on the integrality gap.

Acknowledgements

The author wishes to thank Fred Roberts and James Abello for helpful discussions and encouragement. The author also thanks Austin Murphy for making resources available for computation.

References

1. M. Develin and S. G. Hartke, Fire Containment in Grids of Dimension Three and Higher, manuscript, 2004.
2. J. M. Epstein, D. A. T. Cummings, S. Chakravarty, R. M. Singa, and D. S. Burke, Toward a Containment Strategy for Smallpox Bioterror: An Individual-Based Computational Approach, The Brookings Institute Center on Social and Economic Dynamics Working Paper No. 31, December 2002.
3. S. Eubank, H. Guclu, V. S. A. Kumar, M. V. Marathe, A. Srinivasan, Z. Toroczkai, N. Wang, and the EpiSims Team, `http://episims.lanl.gov`, April 22, 2004.
4. S. Finbow, B. Hartnell, Q. Li, and K. Schmeisser, On Minimizing the Effects of Fire or a Virus on a Network, *J. Combin. Math. Combin. Comput.*, 33 (2000), 311-322.

5. S. Finbow, A. King, G. MacGillivray, and R. Rizzi, The Firefighter Problem for Graphs of Maximum Degree Three, manuscript, 2004.
6. P. Fogarty, *Catching the Fire on Grids*, M.Sc. Thesis, Department of Mathematics, University of Vermont, 2003.
7. B. Hartnell, Firefighter! An Application of Domination, presentation, Twentieth Conference on Numerical Mathematics and Computing, University of Manitoba in Winnipeg, Canada, Sept. 1995.
8. B. Hartnell and Q. Li, Firefighting on Trees: How Bad is the Greedy Algorithm?, *Congressus Numerantium*, 145 (2000), 187-192.
9. G. MacGillivray and P. Wang, On the Firefighter Problem, *J. Combin. Math. Combin. Comput.*, 47 (2003), 83-96.
10. J. M. Read and M. J. Keeling, Disease Evolution on Networks: The Role of Contact Structure, *Proc. Roy. Soc. Lond. B*, 270 (2003), 699-708.
11. P. Wang and S. A. Moeller, Fire Control on Graphs, *J. Combin. Math. Combin. Comput.*, 41 (2002), 19-34.

DEPARTMENT OF MATHEMATICS, UNIVERSITY OF ILLINOIS, URBANA, IL 61801
E-mail address: hartke@math.uiuc.edu
URL: http://www.math.uiuc.edu/~hartke

DIMACS Series in Discrete Mathematics
and Theoretical Computer Science
Volume **70**, 2006

Influences on Breast Cancer Survival via SVM Classification in the SEER Database

Jixin Li, Ilya Muchnik, and Dona Schneider

ABSTRACT. We analyzed factors of survival for breast cancer using SEER data. We have estimated their influences based on their roles in prediction that the survival time is more than 3 years or less. The analysis was done by SVM classifier construction and testing its accuracy changes by perturbations of values of considered factors. We have showed that 40 out of 112 factors demonstrated high statistical significance. Many of them are well known, but few, like marital status, were not known as significant. We interpreted such new statistically significant factors as candidates for further specific epidemiological tests of significance.

1. Introduction

Estimating the influence of epidemiological factors on a disease distribution is central to epidemiology. A typical epidemiologic study compares groups, focusing on person, place and time variables such as age, gender and family history, as well as social and environmental factors. The discipline is also concerned with estimating survival from a given disease. For a disease like cancer, survival estimates aid both physicians and patients in selecting among a series of treatment alternatives. We sought a novel method of estimating short or long survival time for breast cancer based on individual factors available in the Surveillance, Epidemiology and End Results (SEER) data set [**1**]. We use survival time in Boolean format, taking the threshold value for survival as three years. We chose breast cancer because the disease has both high incidence and mortality [**2**], qualities that make it particularly useful for this analysis. Finally, we chose the Support Vector Machine (SVM) classifier design method [**3**] to obtain our estimates[1]. Our method of estimating survival is novel as:

(1) We estimate the accuracy of predicted survival time as a result of factor value perturbations.

2000 *Mathematics Subject Classification.* Primary 68T10 Pattern recognition, speech recognition; Secondary 62P10 Applications to biology and medical sciences.

[1]We use only one classification method here to show that the approach is, in principle, appropriate. Future research requires a large comparative study of classification methods to determine the best approach and standardize the method.

(2) We apply the method to the complete SEER data set for one type of cancer.
(3) Our software allows us to reproduce the analysis for almost all other types of cancers in the SEER data set.

This paper is organized into six sections. The next section describes our classification method for estimating the influences of the different epidemiological factors on survival from breast cancer. The third section characterizes the SEER database in general, the data extracted for breast cancer patients in particular, and the classification space constructed from the original SEER attributes. The fourth section details the procedures of the experiments. In the fifth section we present the results from the experiments and in the last section we discuss the results, limitations of the method and possible extension and improvement of this study.

2. The Classifier Method for Estimating the Influences of the Epidemiologic Factors

Machine learning classification methods allow the building of a classifier-predictor using a group of appropriate parameters (in our case, selected epidemiological factors) and a set of labeled points in space. In our case, labels assign patients by their survival time (greater than or equal to 3 years or "long" is assigned "1"; less than 3 years or "short" is assigned "0"). The space will be called classification space. The classifier is able to label any new "individual" point (a patient) in the space by the categories. This allows for both the recognition of categories of individual points and the comparison of different groups of points by their category distributions.

The classifier is a function over the space of all the considered variables. When one variable is changed and the others are held constant, this change influences the classifier's assignment on patients. In other words, the influence estimate measures how the classifier's function changes when a given input variable changes. We propose to compare the accuracy of a designated classifier on different regions of the classification space with different values of the considered variable. In addition, we test our "predicted" statistics with new data, which was withheld from the classifier design (In the literature, this is referred as a holdout test [**4**].).

We use the term "epidemiological factor" to mean any variable we are able to build from the attributes available in the SEER data set. We represent breast cancer data from SEER by vectors, with the epidemiological factor variables derived from the original SEER attributes. The derived variables are Boolean, which means the estimates from our analysis become both clear for interpretation and statistically robust.

To evaluate the comparative influence of each variable, we first construct a classifier which should be able to predict with a high probability whether the survival time of a given patient will be long or short. Patients with long survival time are labeled as positive, and those with short survival time are labeled as negative. While we derived 112 variables from the original SEER attributes, only 40 were selected by our method as having a significant influence on survival time. Because this is a data mining analysis, we classified those 40 variables as "candidates" for our formative data set of significant influences on survival time. These factors are analyzed for their influence on the survival times of individual patients in the available population.

Classifier accuracy is usually estimated by two criteria (sensitivity and specificity). We can, therefore, estimate factor significance by these criteria and their differences[2]. We assign statistical significance to a variable only when it is significant for both of the criteria. Our notation includes:

p^+(sensitivity)$= |q^+|/|Q^+|$

p^-(specificity) $= |q^-|/|Q^-|$

Q^+ is the subset for which all patients have a long survival time (≥ 3 years), Q^- is the subset for which all patients have a short survival time (< 3 years). $Q = Q^+ \cup Q^-$ is the whole *test* set on which the estimates are calculated. q^+ is the subset in which patients with a long survival time were recognized correctly by the designed classifier; similarly, q^- is the subset in which patients with a short survival time were recognized correctly by the designed classifier. It is clear that $q = q^+ \cup q^-$ is also a subset of the *test* set. The estimates are calculated on a part of data, withheld from the classifier design. In the machine learning literature, this part is called the *test* set [**5**].

Let us say that on a given test data one has received "p^+" and "p^-" estimates, respectively, for sensitivity and specificity. Let us now consider a particular partition of the test data into two subsets of patients. The first subset includes all patients for which the ith variable has a value of "1" and the second subset has a value of "0". If the variable does not have a strong influence on the quality values for designed classifier, then new estimates $p_1^+(x^i)$, $p_0^+(x^i)$, $p_1^-(x^i)$ and $p_0^-(x^i)$ of sensitivity and specificity calculated separately, $(p_1^+(x^i), p_1^-(x^i))$ on the first subset and $(p_0^+(x^i), p_0^+(x^i))$ on the second subset should be very similar. They should also be similar to the estimates "p^+" and "p^-" calculated on the whole data set[3]. This "virtual" condition is our foundation. We can therefore measure significance of a variable by differences of two estimates: $s_{p^+}(x^i) = |p_1^+(x^i) - p_0^+(x^i)|$ and $s_{p^-}(x^i) = |p_1^-(x^i) - p_0^-(x^i)|$. We use absolute values because the signs of the differences do not play a role in the significance estimation.

We propose additionally to determine standard deviations of the estimates. Using these standard deviations we are able to apply t-tests to determine whether the above $s_{p^+}(x^i)$ and $s_{p^-}(x^i)$ are statistically significant or not[4]. We assign a variable as "t-significant", when both sensitivity and specificity are significant.

2.1. Choosing the Classification Method. We sought a classification model that can predict with a high probability whether an individual patient's survival time is long or short based upon the chosen threshold. The SVM method is relevant for our purposes as it can find an optimal hyperplane in the chosen space that maximizes the margin between data samples in two considered classes. Additionally, the SVM method works with very large data sets, gives the widest spectrum for

[2]The classifier for predicting an individual patient's survival time is designed on information which is available after the basic treatment of the disease. We would be extremely interested in repeating this work on data available at intermediate periods during the treatment, but such data are not readily available.

[3]We assume that cardinalities of the subsets are large enough that the estimates would be representative; if the assumption doesn't hold, the significance of the corresponding variable cannot be estimated, in principle, by proposed method.

[4]Our use of the t-test is very different from its common usage, contrasting the "average significance" evaluation from known group data. Our use measures significance from an "individual prediction" prospective.

building different types of classifiers and searches for the most relevance for particular data. The coefficients of variables presented in its optimal hyperplane classifier yield independent information about the corresponding variable significance. Several procedures for variable selection are particular to SVM [**6**]-[**8**]; they give new independent sources for estimating both variable significance and the robustness of the estimated significance. Appendix A provides the methodological background of the method[5]. All experiments were done by applying the SVM light program [**9**].

3. Data Set

3.1. Source of data. The SEER Program is an authoritative source of information on cancer incidence and survival in the United States. From 1973 to 2000, the SEER Program collected and published cancer incidence and survival data from 11 population-based cancer registries and three supplemental registries covering approximately 14 percent of the US population. The 2001 expansion registries increased the population coverage to approximately 26 percent. Information on more than 3 million in situ and invasive cancer cases is included in the SEER database, with approximately 170,000 new cases added from the SEER catchment areas each year. The SEER Registries routinely collect data on patient demographics, primary tumor site, morphology and stage at diagnosis, first course of treatment, and follow-up for vital status.

We chose to work with one segment of the SEER data, breast cancer, although the technology can be easily adapted to other cancers in this database. The database contains 433,272 breast cancer cases for the years 1973-2000. Our current work focuses on a subset of cases ($n = 67,647$), those who died from their disease. This means the information on each case's survival time is fixed in our data set.

The original attributes in the SEER database cannot be used in our classifier design method for two reasons: (1) their values must first be transformed into a unified vector presentation and (2) the percentage of missing data for some variables is high. This brings up a general methodological problem for researchers trying to apply a machine learning classification method to a data set such as that offered by SEER. Often, the original attributes have complex structures not useful for a data mining analysis. These must be transformed into a standard space representation where every object (in our case, a patient) is a point. The transformation can be done in various ways; the problem is how to find a relevant transformation. Transformation is acceptable if it satisfies two conditions: (1) it gives a classification space that yields the construction of a good classifier; (2) it chooses, as much as possible, factors that are interesting for analysis of the problem. In our experiments, we tried to use all possible attributes for breast cancer patients. We eliminated only those that were missing 50 percent or more of their values and those that, after transformation, all had the same value, i.e. were all 1 or all 0.

3.2. Data Space and Class Label. A patient in the SEER data set is represented by 72 original attributes. From these attributes we created 112 variables (106 Boolean and 6 ordinal). Some Boolean variables, if derived from the same original attribute, could introduce redundancy but they yield flexibility for determining whether some possible factors are relevant. For example, we do not know

---

[5]All the appendices can be found at `http://dimacs.rutgers.edu/~muchnik/SEER_Mining/Appendix.html`.

a priori the optimal cutoff point for the age(s) that best influence survival time. Therefore, we created three Boolean variables that employ different cutoff points for age (Appendix B lists the full set of variable names and numbers along with their matching attributes). The ordinal variables are numbers 32, 33, 61, 83, 104 and 105 in the variable list are "year of birth", "age at diagnosis", "date of diagnosis", "morphology (grade)", "age recode", and "historic stage A", respectively. These six were further transformed into Boolean for their influence estimates (value = 1 if the actual value is above or equal to average and value = 0 if the value is less than average). Our coding scheme for the Boolean variables assigns the value of "1" if an attribute is positive or present. Conversely, if an attribute is negative or absent, it is assigned a value of "0". For example, for "marital status" (variable 8), if a patient is married the value is "1", but if other than married, the value is "0". Similarly, for radiation (variable 24), the value "1" means "radiation performed", but the value "0" is used for "radiation not performed". The patient's survival time for this analysis is also in Boolean format.

3.3. Missing data. The SEER database contains a large amount of unknown or missing data. For some variables the situation is of particular concern because these variables are time sensitive. Appendix C lists the number of missing data points for the 64 Boolean variables with missing data.

3.4. Normalization. Since there is a problem with missing data, we chose to unify the data to build the classifier using the simplest normalization method: $z_{ij} = \frac{x_{ij}-\bar{x}_j}{\sigma_j}$, where x_{ij} is the jth variable of the ith case, $\bar{x}_j$ is the sample mean value of the jth variable excluding unknown or missing data. The value $\sigma_j$is the sample standard deviation of the jth variable excluding unknown or missing data; the transformation of the original matrix $\|x_{ij}\|$ into the normalized one $\|z_{ij}\|$ is used on all elements (i,j) for which x_{ij} is not missing. All missing elements are substituted by $z_{ij} = 0$. In other words, before normalization missing elements are substituted by the mean of all known data for that variable. For boolean variables, the mean is equivalent to the probability of the variable being 1.

4. Experiment

We randomly divided the 67647 cases of breast cancer into two approximately equal groups: 33,824 cases (the training set) were used to build the classifier and the other 33,823 cases (the test set) were used to estimate variable influences on survival time. We then extracted 112 variables and used the survival time as our class label. We trained an SVM classifier with linear SVM^{light} with default parameter values given by the software. Based on the training data, we applied the resulting classifier on the test data. We calculated $s_{p^+}(x^i)$ and $s_{p^-}(x^i)$ for every chosen variable x^i. The notation needed for the procedure is presented in Appendix A.

Using the same notation in Appendix A, one can calculate

$$p_1^+(x^i) = |q_1^+(x^i)|/|Q_1^+(x^i)|, \qquad p_0^+(x^i) = |q_0^+(x^i)|/|Q_0^+(x^i)|,$$

$$p_1^-(x^i) = |q_1^-(x^i)|/|Q_1^-(x^i)| \text{ and } p_0^-(x^i) = |q_0^-(x^i)|/|Q_0^-(x^i)|.$$

These coefficients can be interpreted as estimates of probability for the corresponding predicted events as new boolean variables for which $p_1^+(x^i)(1-p_1^+(x^i)))$, $p_0^+(x^i)(1-p_0^+(x^i)))$, $p_1^-(x^i)(1-p_1^-(x^i)))$ and $p_0^-(x^i)(1-p_0^-(x^i)))$ respectively, are variance estimates of the boolean variables.

Based on such probabilistic interpretation for considered predicted event (the boolean variables) we could apply the t-test by taking as null hypotheses H_0^+ : $p_1^+(x^i) = p_0^+(x^i)$ and H_0^- : $p_1^-(x^i) = p_0^-(x^i)$. To do that we have to calculate corresponding t-values[6]

$$t^+(x^i) = \frac{|p_1^+(x^i) - p_0^+(x^i)|}{\sqrt{\left[\frac{n_1+n_2}{n_1 n_2}\right]\left[\frac{(n_1-1)(\sigma_1^+(x^i))^2+(n_2-1)(\sigma_0^+(x^i))^2}{n_1+n_2-2}\right]}}$$

with degree of freedom $n_1 + n_2 - 2 \approx \infty$, where $n_1 = |Q_1^+(x^i)|$ and $n_2 = |Q_0^+(x^i)|$. Similarly,

$$t^-(x^i) = \frac{|p_1^-(x^i) - p_0^-(x^i)|}{\sqrt{\left[\frac{n_1+n_2}{n_1 n_2}\right]\left[\frac{(n_1-1)(\sigma_1^-(x^i))^2+(n_2-1)(\sigma_0^-(x^i))^2}{n_1+n_2-2}\right]}}$$

with degree of freedom $n_1 + n_2 - 2 \approx \infty$, where $n_1 = |Q_1^-(x^i)|$ and $n_2 = |Q_0^-(x^i)|$.

Variables for which both t-values exceeds the corresponding threshold are assigned as having significance for survival time.

5. Results and Analysis

We tested all 112 variables in their Boolean format and found that 40 of them satisfied our two considerations for statistical significance, i.e., hypotheses H_0^+ and H_0^+ were rejected at the 99.9% confidence level. The results for these 40 variables are contained in Appendix D, including information about the values s_{p^+}, s_{p^-}, t^+, t^-, as well as the percentages of correctly classified cases. A subset of these significant variables is presented in Table 1. The first two columns contain the variable idx, or the variable number that allows the reader to link the variable with information to the original attributes in the SEER data set and the variable name. Column 3 of Table 1 lists the number of cases and column 4 denotes the Boolean value. Columns 5 and 6 list the percentages of correctly predicted cases for sensitivity and specificity. Columns 7 and 8 give the corresponding values for the t-criteria.

Table 1 shows a systematic "imbalance" in the total test set. While even the smallest groups had a large cardinality (in the hundreds), the complementary groups were often 5-20 times as large. This difference in the size of the groups did not influence the main t-criteria calculations, but it could have influenced the design classifier quality. Our average accuracy was about 70%, but we assume that it could be improved if we balanced the groups using associated weights. In 3 of the 40 significant variables, the differences in t-criteria values were more than double. In the most cases, however, they were essentially equal. Finally, the range in t-criteria values was very large; between 3.30 (very much close to the critical threshold value) and 133. Moreover, less than 30% of the numbers of significant variables received t-criteria values less than 10 (the critical threshold is 3.29 for the 99.9% confidence limit).

The results for non-significant variables can be found in Appendix E. Most of these variables (72 of the 112) demonstrated non-significance on both t-criteria. Moreover, 30 of them had critical values below 1.45, the threshold for the 90%

[6]Note that since the size of data is large, the degree of freedom can be approximated by infinity and as the degree of freedom goes to infinity, the t-distribution becomes a normal distribution.

confidence level. We did find 17 variables with at least one t-criterion value above 20.

TABLE 1. The results of variables for which the null hypotheses were rejected for both sensitivity and specificity at a confidence level of 0.999 are listed below.

idx	Variable name	n	Boolean value	Sensitivity (%)	Specificity (%)	t^+	t^-
33	Age at diagnosis	16511 17312	1 0	79.58 86.93	61.50 43.86	13.13	22.92
43	Age at diag. in 58-59	1677 32146	1 0	88.70 83.30	45.93 53.47	4.41	3.95
54	Race/Ethnicity white	29095 4689	1 0	84.35 77.95	52.25 57.81	7.33	5.26
55	Race/Ethnicity black	3411 30373	1 0	75.07 84.33	58.61 52.38	8.91	5.28
59	Marital status never married	3176 29618	1 0	79.30 84.41	59.56 52.03	5.05	5.94
60	Marital status married	18469 14325	1 0	87.23 78.79	44.93 61.02	14.70	20.51
61	Year of diagnosis	15937 17886	1 0	75.75 89.09	63.39 41.35	23.82	28.87
83	Morphology grade	8746 3688	1 0	76.16 86.81	57.72 50.22	9.83	5.25
85	Grade (I,II)	3688 8746	1 0	86.81 76.16	50.22 57.72	9.83	5.25
87	Microscopically confirmed	32618 1024	1 0	84.63 3.91	50.44 97.75	29.90	27.44
88	Clinical diagnosis only	531 33111	1 0	1.00 84.27	99.77 51.62	22.87	20.00
89	Surgery performed	28886 898	1 0	86.62 14.72	42.68 94.83	26.82	28.42
97	Surgery not recommended	1207 28819	1 0	15.65 87.05	95.38 41.93	25.65	35.00
101	Radiation after surgery	8107 25519	1 0	85.32 83.03	42.58 56.28	3.55	14.77
102	White non-Hispanic	28115 5669	1 0	84.43 78.67	52.16 57.31	7.22	5.22
103	Age recode	17414 16409	1 0	80.18 86.77	60.89 43.62	11.81	22.33
104	SEER historic stage	23404 8157	1 0	81.19 91.87	56.73 27.58	18.31	27.37
106	Historic stage in situ or localized	8157 23404	1 0	91.87 81.19	27.58 56.73	18.31	27.37
107	In situ localized or regional	24662 6899	1 0	92.28 0.00	23.92 99.98	125.51	133.15
108	ERA position	3573 3735	1 0	83.83 30.79	48.06 87.60	33.57	31.95

6. Discussion

For the purposes of discussion, we divide the significant variables into three groups: (1) those where both t-criteria are above 10 (strong significance), (2) those where both criteria are in the range 9.99-6.1 (intermediate significance) and (3) those where both criteria are less than 6.0 (low significance).

Twenty-eight of the 40 significant variables show strong significance. For instance, rank of morphology grade (No. 83) and SEER's historical stage scale characterize the degree of tumor development (No. 104). While we knew a priori that these two variables would be significant as more advanced disease predicts shorter survival, we were able to correctly predict the threshold where the variables are pushed to statistical significance. For instance, the list of ordinal values for the SEER's historical stage scale is in situ ("1"), localized ("2"), regional ("3"), and distant ("4"). The calculated threshold is between 3 and 4, indicating strong significance for predicting survival as the cancer moves from regional to distant. Our Boolean results conform to SEER's ordinal results. Specifically, variable 107 (Boolean, representing "distant or not") is strongly significant, showing the same very large values of the t-criteria. Variable 106 (Boolean with values "regional or distant" and "in situ or localized") is also estimated as significant, but the correspondent t-criteria are 5-6 times less.

From our point of view the low significant variables are the most interesting because they focus attention on factors whose influence on the survival time is not clear. For example we build a set of variables to characterize each patient's race. Our analysis shows that all variables "white-not white" (No. 54), "black-not black" (No. 55) and "white (but not Hispanic) vs other races" (102) demonstrate low significance. The literature notes that race is a weak risk factor for the breast cancer. Three different modifications of the attribute show consistency in their low degree of significance and this can be interpreted as needing additional systematic investigation. The literature also notes that age factor is a strong risk factor for breast cancer, far stronger than race. Our analysis shows that they have almost the same degree of significance. More precisely, we found that age demonstrates a little bit less influence on the survival time than does race (see variables 40, 43, 52-55).

Even "negative" information about non-significant factors can be also considered from a different perspective. For instance, Appendix E shows that most geographical variables are strongly non-significant. These factors can be presented in many different ways. It is possible that as aggregative factors they might increase in significance because they join "more representative" populations. One could construct that variable in order to get the highest as possible significance. The "optimization approach" to constructing variables for the whole classification space is one of the most interesting and promising future directions for developing a monitoring system for the SEER database.

Our presented work is explorative for both method and results. Several factors must be investigated before we can recommend this work for monitoring the SEER database. First we must determine which type of machine learning classification method is the most relevant for this analysis. We have tested SVM and our results show that it works. It is now necessary to do a comparative study of several other methods to determine if they work as well or better than SVM. Second, we need to determine whether the threshold of a 3 year survival time is optimal for the analysis.

This requires 1) a systematic study to find the threshold which is the most robust to small perturbations in the set of patients used to build a classifier and 2) and an investigation of how the classifier accuracy depends on small changes of the threshold. To date, we have analyzed the factor influences based on a classifier which has an average accuracy around 70%. We need to determine the critical value for accuracy so that the classifier can be used for the influence analysis and for determining how it relates to additional factors.

We see a usefulness in this data mining analysis in "completeness", covering all SEER's attributes (in their many types of representations). Practitioners could consider our tables as a summary of essential information about breast cancer survival time based on the SEER database. Extending this work to other cancers can provide new opportunities for finding significant factors that predict survival time from those diseases. Our already developed software is relatively problem free, allowing for a global study of all data presented in SEER. Moreover, if results of that analysis are recognized as useful by the epidemiological community, the method can be adapted to develop an automatic (or a semi-automatic) system which would be able to continuously monitor the SEER database as it is updated. Many of the cancers listed in Appendix F have sufficient numbers of records so that our method can be used without significant modifications. To determine whether new variables which might be specific to different diseases are needed, intensive collaboration with epidemiological experts is needed.

7. Acknowledgement

We thank anonymous reviewers for significant suggestions. Ilya Muchnik in this research was supported by NSF grant CCR 0325398.

References

1. Surveillance, Epidemiology, and End Results (SEER) Program (www.seer.cancer.gov) Public-Use Data (1973-2000), National Cancer Institute, DCCPS, Surveillance Research Program, Cancer Statistics Branch, released April 2003, based on the November 2002 submission.
2. Ries LAG, Eisner MP, Kosary CL, Hankey BF, Miller BA, Clegg L, Mariotto A, Feuer EJ, Edwards BK (eds), *SEER Cancer Statistics Review, 1975-2001*, National Cancer Institute. Bethesda, MD, http://seer.cancer.gov/csr/1975_2001/, 2004.
3. V. Vapnik, The Nature of Statistical Learning Theory. New York Springer-Verlag, 1995. pp. 188.
4. Kohavi R. A study of cross-validation and bootstrap for accuracy estimation and model selection. International Joint Conference on Artificail Intelligence, San Mateo, CA. 1995. pp. 1137-45. Guyon I and Ellisseeff A. An introduction to variable and feature selection. *Journal of Machine Learning Research* 2003;3;1157-82.
5. Weiss, SM and Kulikowski, CA. Computer Systems That Learn. San Mateo, CA Morgan Kaufmann 1991. 17-49.
6. Guyon, I and Ellisseeff, A., An introduction to variable and feature selection. *Journal of Machine Learning Research* 2003;3;1157-82
7. Guyon, I, Weston, J, Barnhill, S and Vapnik, V. Gene selection for cancer classification using support vector machines. Machine Learning, 2002;46:389-422
8. Hardin, D, Tsamardinos, I Aliferis, CF, A Theoretical characterization of linear SVM-Based Feature Selection. ACM International Conference Proceeding, New York: ACM Press. 2004. p.144-152.
9. T. Joachims, *Making large-Scale SVM Learning Practical. In: Advances in Kernel Methods - Support Vector Learning,* B. Scholkopf and C. Burges and A. Smola (ed.), MIT-Press, 1999. p.169-189.

Department of Computer Science, Rutgers University, Piscataway, NJ 08854
E-mail address: jixli@cs.rutgers.edu

DIMACS, Department of Computer Science, Rutgers University of, Piscataway, NJ 08854
E-mail address: muchnik@dimacs.rutgers.edu

Edward J. Bloustein School of Planning and Public Policy, Rutgers University, New Brunswick, NJ 08901
E-mail address: donas@rci.rutgers.edu

DIMACS Series in Discrete Mathematics
and Theoretical Computer Science
Volume **70**, 2006

Validation of Epidemiological Models: Chicken Epidemiology in the UK

Dmitriy Fradkin, Ilya Muchnik, Patrick Hermans, and Kenton Morgan

ABSTRACT. In epidemiology, a standard way of constructing models is to conduct univariate analysis of independent variables, followed by fitting a multivariate logistic model to the selected features. The main measure for choosing a particular model is a goodness of fit criterion on a given dataset. While this measure indicates how well the model fits the data, it has little relation to the predictive accuracy of the model and therefore may not generalize beyond the given dataset. This aspect is not frequently considered in epidemiology. We suggest using modern machine learning methods for constructing and validating epidemiological models. The resulting models can be used to confirm epidemiologist's models or to suggest possible improvements. These approaches also provide estimates and confidence measures for the parameters and the predictive ability of the model.

1. Overview

In epidemiology, a standard way of constructing models is to conduct univariate analysis of independent variables, followed by manual selection and refinement of the feature set by fitting a multivariate logistic model to the data [**3**]. The model constructed on the final set of variables is seen as the final model. The main measure driving the model selection process is therefore a goodness of fit criterion on a given dataset. While this measure indicates how well the model fits the data, it has little relation to the predictive accuracy of the model and therefore may not generalize beyond the given dataset. However, from the point of view of prevention, it is extremely important to identify the factors responsible for the presence or absence of a disease or a symptom on data that has not yet been observed.

Model validation (estimation of predictive performance) is not frequently done in human epidemiology and medicine, as noted for example in [**11, 14**], despite being recognized as an important part of establishing the usefulness of a model.

2000 *Mathematics Subject Classification.* Primary 62H30 Classification and discrimination; cluster analysis; Secondary 68T05 Learning and adaptive systems.

Key words and phrases. support vector machines, feature selection, cross validation.

Dr. Muchnik's work was supported through NSF grant CCR 0325398.

Dr. Hermans and Dr. Morgan acknowledge Elanco Animal Health and the Engineering and Physical Sciences Research Council (EPSRC) that funded their work.

Validation is even more rare in the field of veterinary epidemiology. A few exceptions ([**5, 12**]) describe models validates using hold-out test sets.

The main goal of our work is to demonstrate how modern machine learning methods can be used to conduct statistical validation of epidemiological models in the absence of an independent test set. We found one publication addressing this issue, [**9**], but the leave-one-out method used there was applied for spectroscopic data, where the measurements are much more accurate than in the standard epidemiological cross-sectional data. It is much harder to have validation based on statistical estimates when one uses noisy cross-sectional data. This paper focuses specifically on such situations.

The principal tool for this task is the cross-validation technique, used in machine learning for obtaining estimates of performance and evaluation of parameters [**10**]. Additionally, we examine a recently proposed feature selection method that was shown to be effective in a number of applications [**6**]. In contrast to univariate feature selection, which is standard in epidemiology, it is a multivariable selection method. This means that it is more general: it will work in the cases where univariate selection works, but it could also work in cases where univariate selection does not. While cross-validation and feature selection methods are not new, they are little known to epidemiologists. We believe that their usage would lead to better models.

We illustrate our suggestions on a dataset describing the occurrences of wet litter in the poultry farms in the UK in the year 2001, collected and investigated using traditional methods by Hermans et. al. [**8**]. The methods discussed, however, can be applied in validation of different classification-based epidemiological models.

We want to emphasize that the logistic models can also be interpreted as classifiers because the data itself is labeled into classes; moreover, frequently only two classes (positive/negative; disease/no disease, etc.) occur. When one estimates a fitness score of the constructed model, the number of errors given by the model on the data should be calculated rather than the quality of the fit.[1]

2. Background

2.1. Wet Litter. Here we present a brief introduction to the significance and causes of wet litter. For a detailed discussion a reader is referred to [**8**].

Wet litter is a term used when the material covering the floors of poultry houses, usually consisting of wood shavings or chopped straw, reaches its saturation threshold and is incapable of holding more moisture. Wet litter prevention and control is important for the health, welfare and productivity of broiler flocks. It has been shown to be associated with the occurrence of foot-pad, breast and hock lesions, and inducing high levels of stress in the birds. A number of risk factors have been identified in the literature.

[1]Strictly speaking, a logistic model assigns to an observation the (estimate of) probability that the observation belongs to one particular class. In practice this estimate is compared with the threshold 0.5. If the estimate is larger than this threshold an instance is assigned to one class, and, if not, then to the other. The probability is given by formula:

$$P(\text{class } 1|x) = \frac{\exp(w \cdot x + b)}{1 + \exp(w \cdot x + b)} \tag{1}$$

where coefficients w and b determine the model [**7**]. It is very important to note that the formula does not give a simple way to measure significance for different variables.

TABLE 1. Notation

Symbol	Meaning
d	dimensionality of the data
$x, y \in X$	data points, belonging to a space X
$x \cdot y$	inner product between two vectors
$\|\|x\|\|$	L_2 norm of vector x
w	a weight vector
b	bias

The analysis of longitudinal data collected from 639 farms (75% of those where the questionnaire was sent) showed that more than half the farmers had wet litter in their most recent flock. This indicates that wet litter is a wide-spread phenomenon and that better understanding of its causes is needed to reduce costs to the poultry industry.

2.2. Notation. Before proceeding further we would like to specify our notation. Symbols are described in Table 1. Throughout this paper we use the words "vector" and "point" interchangeably, depending on which is more suitable in the context of the discussion. Both terms indicate a group of labeled factors. Below we describe instances only by numerical factors. Taken together, these factors form a Euclidean space (the space of numerical variables). The number of factors determines the dimensionality of the space.[2]

2.3. Cross-Validation. The theory of cross-validation [4] is based on two ideas:

- Predictions of the model on new data give the strongest statistical estimates of the model validity.
- There exist re-sampling schemes of the restricted data that can be used to validate a model without use of a hold-out set.

One of the most popular re-sampling schemes is k-fold cross-validation [**10**]. This procedure consists of k identical stages as follows. The set of observations is divided into k equal subsets. Let us choose one of these to be the "test" set. The remaining $k-1$ subsets are then combined to form a "training" set. The training set is used to build a model that is evaluated on the test set. In the next stage, a different subset is chosen to be a test set, and the remaining subsets are combined into a training set. This is repeated k times, using each of the k subsets in turn as the test set. Notice that as a result we obtain a prediction for each available observation, allowing us to estimate the predictive performance of the model built on the whole data, and k estimates of model coefficients. If this procedure is repeated t times (with a different partition into k sets every time), we have kt estimates on the coefficients, and t estimates of the predictive accuracy of the model on all observations.

Note that the cross-validation method estimates an average performance from an ensemble of models and proposes to use them as estimates of performance of a

[2]In practice many factors originally are not numerical, but we transform the original heterogeneous factors in order to be able to represent data as points in a uniform Euclidean space. This type of space has properties which are important for constructing models.

single model identified on the whole set of observations. A proof of the correctness of this approach can be found in [**4**].

This test has several advantages for validation of complex statistical models:

- It is independent of the type of distribution function, and therefore its conclusions about model validity are most rigorous.
- The test directly measures variance of all the coefficients of the model; this is very convenient from the practical point of view.
- If the test confirms that a model has a high validity, the coefficients can be used to numerically compare the significance of variables. Moreover, because the validity is also measured numerically, it is possible to compute confidence of the model validity estimates.

A stratified cross-validation schema differs from regular cross-validation in that the test set is required to have the same distribution of classes as the whole set. Another way to think of this is that each class is partitioned into folds separately and the corresponding folds are then combined.

A number of papers examined the quality of estimates produced by cross-validation. In the experiments reported in [**10**], the k-fold cross-validation was pessimistically biased (that is, true accuracy was higher than the estimate) for $k = 2, 5$, although the estimates improved for k=$10, 20$. Stratified cross-validation behaved similarly, but with a lower bias.

So the recommendation of [**10**] is to use stratified 10-fold cross-validation. In this work we follow that advice.

2.4. Linear Classifiers.

2.4.1. *Classifier Constructed by Logistic Regression.* We have mentioned in the Section 1 that in the epidemiological practice the logistic model is used as a classifier. A standard way to transform logistic regression into a classification model is to consider the logarithm of the ratio of probabilities that an observation belongs to one or the other class. Using formula (1), it is easy to show that this approach results in a linear classifier $f(x)$, given by:

$$f(x) = \begin{cases} 1 & \text{if } w \cdot x + b \geq 0 \\ -1 & \text{otherwise} \end{cases} \tag{2}$$

where $\{-1, +1\}$ are the class labels. This view of has an important advantage over using the original non-linear function of equation (1) to calculate class probabilities. According to formula (2), the vector of coefficients, w, can be directly interpreted as measuring the relative significance of the factors. For instance, the absolute values of the coefficients, $|w_i|$, can be used as significance coefficients.

2.4.2. *Optimal (SVM) Classifier.* A linear classifier can be constructed in ways other than by fitting a logistic model. There are many different methods for doing this [**7**]. In this section we will describe the so-called "support vector machine" (SVM) classifier. The SVM classifier possesses an optimality property: the weight vector w found by this method is perpendicular to the maximal margin between the classes, and this guarantees, in a statistical sense, a low error rate on new observations. These mathematical results are "distribution-free", that is, they do not rely on any assumptions about the distribution of the data. It is the presence of strong and general theoretical foundation, supported by empirical evidence of excellent performance on many applications, that makes SVM such a popular machine learning tool. A detailed discussion of SVM methodology can be found in [**2, 13**]. A short description is contained in the introductory chapter of this volume.

We have to emphasize a particular feature of SVM that is important for practitioners, and particularly, we believe, for epidemiologists, who work with noisy data, i.e., with data containing a lot of missing values, with subjective responses and different scales and types of factors. In the process of constructing a classifier, the SVM method partitions the data into two sets, corresponding to "important" and "not important" observations. The important ones are exactly the so-called "support vectors". They form a boundary for the class margin region. In other words, the support vectors are points from each class that are most similar to the points of the other class. For epidemiologists the "not important" observations should provide prototypical examples of observations and feature ranges in each class.

2.5. SVM-based Feature Selection. This approach [**6**] is based on the observation that the feature i with the smallest absolute value of weight $|w_i|$ is the one that has the least influence on the decision. This suggests the procedure described in Algorithm 1 for recursive feature elimination (RFE). At each step a feature with the smallest weight is removed from all instances, and SVM is retrained on the remaining features. The order in which the variables are removed can be seen as a ranking of the features. Such a ranking can be used in two ways:

(1) It provides means of feature reduction by keeping the most influential features. Of course the phrase "most influential" is not formal because the heuristic procedure does not guarantee finding the subset of features that would result in the best performance. However experiments show that the features selected by this method are important [**6**].
(2) It allows one to interpret the relative influences of the features on the classification. From this perspective, it is interesting to apply Algorithm 1 to ranking the whole set of features.

Algorithm 1 SVM Recursive Feature Elimination (RFE) [**6**]

Require: A set of points W in $\Re^d$; f - number of desired features
1: **for** $i = d, \ldots, f+1$ **do**
2: Construct an SVM on set W. Let w^i be the decision hyperplane of that SVM.
3: Let $k_i = \text{argmin}_j |{w_j}^i|$.
4: Remove feature k_i from all points x in W.
5: **end for**
6: Output resulting classifier with f features and hyperplane w^f.

---

3. Experimental Results of Cross-Validation

The risk factors have been selected manually using the univariate and multivariate analysis described above. We repeated 10-fold stratified cross-validation of each wet litter model 10 times. In our experiments, we used the same 444 observations that were used by epidemiologist to construct final model M1 (248 cases with wet litter and 196 cases without it). We used SVM package called LIBSVM [**1**]. Cross-validation was implemented with a shell script.

TABLE 2. Final Epidemiological Model (M1) [**8**].

Variable	Coefficient	S.E.	O.R.	95% C.I.	p-value
Coccidiosis	1.620	0.654	5.05	1.40-18.19	0.01
Specific breed[4]	-0.794	0.247	0.43	0.27-0.71	0.001
Flock was thinned	1.350	0.402	3.86	1.75-8.49	0.001
Age at slaughter	-0.092	0.022	0.91	0.87-0.95	< 0.001
Side ventilation	0.552	0.236	1.74	1.09-2.76	0.02
Separate farm clothing for each house	-1.116	0.272	0.33	0.19-0.56	< 0.001
Plastic overshoes for each house	0.747	0.235	2.11	1.33-3.34	0.001
Number of rodent baits	0.021	0.007	1.02	1.01-1.04	0.005
Pigs on the farm	1.424	0.665	4.15	1.13-15.29	0.03
Feeding equipment failures	0.701	0.236	2.02	1.27-3.20	0.003
Number of farm workers (quadratic polynomial)	6.162	2.494	474.52	3.57-63012.92	0.01
Number of farm workers (cubic polynomial)	-4.118	1.677	0.016	0.00-0.44	0.01
Constant	2.787	1.019	-	-	-

Table 2 shows the final model constructed by multivariate regression on the set of features M1. Table 3 show the model constructed by SVM on the same set of features. Only two coefficients (of factors "side ventilation" and quadratic polynomial in number of people) have the coefficient of variation (ratio of standard deviation to the mean value) greater than 0.2.[3] The stability of model accuracy estimates is very high.

We would like to make some general observations. One is that the standard deviations of the coefficients and of the predictive accuracy measures are small, indicating high reliability of these estimates. Another observation is that the relative magnitudes and signs of the coefficients match those obtained by fitting multivariate logistic regression to all observations. This observation lends support to the interpretation of the importance of different risk factors. Finally, the estimates of predictive accuracy of the model for wet litter are high, indicating that the factors included in the model are indeed significant, and that the model can be used as a basis for making predictions and recommendations regarding wet litter.

4. Choice of Features

In the previous section we discussed how the quality of a model can be measured with cross-validation. Here we discuss how the choice of features can be compared against other possibilities.

We propose comparing the final features of epidemiological model M1, constructed with traditional methods, against the feature set of the same size (M2) chosen completely by RFE method (Algorithm 1). We also consider the effect of using decreased or increased sets of features (M3 and M4 respectively).

[3]The coefficient of variation is used in statistics to measure fluctuations of a random variable around the variable's mean value.

[4]The name of the breed will be kept anonymous until results are released to the industry.

TABLE 3. Cross-validation of M1 Using SVM.

Features	μ	σ	$\lvert\frac{\sigma}{\mu}\rvert$
Coccidiosis	1.074	0.144	0.134
Specific breed	-0.760	0.136	0.179
Flock was thinned	1.196	0.132	0.110
Age at slaughter	-0.076	0.010	0.137
Side ventilation	0.631	0.144	0.229
Separate farm clothing for each house	-1.120	0.086	0.077
Plastic overshoes for each house	0.796	0.097	0.122
Number of rodent baits	0.023	0.003	0.113
Pigs on the farm	1.106	0.133	0.121
Feeding equipment failures	0.756	0.099	0.131
Number of farm workers (quadratic polynomial)	1.134	0.259	0.228
Number of farm workers (cubic polynomial)	-0.879	0.151	0.172
Model Evaluation			
Sensitivity	0.722	0.007	0.010
Specificity	0.620	0.013	0.020

TABLE 4. RFE Ranking of Features of M1.

Rank	Features	Model size before removal
12	Number of farm workers (quadratic polynomial)	153
11	Coccidiosis	147
10	Side ventilation	18
9	Pigs on the farm	16
8	Number of rodent baits	15
7	Specific breed	14
6	Plastic overshoes for each house	8
5	Feeding equipment failures	6
4	Age at slaughter	5
3	Number of farm workers (cubic polynomial)	3
2	Flock was thinned	2
1	Separate farm clothing for each house	1

In comparing M1 and M2 (or M3), the important aspects are the overlap in the number of features, and the estimates of predictive accuracy. In comparing M1 and M4, the number of features that are "added" into the final set is significant. In both cases, the relative sizes of the coefficients and stability of the results are important.

4.1. Experimental Results. The full feature set (after removing features with more than 10% missing values and "constant" features) is of size 177. Many features still have missing values.

In order to avoid convergence problems with SVM we applied statistical normalization to all features. Each feature is independently transformed to have zero

TABLE 5. Normalized cross-validation of M1.

Features	μ	σ	Rescaled μ	Rescaled σ	$\lvert\frac{\sigma}{\mu}\rvert$
Coccidiosis	0.299	0.053	1.251	0.223	0.178
Specific breed	-0.382	0.065	-0.768	0.131	0.171
Flock was thinned	0.384	0.043	1.298	0.147	0.113
Age at slaughter	-0.425	0.059	-0.076	0.011	0.139
Side ventilation	0.320	0.071	0.660	0.146	0.221
Separate farm clothing for each house	-0.554	0.040	-1.179	0.084	0.071
Plastic overshoes for each house	0.411	0.048	0.862	0.100	0.116
Number of rodent baits	0.391	0.055	0.022	0.003	0.140
Pigs on the farm	0.230	0.029	1.273	0.159	0.125
Feeding equipment failures	0.378	0.049	0.776	0.100	0.129
Number of farm workers (quadratic polynomial)	0.662	0.205	1.192	0.369	0.309
Number of farm workers (cubic polynomial)	-1.431	0.298	-0.882	0.184	0.209
Model Evaluation					
Sensitivity			0.724	0.011	0.015
Specificity			0.629	0.010	0.015

TABLE 6. Normalized cross-validation of M2 - top 12 RFE features.

Features	μ	σ	Rescaled μ	Rescaled σ	$\lvert\frac{\sigma}{\mu}\rvert$
Wall of concrete	0.239	0.032	0.524	0.070	0.134
Number of farm workers	0.521	0.081	0.230	0.036	0.155
Flock was thinned	0.504	0.071	1.704	0.241	0.141
Age at slaughter	-0.470	0.033	-0.084	0.006	0.069
Who cleaned the houses before last crop	-0.322	0.083	-0.387	0.099	0.257
Who disinfected houses before last crop	0.333	0.080	0.385	0.093	0.241
Separate farm clothing for each house	-0.567	0.029	-1.207	0.062	0.051
Plastic overshoes for each house	0.362	0.038	0.759	0.081	0.106
Broiler farm nearby	-0.203	0.037	-0.406	0.073	0.180
Feeding equipment failures	0.396	0.029	0.813	0.061	0.074
Water supply: borehole	-0.347	0.032	-0.790	0.073	0.093
Number of farm workers (cubic polynomial)	-1.407	0.159	-0.867	0.098	0.113
Model Evaluation					
Sensitivity			0.753	0.009	0.011
Specificity			0.525	0.011	0.021

mean and unit variance:

$$x'_{ij} = \frac{x_{ij} - \overline{x_j}}{\sigma_j} \tag{3}$$

TABLE 7. Normalized cross-validation of M3 - top 5 RFE features.

Features	μ	σ	Rescaled μ	Rescaled σ	$\lvert\frac{\sigma}{\mu}\rvert$
Number of farm workers	0.191	0.187	0.084	0.083	0.979
Flock was thinned	0.546	0.119	1.846	0.401	0.217
Age at slaughter	-0.085	0.097	-0.015	0.017	1.145
Separate farm clothing for each house	-0.866	0.090	-1.843	0.192	0.104
Number of farm workers (cubic polynomial)	-0.665	0.387	-0.410	0.238	0.582
Model Evaluation					
Sensitivity			0.679	0.004	0.006
Specificity			0.507	0.012	0.023

where $\overline{x_j}$ is the mean value of the jth coordinate and σ_j is its standard deviation, estimated on the instances where the feature value was present. The missing values were set to 0 (i.e. to the mean feature value).

Since the normalization is "reversible" (i.e. one-to-one), we give the coefficient means and variances for normalized features, and also show their values if scaled back to the original magnitude. Suppose w_i' is the coefficient of feature i after normalization. Since

$$w' \cdot x' + b = \sum_{i=1}^{d} w_i' x_i' + b = \sum_{i=1}^{d} w_i' \frac{x_i - \overline{x_i}}{\sigma_i} + b$$

$$= \sum_{i=1}^{d} \frac{w_i' x_i}{\sigma_i} + (b - \sum_{i=1}^{d} \frac{w_i' \overline{x_i}}{\sigma_i})$$

and the term in parenthesis in the last line is constant, it follows that coefficient w_i for unnormalized ith feature is $w_i = w_i'/\sigma_i$.

Note that the rescaled means and coefficients in Table 5, which shows results with the features of the final model (M1), are very similar to coefficients in the Table 3. The normalized solution differs only very slightly from the unnormalized solution.

We implemented the original feature selection algorithm of [**6**]. As described in Section 2.5, the algorithm removes the least significant features one by one. Therefore, the later the feature is removed, the more important it is for classification. Looking at it from the other direction, the fewer features are left in the model when a given feature is removed, the more important that feature is. Table 4 gives the size of the model each time one of the features from M1 is removed. The most important feature according to this table is "Separate farm clothing for each house", and the least important one is quadratic polynomial of the number of farm workers.

The main comparison is between features of M1 and the top 12 features selected by RFE (M2). Results for the top 12 features (M2), and also for the top 5 (M3) and the top 18 features (M4) are in Tables 6, 7 and 8 respectively.

M1 and M2 have 6 out 12 (in each) features in common. It may seem that combining these features (for total of 18) should give better performance than either one separately. However, we found that this results in sensitivity and specificity of 0.758 and 0.607 respectively and thus is slightly better than M1 in sensitivity and somewhat worse in specificity. (These results are slightly better than M2 in

TABLE 8. Normalized cross-validation of M4 - top 18 RFE features.

Features	μ	σ	Rescaled μ	Rescaled σ	$\lvert\frac{\sigma}{\mu}\rvert$
Wall of concrete	0.330	0.037	0.723	0.080	0.111
Number of farm workers	0.506	0.108	0.224	0.048	0.213
Specific Breed	-0.340	0.052	-0.684	0.105	0.154
Chickens separated by sex	-0.293	0.048	-0.639	0.104	0.163
Flock was thinned	0.443	0.045	1.498	0.151	0.101
Age at slaughter	-0.347	0.052	-0.062	0.009	0.149
Side ventilation	0.255	0.052	0.526	0.106	0.202
Who cleaned the houses before last crop	-0.336	0.090	-0.404	0.108	0.268
Who disinfected houses before last crop	0.250	0.083	0.289	0.096	0.333
Separate farm clothing for each house	-0.568	0.048	-1.209	0.102	0.084
Plastic overshoes for each house	0.425	0.054	0.892	0.114	0.128
Number of rodent baits	0.370	0.042	0.021	0.002	0.112
Pigs on the farm	0.278	0.044	1.539	0.243	0.158
Other poultry farms nearby	0.305	0.064	0.632	0.133	0.210
Broiler farm nearby	-0.316	0.050	-0.632	0.100	0.159
Feeding equipment failures	0.333	0.045	0.684	0.092	0.135
Water supply: borehole	-0.353	0.034	-0.804	0.076	0.095
Number of farm workers (cubic polynomial)	-1.349	0.197	-0.831	0.121	0.146
Model Evaluation					
Sensitivity			0.771	0.010	0.013
Specificity			0.594	0.005	0.009

sensitivity, and much better in specificity). We suspect that the features that are not common between M1 and M2 play roles of "duplicates" to each other. Table 9 displays correlation matrix of these 18 features and finds that some of them correlate strongly.

We also experiment with the model built on the 5 top features (M3) and the top 18 features (M4). These numbers were chosen because they correspond to regions of overlap between features of M1 and the feature ordering produced by RFE. Table 4 demonstrates that the top 18 SVM features include 10 of the 12 M1 features, and considers the other 2 very insignificant. The 5-feature model was chosen because out of these 5 features only 1 does not appear in M1. Therefore models M3 and M4 in some sense "surround" M1. Evaluation of their quality may suggest possible improvements to M1.

Model M3 has 4 out of 5 features in common with M1. Its sensitivity is only somewhat worse than that of M1 (specificity is noticeably worse), but it has only half the features. Model M4 on the other hand has 18 features, and includes 10 top-ranked (by RFE) features of M1. However its results are only slightly better than those of M2, and are comparable (slightly better Sensitivity and slightly worse Specificity) to those of M1.

TABLE 9. Correlation Table of union of M1 and M2 (the two digits after decimal point). Top 6 are the common features, followed by features from M1 only, followed by M2 only.

	1	2	3	4	5	6	7	8	9	10	11	12	13	14	15	16	17	18
1	—	32	12	05	06	02	-01	-13	-07	09	06	03	04	04	09	06	06	04
2	32	—	-07	05	08	02	-02	01	-08	09	05	01	08	03	01	-05	-05	06
3	12	-07	—	16	-10	-03	-04	-32	-18	-26	16	-02	09	-02	25	30	-04	08
4	05	05	16	—	-02	04	01	-01	04	07	03	04	-00	05	-02	-05	03	-08
5	06	08	-10	-02	—	08	09	09	04	24	-05	10	-09	14	-20	-22	04	-20
6	02	02	-03	04	08	—	-02	05	06	06	-01	97	-04	79	-05	-05	05	-02
7	-01	-02	-04	01	09	-02	—	-06	09	04	06	-02	06	-02	-12	-11	-05	-09
8	-13	01	-32	-01	09	05	-06	—	18	22	-07	05	-01	09	-24	-24	08	07
9	-07	-08	-18	04	04	06	09	18	—	10	-09	05	06	05	-15	-13	03	04
10	09	09	-26	07	24	06	04	22	10	—	-07	08	-16	14	-17	-17	01	-08
11	06	05	16	03	-05	-01	06	-07	-09	-07	—	-02	02	-04	06	06	-06	00
12	03	01	-02	04	10	97	-02	05	05	08	-02	—	-05	90	-07	-08	04	-01
13	04	08	09	-00	-09	-04	06	-01	06	-16	02	-05	—	-06	01	01	-00	15
14	04	03	-02	05	14	79	-02	09	05	14	-04	90	-06	—	-11	-13	02	02
15	09	01	25	-02	-20	-05	-12	-24	-15	-17	06	-07	01	-11	—	81	-03	10
16	06	-05	30	-05	-22	-05	-11	-24	-13	-17	06	-08	01	-13	81	—	00	14
17	06	-05	-04	03	04	05	-05	08	03	01	-06	04	-00	02	-03	00	—	01
18	04	06	08	-08	-20	-02	-09	07	04	-08	00	-01	15	02	10	14	01	—

TABLE 10. Features in Table 9.

ID	Feature
1	Flock was thinned
2	Age at slaughter
3	Separate farm clothing for each house
4	Plastic overshoes for each house
5	Feeding equipment failures
6	Number of farm workers (cubic polynomial)
7	Coccidiosis
8	Specific breed
9	Side ventilation
10	Number of rodent baits
11	Pigs on the farm
12	Number of farm workers (quadratic polynomial)
13	Wall of concrete
14	Number of farm workers
15	Who cleaned the houses before last crop
16	Who disinfected houses before last crop
17	Broiler farm nearby
18	Water supply: borehole

We note that when using all features, the sensitivity and specificity averages are 0.599 and 0.515 respectively. Therefore, all three selected feature sets perform much better than the whole feature set.

These experiments suggest that M1 is a very good set of features that balances off a reasonable model size with a good predictive performance. On the other hand, our results suggest that RFE method is capable of finding interesting features, many of which match those selected by epidemiologist. It may be interesting to examine some additional features in M4 and to consider effects of possible strong correlations between features in M1 and in M2. The importance of these experiments is that they show how cross-validation should be used to determine predictive power of the selected set of features and the confidence in the parameters of the model. These considerations, rather than goodness of fit should be the driving force in model design.

5. Conclusion

In this work we have shown how machine learning methods can be used to validate epidemiological models (via cross-validation) and to aid in their construction by suggesting features of interest (via feature selection methods). We plan to continue exploring potential applications of machine learning methods in epidemiology with more sophisticated methods and new real-life data.

References

1. C.-C. Chang and C.-J. Lin. *LIBSVM: a library for support vector machines*, 2001. Software available at `http://www.csie.ntu.edu.tw/~cjlin/libsvm`.
2. N. Cristianini and J. Shawe-Taylor. *An Introduction to Support Vector Machines and Other Kernel-Based Learning Methods*. Cambridge University Press, 2000.

3. I. Dohoo, C. Ducrot, C. Fourichon, A. Donald, and D. Hurnik. An overview of techniques for dealing with large numbers of independent variables in epidemiologic studies. *Preventive Veterinary Medicine*, 29:221–239, 1996.
4. B. Efron. *The Jackknife, the Bootstrap and Other Resampling Plans.* Monograph 38 in CBMS-NSF Regional Conference Series in Applied Mathematics. SIAM, Philadelphia, 1982.
5. N. M. Ferguson, C. A. Donnelly, M. E. J. Woolhouse, and R. M. Anderson. The epidemiology of BSE in cattle herds in Great Britain. II. Model construction and analysis of transmission dynamics. *Philosophical Transactions of the Royal Society of London*, 352(1355):803–838, July 1997.
6. I. Guyon, J. Weston, S. Barnhill, and V. Vapnik. Gene selection for cancer classification using support vector machines. *Machine Learning*, 46(1-3):389–422, 2002.
7. T. Hastie, R. Tibshirani, and J. Friedman. *The Elements of Statistical Learning. Data Mining, Inference, and Prediction.* Springer, New York, 2001.
8. P. Hermans, D. Fradkin, I. Muchnik, and K. Morgan. Prevalence of wet litter and associated risk factors in broiler flocks in the UK. Submitted, 2004.
9. C. Heuer, H. Luinge, E. Lutz, Y. Schukken, J. van der Maas, H. Wilmink, and J. Noordhuizen. Determination of acetone in cow milk by Fourier transform infrared spectroscopy for the detection of subclinical ketosis. *Journal of Dairy Science*, 84:575–582, 2001.
10. R. Kohavi. A study of cross-validation and bootstrap for accuracy estimation and model selection. In *Proceedings of Fourteenth International Joint Conference on Artificial Intelligence*, pages 1137–1143, 1995.
11. B. Rockhill, D. Spiegelman, C. Byrne, and D. J. H. G. A. Golditz. Validation of the Gail et al. model of breast cancer risk prediction and implications for chemoprevention. *Journal of the National Cancer Institute*, 93(5):358–366, March 2001.
12. N. Rose, J. Mariani, P. Drouin, J. Toux, V. Rose, and O. Colin. A decision-support system for salmonella in broiler-chicken flocks. *Preventive Veterinary Medicine*, 59:27–42, 2003.
13. V. Vapnik. *The Nature of Statistical Learning Theory.* Springer-Verlag, 2nd edition, 1998.
14. A. Wade. Derivation versus validation. *Archives of Disease in Childhood*, 83:459–460, 200.

Department of Computer Science, Rutgers University, Piscataway, New Jersey 08854, USA
E-mail address: `dfradkin@cs.rutgers.edu`

DIMACS, Rutgers University, Piscataway, New Jersey 08854, USA
E-mail address: `muchnik@dimacs.rutgers.edu`

University of Liverpool, Faculty of Veterinary Science, Leahurst Veterinary Field Station, Neston, CH64 7TE, United Kingdom
E-mail address: `hermans@liverpool.ac.uk`

University of Liverpool, Faculty of Veterinary Science, Leahurst Veterinary Field Station, Neston, CH64 7TE, United Kingdom
E-mail address: `K.L.Morgan@liverpool.ac.uk`

Index